Behavior Analysis and Treatment

APPLIED CLINICAL PSYCHOLOGY

Series Editors:
Alan S. Bellack, *Medical College of Pennsylvania at EPPI, Philadelphia, Pennsylvania,*
and Michel Hersen, *Nova University School of Psychology, Fort Lauderdale, Florida*

A Continuation Order Plan is available for this series. A continuation order will bring delivery of each new volume immediately upon publication. Volumes are billed only upon actual shipment. For further information please contact the publisher.

Behavior Analysis and Treatment

Edited by

RON VAN HOUTEN

Mount Saint Vincent University
Halifax, Nova Scotia
Canada

and

SAUL AXELROD

Temple University
Philadelphia, Pennsylvania

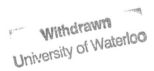

Plenum Press • New York and London

Library of Congress Cataloging-in-Publication Data

Behavior analysis and treatment / edited by Ron Van Houten, Saul
  Axelrod.
      p.   cm. -- (Applies clinical psychology)
    Includes bibliographical references and index.
    ISBN 0-306-44371-6
    1. Behavior therapy. 2. Behavioral assessment. 3. Behavior
  modification.   I. Van Houten, Ron.   II. Axelrod, Saul.
  III. Series.
    [DNLM: 1. Behavior Therapy--methods.   WM 425 B1485 1993]
  RC489.B4B426   1993
  616.89'142--dc20
  DNLM/DLC
  for Library of Congress   93-4431
                                                                CIP

ISBN 0-306-44371-6

© 1993 Plenum Press, New York
A Division of Plenum Publishing Corporation
233 Spring Street, New York, N.Y. 10013

Printed in the United States of America

To behavior analysis researchers,
who have advanced our understanding of the
causes and solutions of social and personal problems

Contributors

SAUL AXELROD, Special Education Program, Temple University, Philadelphia, Pennsylvania 19122

BRIAN BERRY, Special Education Program, Temple University, Philadelphia, Pennsylvania 19122

EDWARD G. CARR, Department of Psychology, State University of New York at Stony Brook, Stony Brook, New York 11794

GLEN DUNLAP, Florida Mental Health Institute, University of South Florida, Tampa, Florida 33612

JUDITH E. FAVELL, AuClair Program, Mount Dora, Florida 32757

K. BRIGID FLANNERY, College of Education, University of Oregon, Eugene, Oregon 97403

ROBERT H. HORNER, College of Educaton, University of Oregon, Eugene, Oregon 97403

BRIAN A. IWATA, Psychology Department, University of Florida, Gainesville, Florida 32611

J. M. JOHNSTON, Department of Psychology, Auburn University, Auburn, Alabama 36849

DUANE C. KEMP, Department of Psychology, State University of New York at Stony Brook, Stony Brook, New York 11794

ELIZABETH PINTER LALLI, Council Rock School District, Langhorne, Pennsylvania 18940

JOSEPH S. LALLI, Department of Pediatrics, University of Pennsylvania School of Medicine, Philadelphia, Pennsylvania 19104

LEN LEVIN, Department of Psychology, State University of New York at Stony Brook, Stony Brook, New York 11794

THOMAS R. LINSCHEID, Ohio State University and Columbus Children's Hospital, Columbus, Ohio 43205

F. CHARLES MACE, Department of Pediatrics, University of Pennsylvania School of Medicine, Philadelphia, Pennsylvania 19104

JOHNNY L. MATSON, Department of Psychology, Louisiana State University, Baton Rouge, Louisiana 70803

GENE McCONNACHIE, Department of Psychology, State University of New York at Stony Brook, Stony Brook, New York 11794

JAMES F. McGIMSEY, AuClair Program, Mount Dora, Florida 32757

LYNN MOYER, Special Education Program, Temple University, Philadelphia, Pennsylvania 19122

TERESA A. RODGERS, Psychology Department, University of Florida, Gainesville, Florida 32611

AHMOS ROLIDER, Department of Psychiatry, McMaster University, Hamilton, Ontario L8N 3Z5

MICHAEL C. SHEA, Graduate School of Applied and Professional Psychology, Rutgers University, Piscataway, New Jersey 08855

GERALD L. SHOOK, Shook and Associates, Community Enviroments, 310 East College Avenue, Tallahassee, Florida 32301

JEFFERY R. SPRAGUE, College of Education, University of Oregon, Eugene, Oregon 97403

SCOTT SPREAT, The Woods School, Langhorne, Pennsylvania 19047

MARK W. STEEGE, School Psychology Program, University of Southern Maine, Gorham, Maine 04038

NAOMI B. SWIEZY, Department of Psychology, Louisiana State University, Baton Rouge, Louisiana 70803

RON VAN HOUTEN, Psychology Department, Mount Saint Vincent University, Halifax, Nova Scotia B3M 2J6

TIMOTHY R. VOLLMER, Psychology Department, University of Florida, Gainesville, Florida 32611

DAVID P. WACKER, Department of Pediatrics, University Hospital School, University of Iowa, Iowa City, Iowa 52242

JENNIFER R. ZARCONE, Psychology Department, University of Florida, Gainesville, Florida 32611

Preface

In May 1986, the Association for Behavior Analysis (ABA) established a task force on the right to effective behavioral treatment. The mandate of this task force was to identify and delineate specific rights as they apply to behavioral treatment. Impetus for this project came in part from the controversy over the use of aversive procedures, which some held had no place in treatment and, with evolution of the treatment process, were no longer necessary. In contrast, others cited evidence that programs based on positive reinforcement alone were sometimes not effective in treating severe problems. These researchers and practitioners desired to ensure that clients and guardians be permitted to choose treatments that included punishment procedures when assessments warranted their use.

The first editor approached Ogden Lindsley, president of ABA, about establishing a task force to examine this isuse. The ABA council decided to broaden the mandate to include an examination of clients' right to effective behavioral treatment in general. The first editor was asked to chair the task force and appointed Saul Axelrod, Jon S. Bailey, Judith F. Favell, Richard M. Foxx, and O. Ivar Lovaas as members. Brian A. Iwata was appointed liaison by the ABA council.

The task force issued a report delineating six client rights, which was accepted by the ABA council and later published simultaneously in the *Journal of Applied Behavior Analysis* and *The Behavior Analyst*. A summary of these rights was later endorsed as an official ABA position statement by a vote of the general membership. *Behavior Analysis and Treatment* provides an in-depth examination of some of the issues raised in the task force report. We hope that the information presented in this book will help promote clients' rights to effective behavioral treatment.

Two weaknesses that should be acknowledged are the overreliance in most chapters on data obtained with people exhibiting developmental disabilities, and reliance on examples pertaining to the treatment of challenging behaviors. These emphases are to be expected given the areas of specialization of the authors. The reader is cautioned, however, that in most cases the rights mentioned apply equally to individuals from other populations recieving direct individual therapy, regardless of the relative seriousness of the problem.

One area that receives a good deal of attention in this book is the behavioral analysis of targeted behaviors. Many of the authors examine how an analysis of contingencies maintaining behavior and the stimuli controlling that behavior can improve treatment efficacy. This increased emphasis on the full range of variables controlling and maintaining behavior represents a significant development in the field of behavior analysis. Traditionally, measurement techniques were employed in order to obtain a baseline and to determine the efficacy of particular treatment. Although long recognized as important from a theoretical perspective, the empirical identification of controlling stimuli and maintaining variables was rarely attempted in applied settings. Once identified, these factors explain the occurrence of a behavior and provide information useful in developing a treatment plan. Although it may often prove fruitful to change behavior by altering the direct consequences of the behavior without addressing its function, there is little question that an analysis of controlling factors will frequently be helpful in designing an effective treatment plan.

Those interested in the use of a functional analysis will find much of interest in *Behavior Analysis and Treatment*. Other issues addressed in this book include examining the factors that contribute to an effective treatment environment, selecting the right treatment curriculum, making treatment decisions, coordinating the efforts of professionals, disseminating new treatment technology, and promoting generalization and transfer of treatment gains.

RON VAN HOUTEN
SAUL AXELROD

Contents

PART I CREATING AN OPTIMAL
LEARNING ENVIRONMENT

BRIAN A. IWATA, TIMOTHY R. VOLLMER, JENNIFER R. ZARCONE, AND
TERESA A. RODGERS

Chapter 8.   A Decision-Making Model for Selecting the Optimal Treatment Procedure

Saul Axelrod, Scott Spreat, Brian Berry, and Lynn Moyer

Naomi B. Swiezy and Johnny L. Matson

PART IV PROMOTING GENERALIZATION AND MAINTENANCE OF TREATMENT GAINS

PART V ADVANCING THE STATE OF THE ART

1

Introduction

RON VAN HOUTEN AND SAUL AXELROD

During the 1980s, there was a perceived need to define more clearly the rights of people receiving behavioral treatment. This need arose from abundant controversies involving the courts, legislatures, professional groups, and advocacy organizations. In response to this need, (the Association for Behavior Analysis (ABA) commissioned a task force to examine issues concerning people's right to effective treatment.) The final report was accepted by the executive council of ABA at its October 1987 meeting. An abbreviated version of the task force report subsequently was overwhelmingly endorsed as a position statement by the voting members of ABA and became official ABA policy. A copy of the final task force report, and the position statement endorsed by the ABA membership, are included in Appendices A and B.

The ABA position statement on clients' rights to effective behavioral treatment delineated six rights to which individuals receiving behavioral treatment are entitled (The first right is to a therapeutic physical and social environment. Thus, treatment should not proceed unless an individual is provided with a stimulating and educational environment. In a situation where the behavior analyst does not judge that the individual is living in a therapeutic physical and social environment, he or she must decide either to withhold treatment until the environment is sufficiently improved or to provide treatment while advocating an improved environment. The appropriate decision in each specific case is the one that takes into account the individual's long-term best interest.)

(The second right specifies that the overriding goal of treatment is the

RON VAN HOUTEN • Psychology Department, Mount Saint Vincent University, Halifax, Nova Scotia, Canada B3M 2J6. SAUL AXELROD • Special Education Program, Temple University, Philadelphia, Pennsylvania 19122.

Behavior Analysis and Treatment, edited by R. Van Houten & S. Axelrod. Plenum Press, New York, 1993.

personal welfare of the individual. Thus, an individual's program should not be based on the comfort or convenience of others; rather, there should be evidence that the program is in the individual's long-term interest. When the implementation of the program involves potential risk and the individual is not capable of providing consent, the individual's rights are ensured through peer review and human rights committees. It is important that only the peer review committee be permitted to make judgments on the selection or parameters of treatment.

The third right states that the treatment program should be devised and directed by a competent behavior analyst, who must have suitable training and experience. The statement emphasizes the need for the direct involvement of a doctoral-level behavior analyst in cases where a problem or treatment may be complex or cause risk. In these situations, the functions of the behavior analyst include modeling the appropriate implementation of the treatment procedures, determining that data are being collected and depicted correctly, interpreting the data, and making future treatment decisions.

The fourth right is the right to programs that teach functional skills. Skill development should be directed toward community integration and independence, as well as the elimination of behaviors that are dangerous or impede integration or independence. If behaviors need to be eliminated, the process must involve the collateral development of any skills that are necessary and lacking.

The fifth right specifies that the individual has a right to assessment and ongoing evaluation. The behavior analyst must not only collect data to assess the effectiveness of treatment, but also attempt to identify factors relevant to behavioral maintenance and treatment prior to initiating the treatment. Pre-treatment assessment may include interviews, measurement of ongoing behavior, and experimental manipulations. One purpose of such practices is to identify relevant antecedents or consequences that may play a role in maintaining the behavior.

The sixth right states that the client should receive the most effective treatment procedures available. In making treatment decisions, the urgency with which the behavior must be altered should be taken into account. It is also important to consider the amount of time needed to produce a clinically significant outcome and any lost habilitative opportunities associated with the use of a slow-acting treatment. Thus, a procedure's overall level of restrictiveness is viewed as a product of its absolute level of restrictiveness and the number of times it needs to be employed. Given the complexity of the decision-making process, clinical judgment is a crucial and necessary factor.

Each of the chapters in this book elaborate on at least one of the six rights to effective treatment mentioned above. The views expressed by the authors are their own and do not reflect the official position of the ABA.

PART I: CREATING AN OPTIMAL LEARNING ENVIRONMENT

In the second chapter, Judith E. Favell and James McGimsey address the right to an acceptable treatment environment by defining seven components of a therapeutic environment. First, the authors indicate that the environment must be engaging. This means that people are active participants in their environment, use interesting materials, interact with others at high rates, and are receiving high levels of reinforcement. People living in such an environment are also less likely to behave inappropriately and are more likely to learn incidentally (Horner, 1980).

Next, Favell and McGimsey indicate that an environment should teach and maintain functional skills (those that will enhance independence and quality of life). Past indicators of a functional environment (program plans and progress graphs) did not guarantee habilitative programs (Repp & Barton, 1980), partly because of the large amount of staff time consumed in their preparation. Thus, the authors point to the need to validate the components of program plans experimentally in a manner that leads to superior outcomes and takes into account the cost (e.g., staff time) versus the benefit to the individual. The authors also describe the nonfunctional, nongeneralizable manner in which skills were taught in the past. This was typically done in discrete training sessions apart from ongoing activities. Presently, the focus of training is on increasing independence and on practicing generalized skills in everyday environments. The authors also discuss the question of whether people with handicaps should be taught only with normalized methods. Although they affirm the preference for such an approach when feasible, they also indicate that this is not always possible and that more powerful procedures employing contrived consequences must sometimes be used.

The third component of an acceptable treatment environment is that it ameliorates problem behaviors (e.g., self-injury and aggression). The authors describe the ongoing debate on the use of restrictive procedures to deal with aberrant behaviors. They oppose current methods of ranking the restrictiveness of procedures according to their category; instead, they propose conducting a careful evaluation of a procedure's properties in the behavior change process. Thus, a given category of behavior, such as a reprimand, can be delivered in a humane or inhumane manner, can punish or reinforce behavior, and can vary in topography from a raised eyebrow to a verbal diatribe that demeans one's character. The authors also state that in making treatment decisions, one must take into account the harm arising from procedures that do not work. Favell and McGimsey also call for the measurement of the side effects, generality, and duration of interventions.

The next element of an acceptable treatment environment is that it is the least restrictive of the alternatives. Presently, location is a major determinant of whether environments are considered restrictive: Large-scale institutions are considered the most restrictive, whereas community placement is regarded as the least restrictive. The authors argue for more functional measures of restrictiveness. They propose that professionals measure the degree to which various placements lead to increased freedom and engagement in appealing activities.

The fifth and sixth components of an acceptable environment are that it be stable and safe. A stable environment is one characterized by predictability and continuity (Favell & Reid, 1988), rather than frequent changes in schedules, activities, staff, and housemates. To deal with the problem of staff turnover, the authors suggest not simply providing increased salaries, but also making use of social reinforcers that increase work satisfaction, performance, and stability. A safe environment is one in which people are free from the threat of physical and psychological harm caused by themselves or others. The problem of safety is compounded by the fact that some practitioners are first required to use benign (but weak) treatment procedures, some of which result in safety problems. The problem cannot be solved through policies and philosophies alone, but rather by devising improved procedures and allowing pragmatism to prevail in decision making. Favell and McGimsey also indicate that protective devices such as helmets are often criticized because they are nonnormalized, yet such items may be necessary given the realities of imperfect behavioral control. Finally, the authors state that human rights and peer review committees often protect clients' rights, but should not require cumbersome review processes or enter into clinical decision making.

The seventh component of an acceptable learning environment is that a person chooses to live in it. Favell and McGimsey propose that it is important to develop better means of assessing client preference for living environments; when professionals make choices for other people, the former may be insensitive to the latter's preferences. In closing, the authors suggest that indicators of an acceptable environment are increases in skill development and social activity and decreases in aberrant behaviors.

In the third chapter, Robert H. Horner, Jeffery R. Sprague, and K. Brigid Flannery address the right to programs that teach functional skills. The authors point out that applied behavior analysts are reevaluating the means by which they deal with dangerous behaviors (Wacker, 1989). In particular, behavior analysts are using individualized assessments (Iwata, Dorsey, Slifer, Bauman, & Richman, 1982) to teach appropriate behaviors that are functionally equivalent to dangerous behaviors (i.e., that produce the same consequences). Horner et al. stress that an appropriate instructional program can reduce the occurrence of problem behaviors.

The authors' approach is to merge general curriculum changes in education with the idiosyncratic curricular needs of people who perform dangerous behaviors. They discuss three developments that are changing the manner in which teachers build curricula: (a) the move to measure broader response classes (often termed life-style changes), rather than frequency counts of limited numbers of narrowly defined behaviors; (b) the recognition that activities (more comprehensive response classes) constitute a more sensitive measure of progress than discrete skills; and (c) recent developments in functional analysis research that help to define curricula.

Horner et al. stress the need to expand the measures of program success. Rather than devising procedures to decrease dangerous behaviors, there is a need to produce more comprehensive life-style changes (Evans & Meyer, 1987). The authors propose behavior support programs that improve all aspects of a person's daily life. Included are social, recreational, learning, and living opportunities, as well as the freedom to express preferences. The authors also recommend that studies include measures of physical and social integration, the variety of tasks in which a person participates, and the number of opportunities to express preference and engage in different social roles. Researchers would then look for relationships between the dependent variables. Use of these expanded measures should increase the range of possible interventions program developers use and shift the focus to broader life-style activities.

The authors next discuss the means of moving from skills-based to activity-based curricula (Brown et al., 1979). In the past, curriculum development consisted of isolated skills that were regarded as important either for future development or because people without handicaps performed them. The Horner et al. curriculum centers on the functions of behavior and is sequenced so that the cluster of behaviors to achieve an outcome is taught as a group (so that the person achieves the function, rather than simply performs a skill). The approach does not require people with and without handicaps to perform activities in the same manner; rather, the aim is to achieve the same outcome (e.g., eating food with a prosthetic device achieves the same goal of putting food in a person's mouth). The activities-based curriculum that the authors describe (a) produces immediate benefits to the student, (b) teaches activities valued by both the student and society, (c) stresses behaviors that are meaningful locally, and (d) is age appropriate.

With respect to assessment in functional analysis, the authors point out that the field has moved from only manipulating hypothesized antecedents and consequences suspected of producing inappropriate behavior to also using interview procedures (Durand & Crimmins, 1987) and systematic observation (Touchette, MacDonald, & Langer, 1985). These approaches may be less definitive, but are also less time-consuming and intrusive. The information that results has implications for curriculum development. First, if the analysis indicates that the person performs an inappropriate behavior in order to acquire a reinforcer, the curriculum might specify an appropriate behavior that achieves the same outcome. Second, it is important that the new behavior becomes as efficient as the existing, undesirable behavior. The authors speculate that the functional analysis approach is not useful for behaviors with a physiological basis. They also point out that the technology does not remove the need for all behavior-reducing procedures.

Horner et al. stipulate that modifying an existing behavior does not always involve the manipulation of consequences. It is also possible to alter antecedent instructional stimuli by (a) making the curriculum more functional, (b) removing stimuli that occasion problem behavior, (c) using superior teaching methods, and (d) embedding mastered tasks with those that must be learned.

In selecting functional reinforcers, the authors employ the principle of functional equivalence. The idea is to isolate the reinforcers maintaining aberrant behavior and use them to reinforce desirable behavior. Finally, the authors stress the need to identify setting events that affect the occurrence of behavior. Some of these events may be easy to manipulate (e.g., room temperature), whereas others are more difficult (e.g., a medical problem).

PART II: THE ROLE OF BEHAVIORAL ASSESSMENT IN PROVIDING QUALITY CARE

Chapters 4, 5, and 6 each address the client's right to assessment and ongoing evaluation. In Chapter 4, F. Charles Mace, Joseph S. Lalli, Elizabeth Pinter Lalli, and Michael C. Shea review the literature on functional analysis in the treatment of aberrant behavior. They classify controlling variables with regard to the following types of reinforcers: attention (Ayllon & Michael, 1959), sensory and perceptual consequences (Lovaas, Newsom, & Hickman, 1987), access to materials or activities, and escape-avoidance of aversive demand condition (Carr & Newsom, 1985). In each instance, numerous examples are provided to illustrate the specific identification of reinforcers from the classes. In addition, Mace et al. mention the important role that antecedent and concurrent stimuli can play in the treatment of maladaptive behavior.

Next the authors describe the following steps in performing a functional analysis based intervention: (a) a descriptive analysis of natural conditions, (b) formulation of hypotheses about functional relationships, (c) performing an experimental analysis under analogue conditions (Iwata et al., 1982), (d) intervention development based on the results of the functional analysis, and (e) maintenance and generalization of intervention effects. In this section, Mace et al. make the excellent point that conditions presented in any analogue assessment should parallel those in the person's natural environment. If significant variables active in the natural setting are not tested in the analog setting, the results of the analog analysis may prove incomplete. The authors recommend unstructured observation in the natural setting, followed by the collection of data on antecedents, responses, and consequences using a partial interval recording procedure. Next they describe how the data obtained from this assessment provide the information needed to formulate hypotheses about possible functional relationships, and how one designs analog conditions to test these hypotheses. In this phase, the authors point out that it is essential that behavior analysts hold constant or eliminate as many extraneous factors as possible, in order to test one possible function at a time.

Once the function of the behavior is identified, Mace et al. recommend using this information in designing a treatment plan. It is suggested that following this advice will lead to more effective treatment plans and should reduce the need to incorporate aversive components in the treatment plan.

In Chapter 5, Brian A. Iwata, Timothy R. Vollmer, Jennifer R. Zarcone, and Teresa A. Rodgers further discuss treatment classification and selection based on behavioral function. The chapter begins by classifying the learned functional characteristics of behavioral disorders along two dimensions: positive versus negative reinforcement, and socially mediated versus automatic reinforcement (Iwata, Vollmer, & Zarcone, 1990). The authors reject classifying function by specific reinforcer type, because reinforcers have been found to be highly idiosyncratic (e.g., a form of attention could function as a punishing stimulus for one individual and a reinforcer for another), and because an analysis of all reinforcing stimuli will never be complete. The proposed method of classification is appealing because it is both comprehensive and uncomplicated.

Next, Iwata et al. examine each of the four categories resulting from their schema. Although most of the examples provided for each of these categories involve self-injurious behaviors, it should be noted that this classification system works equally well for a wide variety of behaviors and populations. The authors identify several advantages served by identifying which of the four functions apply in a particular case: (a) it helps to identify the conditions that will make the behavior more or less probable; (b) it indicates the source of reinforcement that could be eliminated by extinction; (c) it suggests the type of contingency and reinforcer that should be employed in treatment; and (d) it should provide information on which treatments would likely prove effective.

Before providing a more detailed examination of how the proposed model can be employed, the authors review the range of alternative approaches to treatment classification and selection. Approaches included are arbitrary selection, classification by treatment topography, selection based on the least restrictive alternative, selection based on differential effectiveness, selection based on the topography of the target behavior, and the communication model. In the case of each of these alternative methods of classification, the authors raise cogent points about their limitations.

In the next section of the chapter, Iwata et al. examine the functional analysis model of assessment and treatment. They provide data showing the

weakness of the questionnaires and descriptive analysis often used to determine the function of a problem behavior (Zarcone, Rodgers, Iwata, Rourke, &
Dorsey, in press), and they reveal the power of a direct functional analysis
(Iwata, et al., 1982). Only by directly testing for each suspected contingency
with adequate control conditions can the function of a behavior be identified
with any degree of certainty. Although the model accounts well for the four
categories of operant behavior, it does not address the issue of possible
respondent processes that may influence behavior.

One of the most attractive features of the model proposed by Iwata et al.
is how treatment selection is logically related to assessment results. In each
case the identification of the reinforcing function of the behavior by the
functional analysis leads to the application of three intervention components.
First, motivation (or the establishing operation for the inappropriate behavior)
is reduced. Second, the behavior is placed on extinction. Third, a differential
reinforcement of other behaviors (or reinforcement of alternative behaviors)
procedure is implemented. It is argued that each of these three treatment
components depend on a correct functional analysis to be consistently
effective. In this portion of the chapter, the authors provide many excellent
examples for each of the four functions. They describe how establishing
operations for the target behavior can be weakened, how extinction can be
applied (it is pointed out that this component is not applicable for behavior
maintained by automatic negative reinforcement), and how differential reinforcement procedures can be employed to form a comprehensive treatment
package based upon the functional analysis of the behavior.

In Chapter 6, Ahmos Rolider and Ron Van Houten examine the role of
antecedent variables in regulating inappropriate and appropriate behavior
and describe the role that the assessment of these factors can play in the
treatment process. Since the advent of the behavioral revolution, behavior
analysts have emphasized the use of operant conditioning processes in order
to effect changes in human behavior. The chapter by Rolider and Van Houten
breaks ground in at least two areas. First, the authors point out the effect that
respondent processes have on aberrant behavior. Second, they present their
interpersonal stimulus control model, which takes advantage of the fact that
some people consistently behave appropriately in the presence of some
people but not others.

In the initial step of the Rolider and Van Houten model, the practitioner
conducts an analysis of behavior that not only isolates the function (i.e.,
consequences) of a behavior, but also seeks antecedent discriminative and
eliciting stimuli associated with problem behaviors. Thus, emotional responses to delayed, terminated, and denied reinforcers—as well as responses to certain schedules of reinforcement and extinction (Azrin,
Hutchinson, & Hake, 1966)—are considered as part of a comprehensive
analysis that also takes operant factors into account. Identifying both ante-

cedent and consequent factors associated with a behavior problem is initiated by interviewing people who are familiar with the client. The assessment might suggest several factors associated with the problem behavior. The factors can range from being operant in nature (e.g., attention) to being respondent (e.g., waiting for a positive reinforcer). Once the evaluation is complete, the suspected factors are systematically manipulated to determine whether, in fact, they do occasion or elicit the problem behavior.

The second stage of the Rolider and Van Houten model is to devise an appropriate curriculum. This process can take the form of either graded exposure to various stimuli that elicit inappropriate social behavior or teaching an appropriate behavior that is functionally equivalent to the behavior of concern. In establishing treatment priorities, it is necessary to evaluate the seriousness of the behavior problem. The general operating principle is to begin treatment with the precursor, mediator, and environment that elicit the least serious response from the individual and then gradually introduce situations causing more extreme reactions. In teaching new behaviors to stimuli that formerly elicited inappropriate responses, it is important that the new behavior be at least as efficient as the inappropriate behavior in producing desirable consequences.

In the third stage of the model, teaching takes place. Initially training occurs in a highly structured environment in which the student and teacher sit opposite each other, and in which there are a minimal number of distractions. As progress occurs, the environment becomes less structured. The teacher works from scripts that specify how the antecedents will be presented. The script also informs the teacher how to respond to each of the student's behaviors. In the process, a student might learn how to wait for progressively longer periods of time for a reinforcer, or that a reinforcing activity must come to an end. Crucial factors in the success of the teaching process are (a) that treatment begins with a trainer who elicits the smallest number of inappropriate interactions from the person (Schloss, Smith, Santora, & Bryant, 1989), (b) that the teacher builds rapport with a student, and that shaping procedures be employed. At times of crisis, intervention consists of procedures that prevent injuries and escape and that do not reinforce the misbehaviors of the student.

Once the behavior is brought under the control of the teacher, the final step is to transfer control to people who are more naturally a part of the student's environment and to situations that the person will normally encounter. New mediators will include parents, siblings, and classroom teachers, whereas new situations will include noisy, crowded, and less structured environments. Procedures for bringing about generalization include gradually introducing untrained mediators, time-delay procedure (Charlop, Schreibman, & Thibodeau, 1985), and recreating a situation in which a misbehavior had earlier occurred.

Part III: Providing State-of-the-Art Treatment

The third right stipulated in the ABA task force report was that each person receiving treatment have a competent behavior analyst. In Chapter 7, Gerald L. Shook and Ron Van Houten specify the means of fulfilling this right. The authors compare a competent behavior analyst to a qualified surgeon, in that both must be sensitive to the factors affecting the problem, both work directly with people until successful, and both are bound by the outcomes of scientific research. They point out that a problem in behavior analysis is that the standards of surgeons are not always upheld, insofar as untrained people are attempting complex operations. To overcome this difficulty, the authors suggest that at the beginning of an intervention, it may be necessary to restrict who is permitted to provide services; when success is established, other people may become involved.

The training process Shook and Van Houten promote involves observing a practitioner's progress, testing her or his practical skills, and collecting data on performance. They also suggest that behavior analysts train only a few people at a time (Lovaas & Favell, 1987) and that the former be available for consultation when difficulties arise. The authors propose that if behavior analysts are to achieve the same regard that physicians have, they must develop a professional discipline with uniform standards of competence. In addition to the appropriate educational background and programmatic skills, behavior analysts must also have diagnostic skills and be in contact with emerging literature and colleagues. Finally, they must operate within a scientific framework and be responsive to data.

A problem that Shook and Van Houten see is that behavior analysts are dispersed among many disciplines and, therefore, must depend on the benevolence of others to further their field (Fraley & Vargas, 1986). This situation is often unacceptable given the hostility of many professionals to behavior analytic principles and practices. The authors, therefore, raise the question of whether behavior analysis should become an autonomous discipline. As an alternative to separating from other disciplines, they also suggest that behavior analysis might concurrently promote itself as a separate entity and continue to develop as a subdiscipline of psychology.

The authors also describe ways in which behavior analysts can ensure the training of competent professionals. These include consistent standards of graduate training, licensure of behavior analysts, and education of professionals through the ABA. Shook and Van Houten support the regulation of the profession of behavior analysis through the accreditation process (Johnston & Shook, 1987). This would have the benefits of gaining professional recognition for behavior analysts, helping to establish behavior analysis as an independent discipline, achieving quality control, and providing consistency in licensing practices. The authors describe the work of an ABA task force that proposed standards for accrediting masters and doctoral programs. Programs would be approved if they provided appropriate coursework and competency standards for students and satisfied the terms of a site visit. Approval would be for 5 years, with an annual review to maintain quality control. Shook and Van Houten point out that ABA requirements do not include the demonstration of hands-on skills, but they still see the process as advancing the field.

In addition to accrediting training programs, the authors propose the licensing of individual behavior analysts. This would have the benefit of providing a list of behavior analysts that would be available to the public, government agencies, and insurance companies.

The third form of accreditation is through a government act regulating which practices qualify as behavior analysis and who can engage in such practices (Johnston & Shook, 1987). The authors point out that a title act specifies who can identify themselves as behavior analysts, whereas a practice act includes both the title provision and the acts that can be characterized as behavior analysis. The conditions for governmental accreditation include education requirements, professional experience, and satisfactory completion of written tests. Again, the authors make a case for requiring actual demonstrations of competence through work with clients.

Finally, Shook and Van Houten summarize the reasons why there should be a credential in behavior analysis. These include (a) protection of the public against inappropriate practices, (b) the production of sufficient numbers of competent practitioners, (c) protection of the profession from the adverse publicity associated with malpractice, (d) assistance to employers and government agencies in hiring qualified behavior analysts, and (e) protection against other professionals who might usurp the role of behavior analysts without possessing the necessary skills.

In Chapter 8, Saul Axelrod, Scott Spreat, Brian Berry, and Lynn Moyer present a decision-making model for selecting the optimal treatment procedure. The model addresses the issue of ensuring that a treatment plan conforms with an individual's right to services whose overriding goal is the client's personal welfare. The authors point out five important advantages of the proposed model: (a) it is simple; (b) it is based on a scientific approach; (c) it recognizes the importance of professional judgment; (d) it ensures equal protection for the client whether the procedures are termed restrictive or nonrestrictive; and (e) it does not rule out procedures on an *a priori* basis.

The first step in the Axelrod et al. model is to determine whether an important performance discrepancy exists between actual and expected performance. The existence of a discrepancy does not in and of itself dictate that an intervention should take place. Factors to be considered include whether the discrepancies detract from the person's quality of life (or, in some cases, the quality of life of others), and whether the discrepancy is based on personal preference or deficits. It is also recommended that discrepancies be ranked in regard to the negative impact on the quality of life and that the most serious problem be treated first.

The second step in the model is to perform a structural and functional analysis of behaviors selected for treatment. This step allows the therapist to identify the antecedents and consequences that are related to the behavior's occurrence. This information is critical to the development of a treatment plan.

The third step is to conduct a historical analysis of the client, behavior, and procedures under consideration. This should include reviewing the behavioral and medical records of the client, as well as interviewing people who know the client. The authors also make the important point that the practitioner should directly interact with the client. A complete review of all historical information, coupled with a hands-on assessment, should give the behavioral clinician the information required to select the treatment most likely to be effective. If a treatment is to be employed that has not been applied by the behavior analyst in the past, then the behavior analyst should peruse the relevant literature for its likely effects and side effects. Based on the historical review, predictions should be made about these effects, as well as the risks and benefits that might be expected.

The fourth step is to select the least restrictive effective treatment. Axelrod et al. point out that the behavior analyst has an obligation to select only treatments that have a reasonable probability of being effective when treating serious problems. After describing the difficult questions that need to be addressed in order to evaluate the intrusiveness of a procedure, the authors list nine factors that should be considered. Addressing these questions should make it easier for behavioral clinicians to make important decisions about the relative intrusiveness of alternative procedures.

The fifth step is to perform a risk-benefit analysis. The authors point out the deficiencies of the traditional fixed hierarchy approach and make a convincing argument for performing a careful and measured risk-benefit analysis before selecting the treatment of choice (Spreat, Lipinski, Dickerson, Nass, & Dorsey, 1989). This analysis involves evaluating the probability of treatment success, estimating the period of time required to produce the desired change in behavior, assessing the distress that might be associated with the procedure, and evaluating the distress caused by the behavior.

The sixth proposed step is to complete a checklist to safeguard the rights of the person receiving treatment. This checklist is divided into the following groupings: determining the target behavior, treatment environments, and procedures; reviewing the proposed procedures; informed consent; implementation; documentation and reporting; and evaluation of procedures. The use of this checklist is an excellent way to ensure that important considerations are not overlooked.

The final step suggested by Axelrod et al. is to obtain appropriate authorization for all programs. This section of the chapter addresses the issue of interdisciplinary development with the behavior analyst as the team leader. The role of peer review and human rights committee review is also discussed in some detail. In this section the authors make the important point that the sole domain of human rights committees is to address human rights issues; it is not appropriate for such committees to exercise clinical judgment (Spreat & Lanzi, 1989).

Because behavioral treatment often involves the active participation of other professionals, coordinating the efforts of various specialties is crucial for optimizing treatment. Chapter 9, by Naomi B. Swiezy and Johnny L. Matson, describes how such coordination can be achieved.

In specifying changes in professional roles, the authors begin with a description of recent changes in treatment goals. The evolution in treatment goals may result, in part, from the current debate concerning the ethics of using punishment procedures to reduce aberrant behavior. Thus, in addition to treatment efficacy, treatment acceptability is a factor in selecting a corrective procedure. Other goals include early detection and intervention, minimizing undesirable side effects of treatment, and achieving maintenance and generalization of gains. In selecting a procedure, Swiezy and Matson propose using the least restrictive alternative model, employing restrictive procedures only when nonrestrictive alternatives have proven ineffective.

Next, the authors discuss the changing role of behavior analysts in providing treatment, which has evolved from intervening directly with client behavior to acting as behavioral consultants to various personnel who will carry out the procedures. Swiezy and Matson describe, in turn, procedures for training parents, school personnel, residential staff, peers, and the clients themselves.

There is much commonality in the training procedures the authors recommend. A major point they make is that practical, interactive training is superior to didactic teaching methods. Thus, they support a competency-based approach in which people actually demonstrate that they have mastered various skills. In order to achieve maintenance of skill development, the authors suggest periodic contact with the behavior analyst. They also warn that teaching one skill will not necessarily result in related skill acquisition. Therefore, it may be necessary to teach each skill sequentially. The authors also claim that an important factor in recommending a procedure is its acceptability to the program implementer, and they make numerous specific suggestions on how to increase treatment acceptability.

Swiezy and Matson next discuss the issue of coordinating the efforts of different professionals in order to establish a team effort. They concur with Kazdin (1984) that the involvement of paraprofessionals is often essential for successful program implementation. Therefore, the skills of paraprofessionals are crucial to program success, because most problems exist in the natural setting rather than the therapist's office. In determining the members of a team, it is necessary to establish whether there are any gaps in necessary skills (e.g., speech). If there are deficits, a new member should be appointed to the team.

To increase the chances of coordinated efforts, the professional in charge should be made aware of the similarity in goals for all team members. Also, it is important that all people involved in the program be familiar with behavior analysis principles. This is particularly true of psychiatrists who may prescribe drugs for behavior control. Next, there should be a legal professional available to the team to inform members of any litigious issues raised by their treatment protocol. With sufficient coordination of team efforts, behavioral consultants can have a major impact on client behavior. Finally, Swiezy and Matson point out the four stages of behavioral consultation, which include problem identification, problem analysis, plan implementation, and program evaluation.

Part IV: Promoting Generalization and Maintenance of Treatment Gains

In Chapter 10, Edward G. Carr, Gene McConnachie, Len Levin, and Duane C. Kemp address two individual rights specified in the ABA task force report: the right to programs that teach functional skills and the right to behavioral assessment and ongoing evaluation. More specifically, the chapter describes assessment procedures that isolate the communicative function of aberrant behaviors (Carr, 1985). The information is then used to teach the individual an appropriate means of communicating needs. The authors point out that there is often an inverse relationship between behavior problems and a person's communication skills. Thus, some behavior problems might serve as a form of nonverbal communication. The functional communication strategy involves teaching the client appropriate and functionally equivalent behavior to communicate the same message.

The initial step in teaching communication skills is to conduct a functional analysis of problem behaviors. Carr et al. describe three components of the process. The first is to describe the various situations in which the behavior occurs; this is done through interview and observation. The information is then categorized according to whether it is attention seeking, escape motivated, tangible seeking, or associated with other factors. Situations that are suspected of producing aberrant behavior are then verified by exposing the individual to the condition and determining whether the behavior reliably occurs.

A successfully conducted functional analysis allows training to begin. A crucial step is to develop rapport between the teacher and the student, which can be done by playing games and joking. Initially, the student receives noncontingent reinforcement; only gradually does the teacher make demands. In the beginning, it is acceptable for the student to use any appropriate form of communication (e.g., grunting or pointing).

Carr et al. stress that aberrant behavior serves a function: The behaviors themselves can be eliminated, but the functions remain. Not only can the functions not be eliminated, but often there is no reason to eliminate them. Rather, the goal is to teach a functionally equivalent behavior (Carr & Durand, 1985). Thus, if a student self-injures for attention, it may be possible to teach the person to communicate a need for attention appropriately.

In teaching functionally equivalent behavior, practical issues emerge. It is essential that the new behavior be more efficient than the one it is replacing (Horner & Billingsley, 1988). Carr et al. describe two variables influencing response efficiency—ease of performance and ease of interpretability. In teaching a new form of communication, it is necessary to teach it to a level of competence that makes it as easy to perform as the aberrant behavior. To deal with interpretability problems, the authors suggest using the most general form of communication whenever possible. If this is not feasible, they suggest using a form of communication that is less general, but easier to interpret. Therefore, if speech results in insurmountable interpretability problems, using cards with words is appropriate.

Once the teacher determines the most desirable mode of communication, it is necessary to provide opportunities to practice the new skill. This should be done in an educational, integrated environment where the curriculum is functional and age appropriate. Given these conditions, Carr et al. suggest that teachers not wait for natural conditions to create opportunities to respond, but that they create such conditions themselves. As a student progresses, the teacher should build a tolerance for delay of reinforcement by requiring progressively more work before dispensing reinforcers. In order to increase the likelihood of compliance, the authors recommend embedding stimuli associated with high rates of disruptive behavior among stimuli that are associated with low rates of disruptive behavior. Carr et al. have also found that teachers can diminish disruptive behavior by providing students with the choice of where and with whom a task will be performed and what the reinforcers will be. To produce generalized gains across stimuli, Carr et al. use a two-step process: Training takes place first in a controlled environment (e.g., a classroom) and then in a less controlled environment (e.g., a shopping mall). In closing, the authors speculate that communication programs may be effective because they give people greater control over their environments. This may be a particularly strong reinforcer for people whose disabilities have historically afforded them little control over their lives.

In Chapter 11, Glen Dunlap addresses the issue of promoting generalization. The chapter begins by defining the concepts most closely involved in the issue of generalization: stimulus control, stimulus generalization, maintenance, and enlarging the size of the response class. Factors that may be related to the failure to develop stimulus control are listed; these include the discriminative stimulus not being present in the nontraining setting, the discriminative stimulus being blocked or overshadowed by other stimuli in the nontraining setting, another stimulus evoking a competing response, and the conditioning history of the training stimulus in the nontraining setting. Response generalization is acknowledged to involve response classes and response covariation.

Next, the technology of generalization is summarized in terms of three tactics: exploiting current functional contingencies, training diversity, and incorporating functional mediators. The contribution of Stokes and Baer (1977) in this area is acknowledged, and numerous examples are provided to illustrate each tactic. Although these tactics are often useful, Dunlap argues for the development of a technology of behavior change with enough authority and precision to assure generalization. To this end he describes three areas of importance for generalization programming. First, he presents the general case programming strategy described by Horner, McDonald, and Bellamy (1986). The first step in employing general case programming is to define the set of stimulus conditions that should occasion the occurrence of the trained response. A minimum number of examples are then selected that sample the range of stimulus variations and response variations required. Negative examples are also included.

Second, Dunlap examines contextual factors and competing events that interfere with the occurrence of the desired behavior in the natural setting. It is recommended that these factors be identified and ameliorated whenever possible in order to promote generalization. Third, the author examines response generalization and functional equivalence.

In the final section of this chapter, Dunlap presents seven guidelines for promoting functional behaviors that are likely to be exhibited in a variety of natural settings. The first guideline involves planning for generalization from the beginning. By carefully specifying the circumstances that should occasion the behavior, the probability of generalization can be promoted when designing the initial program. The second is to assess the relevant stimulus and reinforcement conditions in the identified contexts. The identification of these factors can allow one to adapt the training setting to resemble the natural setting, or to plan relevant changes in the natural setting.

The third guideline is to provide intervention in relevant settings under naturally occurring conditions, when feasible. The fourth is to make use of the existing technology of generalization mentioned in the earlier portion of the chapter. The fifth guideline is to attend to the functions of stimulus control when addressing questions of stimulus generalization; the sixth is to attend to the functions of reinforcer schedules when attending to questions of maintenance. The seventh guideline states that one should attend to the generalization of functional alternatives when generalized response suppression is a treatment goal. Following these guidelines should markedly increase the likelihood that behavioral changes will generalize to new settings.

In Chapter 12, David P. Wacker and Mark W. Steege provide an excellent model for providing outclinic services that is in accord with the client's right to effective treatment. They point out in their introductory remarks that practitioners working in outpatient settings typically rely upon indirect measures in order to identify target behaviors and to assess functional control of these behaviors. The authors then present a model that allows practitioners to determine empirically the function of the target behavior in the natural setting.

The first step in the Wacker and Steege model is to collect historical and descriptive information from parents and teachers prior to the first clinic session. Two or more examiners read the descriptive information and present the information at a morning staff meeting on the day of the clinic session. At this meeting, the primary target behavior is selected, and several possible maintaining conditions are identified.

Second, a two-part evaluation is performed during a 90- to 120-minute assessment session in order to verify or reject these hypotheses. A functional analysis is performed with the parent or a therapist interacting with the child, and a behavioral interview is conducted to verify the historical information provided to the clinic. Following this assessment a multidisciplinary staff meeting occurs, treatment recommendations are generated, and parents receive training to facilitate the integrity and acceptability of the treatment plan selected. Third, staff provide follow-up on treatment integrity. This follow-up involves phone calls, outreach visits, and videotaping.

The functional analysis employed by Wacker and Steege involves the rapid alternation of 10-minute conditions and is based on the research reported by Iwata et al. (1982). Wacker and Steege have modified the procedure to allow it to be carried out within the time constraints of the outpatient setting. The conditions evaluated can include high or low parental attention, high or low demand, and high or low levels of social and sensory consequences provided for stereotypic behavior. Each condition is presented once; conditions that lead to differential results are then presented a second time in order to replicate the results obtained the first time. Contextual variables relevant to each client are employed in each analogue condition.

Once a treatment has been selected that addresses the function of the target behavior, Wacker and Steege obtain long-term data on treatment acceptability. Data are collected on the acceptability of the various aspects of the treatment and the acceptability of the logistics of implementation (e.g., who is to apply it, when it is to be applied, and for how long it is to be applied).

In the next section of the chapter, Wacker and Steege present several case examples to illustrate how the model is used. These three examples illustrate how the initial analogue conditions are selected, as well as how factors identified in the first presentation of conditions are validated during the replication presentation. The authors point out the advantages of identifying the function of a behavior as well as the need to validate the reliability of results obtained in a brief session against those obtained using a longer-duration functional assessment.

Part V: Advancing the State of the Art

In order to ensure that clients receive the most effective treatment possible, it is critical that behavior analysts promote research designed to advance the state of the art. Chapters 13 and 14, written by J. M. Johnston and Thomas R. Linscheid, respectively, address this important question from two important perspectives. Johnston examines the issues related to the development of behavior technology, whereas Linscheid describes how political issues can sometimes impede the development of innovative treatment procedures.

In Chapter 13, J. M. Johnston provides a model for developing and evaluating behavioral technology. The author begins by distinguishing between technology and craft and presents an excellent definition of *behavioral technology*—change procedures whose influence has been established by experimental analysis in terms of the science of behavior. He further states that to qualify as technology, such procedures must produce reliable and general effects that have been empirically evaluated in the applied setting. In order to produce reliable and general effects, the researcher must isolate and evaluate the important components and parameters of the intervention in isolation as well as collectively. This point is well illustrated by an example from the author's own work on rumination (Rast & Johnston, 1988; Rast, Johnston, Ellinger-Allen, & Drum, 1985). Johnston also points out the advantage of developing a complete behavioral technology that can produce predictable results under routine conditions.

In the next section, Johnston examines the strategies of technological change and provides a list of 13 points to help guide applied researchers involved in developing new technology. As he mentions, these points need not be pursued in a fixed sequence, although many depend on previous steps. The first step involves the researcher defining the nature of the problem; Johnston urges the reader to examine problems from a variety of perspectives and to consider the different environments that may be involved in the future. The second step involves defining the goals for the procedure. Goals should be specific, and they should reflect the multifaceted features of the problem defined in the first step.

The third step is to define the behaviors of interest. Johnston points out that it is necessary to identify all of the participants' behaviors that need to be modified in order to attain the goal. The fourth step involves identifying the controlling variables; this is a complex question that is central to a comprehensive behavioral analysis. In step five, the applied researcher must identify the relevant principles and procedures, and the sixth step is to identify the procedures' effects. The author points out that the failure to examine all of the effects of an intervention on the individuals involved can lead to the development of a technology that produces a worse problem than it solves.

Step seven involves identifying the relevant components of the treatment. This step allows the researcher to improve the power and efficiency of the intervention. In step eight, the applied researcher examines how the components produce their effects. Research activity to address this question can provide clues about how to make the treatment more effective and will also help delineate the limitations of the technology. The ninth step is to ask how the procedure can be improved; the next four steps involve evaluating and further refining procedures. Step ten is to determine the effects under applied conditions. The eleventh step is to add and evaluate refinements that are required in the natural setting. The twelfth step is to determine whether the conditions of application maintain the procedure, and the thirteenth step is to examine whether the procedure meets the original goals.

Johnston then examines the relationship between research and practice. He argues for a division of labor between technological research and technological application, pointing out that the conditions and contingencies of the natural setting are often in conflict with the requirements of careful measurement and control required for effective research. Johnston argues that persons training to be applied researchers have somewhat different educational requirements than persons training to be practitioners. He closes the chapter by asking behavior analysts to apply their skills to manage their own behavior and redefine their concepts of behavioral technology.

In Chapter 14, Thomas R. Linscheid provides a personal history related to the development and evaluation of a new treatment technology, the self-injurious behavior inhibiting system (SIBIS; Linscheid, Iwata, Ricketts, Williams, & Griffin, 1990). The chapter also reveals an added dimension in the development of new behavioral technology not mentioned in the preceding chapter—politics. Linscheid shows how proponents of a particular belief will use disinformation, distortion, and ad hominem attacks in order to achieve their ends. Although he makes an appeal for scientific integrity, the open exchange of information, and open-mindedness in evaluating new treatment options, it is doubtful that one can completely eliminate political considerations when people have strong philosophical commitments and beliefs that are not dependent on scientific evidence.

Linscheid also illustrates the human qualities involved in the development of new technology designed to benefit persons in need of treatment: the concern for the individuals being treated, the careful weighing of potential harm versus benefit involved in the development of new treatment options, and the overriding concern for the client's personal welfare. Linscheid describes how his initial assumptions about what electric shock treatment entailed were somewhat negative and incorrect. The reader can see, however, that Linscheid's dedication to scientific skepticism and his commitment to remain objective about the data led him to change his view about the effects and side effects of shock. One of the strengths of a scientific approach is that one can learn from other people's work. It surely would not be possible to progress very far in one lifetime without such an interactive and cumulative approach. The denial or distortion of research findings thus is clearly not in accord with an evolutionary approach to science.

Linscheid also informs the reader on the activities of those who would oppose the free exchange of information in order to manipulate others to support their position. The use of disinformation and censorship techniques has no place in the selection of treatment methods to meet the needs of any client population. It is certainly unfortunate that a dedicated clinical researcher should be subjected to the personal attacks of the type mentioned in this chapter.

In his summary, Linscheid states that in the

> nearly 20 years of providing clinical service to individuals with developmental disabilities and various medical problems and teaching operant conditioning procedures to students, I have met very few, if any, people in professional positions who truly do not care about their clients' welfare. The emotional intensity that this controversy has engendered, however, has led educated people to disregard or distort the scientific literature, to make proclamations in the absence of proper knowledge, and to attempt to manipulate the free exchange of information.

In support of this position, he points out that the American Association on Mental Retardation denied exhibit space at its national convention to the manufacturer of SIBIS, and that it refused to sell its mailing list to an organization sponsoring a conference because one of the speakers would be describing research on SIBIS. This type of censorship is unprofessional and shameful.

The information presented in this book should help promote the right of clients to effective treatment. One weakness that should be acknowledged, however, is the overreliance in most chapters on data obtained in the area of developmental disabilities. This restricted focus may reduce the generality of many of the points made in that they may not apply equally to work with other populations, such as school applications with nondelayed pupils, clinical applications with nonhandicapped persons, or community applications of behavior analysis.

For example, it may not always be possible to tailor all treatments to the individual if the intervention is to produce a change in the behavior of a large proportion of the community (e.g., reducing highway speeding, increasing condom use in populations at risk for AIDS, or improving the academic performance of disadvantaged children in Head Start programs). In these cases, the use of a treatment package designed to cover many possible factors would likely prove a more effective strategy. Even with this important limitation in mind, the suggestions made in this book should assist behavioral practitioners providing services to individual clients to meet the latter's right to effective treatment.

REFERENCES

Ayllon, T., & Michael, J. (1959). The psychiatric nurse as a behavioral engineer. *Journal of the Experimental Analysis of Behavior, 2*, 323–334.

Azrin, N. H., Hutchinson, R. R., & Hake, D. F. (1966). Extinction induced aggression. *Journal of the Experimental Analysis of Behavior, 9*, 191–204.

Brown, L., Bronston, M. B., Hamre-Neitupski, S., Pumpian, I., Certo, N., & Greunwald, L. A. (1979). A strategy for developing chronological age appropriate and functional curricula content for severely handicapped adolescents and young adults. *Journal of Special Education, 13*, 81–90.

Carr, E. G. (1985). Behavioral approaches to language and communication. In E. Schopler & G. Mesibov (Eds.), *Current issues in autism, Vol. 3: Communication problems in autism* (pp. 37–57). New York: Plenum.

Carr, E. G., & Durand, V. M. (1985). The social-communicative basis of severe behavior problems in children. In S. Reiss & R. Bootzin (Eds.), *Theoretical issues in behavior therapy* (pp. 219–254). New York: Academic Press.

Carr, E. G., & Newsom, C. (1985). Demand-related tantrums. *Behavior Modification, 9*, 403–426.

Charlop, M. H., Schreibman, L., & Thibodeau, M. G. (1985). Increasing spontaneous verbal responding in autistic children using a time delay procedure. *Journal of Applied Behavior Analysis, 18*, 155–166.

Durand, V. M., & Crimmins, D. B. (1987). Assessment and treatment of psychotic speech in an autistic child. *Journal of Autism and Developmental Disorders, 17*, 17–28.

Evans, I. M., & Meyer, L. H. (1987). Moving to educational validity: A reply to Test, Spooner, and Cooke. *Journal of the Association for Persons With Severe Handicaps, 12*, 103–106.

Favell, J. E., & Reid, D. H. (1988). Generalizing and maintaining improvement in problem behavior. In R. H. Horner, G. Dunlap, & R. L. Koegel (Eds.), *Generalization and maintenance: Lifestyle changes in applied settings.* Baltimore: Paul H. Brookes.

Fraley, L. E., & Vargas, E. A. (1986). Separate disciplines: The study of behavior and the study of psyche. *Behavior Analyst, 9*, 47–59.

Horner, R. D. (1980). The effects of an environmental "enrichment" program on the behavior of institutionalized profoundly retarded children. *Journal of Applied Behavior Analysis, 13*, 473–491.

Horner, R. H., & Billingsley, F. F. (1988). The effect of competing behavior on the generalization and maintenance of adaptive behavior in applied settings. In R. H. Horner, R. L. Koegel, & G. Dunlap (Eds.), *Generalization and maintenance: Lifestyle changes in applied settings* (pp. 197–220). Baltimore: Paul H. Brookes.

Horner, R. H., McDonald, R. F., & Bellamy, G. T. (1986). Teaching generalized skills: General case instruction in simulation and community settings. In R. H. Horner, L. H. Meyer & H. D. B. Fredericks (Eds.), *Education of learners with severe handicaps: Exemplary service strategies* (pp. 289–314). Baltimore: Paul H. Brookes.

Iwata, B. A., Dorsey, M. F., Slifer, K. J., Bauman, K. E., & Richman, G. S. (1982). Toward a functional analysis of self-injury. *Analysis and Intervention in Developmental Disabilities, 2*, 3–20.

Iwata, B. A., Vollmer, T. R., & Zarcone, I. R. (1990). The experimental functional/analysis of behavior disorders: Methodology, applications, and limitations. In A. C. Repp & N. N. Singh, *Perspectives on the use of nonaversive and aversive interventions for persons with developmental disabilities* (pp. 301–330). Sycamore, IL: Sycamore.

Johnston, J. M., & Shook, G. L. (1987). Developing behavior analysis at the state level. *Behavior Analyst, 10,* 199–233.

Kazdin, A. E. (1984). *Behavior modification in applied settings* (3rd ed.). Homewood, IL: Dorsey.

Linscheid, T. R., Iwata, B. A., Ricketts, R. W., Williams, D. E., & Griffin, J. C. (1990). Clinical evaluation of the self-injurious behavior inhibiting system (SIBIS). *Journal of Applied Behavior Analysis, 23,* 53–78.

Lovaas, I. O., & Favell, J. E. (1987). Protection for clients undergoing aversive restrictive interventions. *Education and Treatment of Children, 10,* 311–325.

Lovaas, I., Newsom, C., & Hickman, C. (1987). Self-stimulating behavior and perceptual reinforcement. *Journal of Applied Behavior Analysis, 20,* 45–68.

Rast, J., & Johnston, J. M. (1988). Effects of pre-meal chewing on ruminative behavior. *American Journal of Mental Retardation, 93,* 67–74.

Rast, J., Johnston, J. M., Ellinger-Allen, J., & Drum, C. (1985). Effects of nutritional and mechanical properties of food on ruminative behavior. *Journal of the Experimental Analysis of Behavior, 44,* 195–206.

Repp, A. C., & Barton, L. E. (1980). Naturalistic observations of institutionalized retarded persons: A comparison of licensure decisions and behavioral observations. *Journal of Applied Behavior Analysis, 13,* 333–341.

Schloss, P. J., Smith, M., Santora, C., & Bryant, R. (1989). A respondent conditioning approach to reducing anger responses of a dually diagnosed man with mild mental retardation. *Behavior Therapy, 20,* 459–464.

Spreat, S., & Lanzi, F. L. (1989). The role of human rights committees in the review of restrictive/ aversive behavior modification procedures: Results of national survey. *Mental Retardation, 27,* 375–382.

Spreat, S., Lipinski, D., Dickerson, R., Nass, R., & Dorsey, M. (1989). A paramorphic representation of the acceptability of behavioral programming. *Behavioral Residential Treatment, 4,* 1–13.

Stokes, T. F., & Baer, D. M. (1977). An implicit technology of generalization. *Journal of Applied Behavior Analysis, 10,* 349–367.

Touchette, P. E., MacDonald, R. F., & Langer, S. N. (1985). A scatter plot for identifying stimulus control of problem behavior. *Journal of Applied Behavior Analysis, 18,* 343–351.

Wacker, D. P. (1989). Further evaluation of functional communication training: An analysis of active treatment components. In *Treatment of destructive behaviors in persons with developmental disabilities* (pp. 57–58). Washington, DC: National Institutes of Health.

Zarcone, J. R., Rodgers, T. A., Iwata, B. A., Rourke, D., & Dorsey, M. F. (in press). Reliability analysis of the Motivation Assessment Scale: A failure to replicate. *Research in Developmental Disabilities.*

I

Creating an Optimal Learning Environment

2

Defining an Acceptable Treatment Environment

Judith E. Favell and James F. McGimsey

"Our knowledge of the characteristics of effective treatment environments for severely and profoundly retarded people is only in an emergent state of development" (Bruinicks, Rotegard, Lakin, & Hill, 1987, p. 37).

This statement is both true and remarkable. Services for people with developmental disabilities have steadily evolved over the last decades. The methods of habilitation and treatment have advanced, as have the overall service delivery systems of which they are a part. The primitive methods of teaching skills and treating behavioral problems applied within custodial, institutional environments have been steadily replaced by more finesseful, systematic, and sophisticated strategies of active treatment provided in more humane and therapeutic living environments. Despite the unarguable progress seen, the definition of the precise elements that constitute an acceptable treatment environment remain very much an issue of discussion and debate.

Such a perspective may seem uninformed and untrue in light of the vast array of standards that have been promulgated to define and regulate quality in service delivery settings (Holburn, 1990). These standards, including those from the Title XIX Medicaid Reimbursement Program for Intermediate Care Facilities for the Mentally Retarded (ICF/MR), the Accreditation Council for Developmental Disabilities (ACDD), and those developed by individual states and agencies, specify a comprehensive array of dimensions that are deemed necessary in providing adequate services and judged to be reflective of their quality. Such standards have been developed and revised through a

Judith E. Favell and James F. McGimsey • Au Clair Program, Mount Dora, Florida 32757.

Behavior Analysis and Treatment, edited by R. Van Houten & S. Axelrod. Plenum Press, New York, 1993.

process that reflects both competence and experience in provision of active treatment, and they have been of undeniable benefit in increasing the level of services to people with developmental disabilities (Sparr & Smith, 1990). Most agree, however, that much more needs to be done to validate empirically the characteristics of an effective and acceptable therapeutic environment.

Empirical tests of current standards and definitions of an acceptable treatment environment are likely to result in improvements in the efficiency and effectiveness of many dimensions of services. For example, when evaluating the acceptability of an environment, an issue commonly raised relates to the age appropriateness of the materials available in that environment. This quite legitimate issue should not, however, eclipse an equally vital question of whether leisure and habilitative materials are actually used and whether they actually teach functional skills. Regardless of their apparent social appropriateness and instructional potential, materials should not be considered acceptable unless they are actually engaging to clients. Thus, appearance alone cannot define appropriate materials; their functional use must be empirically assessed.

As a further example, adequate staff training constitutes another ingredient of services considered essential in defining an acceptable program. Too often, however, the adequacy of staff training is judged on such dimensions as the number of hours spent in didactic instruction or the written material read. Most agree that these indirect barometers of quality must be replaced by a focus on validating staff training methods against their effectiveness and efficiency in changing client behavior (Christian & Hannah, 1983). Though the point has been made repeatedly, staff training efforts continue to feature methods and content that do not optimally teach caregivers skills that affect clients.

For example, research has shown the power and efficiency of teaching staff through the use of checklists that define tasks such as how to complete client health care routines (Lattimore, Stephens, Favell, & Risley, 1984). Despite convincing effects, in common practice most of these caregiver skills continue to be taught in workshop or didactic formats, often with lengthy verbal and written presentations. These methods are often not effective in ensuring correct staff performance and thus are of dubious benefit. Further, their inefficiency often constitutes a direct interference with client services, as staff spend hours in training and away from their clients. The reluctance to change to more efficient and effective methods of training staff is caused by many factors. Among these is the continued premium placed on documented amount of staff training as a valued barometer of the adequacy of a treatment environment. As standards of staff training are subjected to an empirical analysis of their actual impact on client care, a variety of practices are likely to be changed, and standards redefined.

In a similar fashion, every structural or procedural component currently used to define an acceptable treatment environment can be improved through empirical evaluation. Regardless of their face validity, all dimensions of a program's adequacy must be analyzed for effectiveness and efficiency in benefiting clients. The habilitation planning process, the number and credentials of staff, the due process system whereby treatment plans are reviewed, the monitoring and documentation of services—each element of a treatment environment warrants analysis.

In short, the definition of an effective treatment environment must be *functional*, specifying how its individual aspects and composite milieu actually affect the behavior of individuals within it. Thus, the question of what defines an acceptable treatment environment may be productively addressed by defining a process of analyzing the functional impact of an environment in an individual case and, where effects are found wanting, examining and reordering the means. The examples that follow focus on how an emphasis on functional effects alters the way an acceptable treatment environment is defined, and how it changes the practices in that environment that are designed to promote acceptable and effective treatment.

An Acceptable Environment Is an Engaging Environment

Of the literally hundreds of elements and indicators that might constitute a definition of an acceptable and effective treatment environment, *client engagement* may be the most fundamental measure of whether an environment is responsive to individual needs. Engagement means the active participation of clients in the activities provided in the living environment. Active interaction with the environment, including using materials and interacting with others, may arguably be the least common denominator in defining the adequacy of a therapeutic setting. High levels of engagement denote high levels of reinforcement. Indeed, the "Premack principle" defines high-frequency behavior (i.e., engagement) as reinforcement (Premack, 1959). Thus, frequent engagement with an environment reflects and even defines the extent of reinforcement in that environment.

Dr. Todd Risley (1990), who has articulated and advanced this concept, has discussed the important benefits of engagement in six pivotal areas. First, many studies have shown a negative correlation between engagement and occurrences of problem behavior (Horner, 1980). In short, people who are actively occupied in activities are less likely to exhibit behavior problems. Second, behavior problems are less likely to develop in highly engaging environments. In nonreinforcing environments, behavior problems may emerge as the only reliable means of producing reinforcement of any sort (Steege, Wacker, Berg, Cigrand, & Cooper, 1989). In contrast, in environments in which reinforcement is abundantly available for many behaviors, occasional reinforcement for problems will be less salient and potent, and thus less likely to differentially shape problems relative to other appropriate behavior.

Third, successful management of behavior problems typically depends directly on high levels of reinforcement for appropriate behavior and reduced levels of reinforcement for undesirable behavior. In highly engaging environments, even brief and benign methods of reducing reinforcement contingent upon behavior problems can be expected to have substantial effects, because the period in "time-out" will contrast markedly with higher relative rates of reinforcement in the ongoing "time-in" environment. Conversely, in environments in which engagement in reinforcing activities is low, methods of further reducing reinforcement as a time-out consequence for problem behavior will have to be very depriving and restrictive, if effective at all.

Further, engagement sets the occasion for natural teaching and exploratory play and practice. The best time to teach skills is in the context of activities in which an individual has demonstrated an interest. For example, communication training can effectively be focused on words and signs pertaining to a leisure material the individual has selected and is engaged with (Hart & Risley, 1974; Koegel, O'Dell, & Koegel, 1987). Using engagement as an opportunity for incidental teaching stands in contrast to attempting training with arbitrarily selected and imposed tasks that may have no inherent reinforcing properties.

Aside from the benefits of formal incidental teaching strategies, engagement per se may teach and elaborate skills through exploration and practice. One learns from interacting with the environment, and with sustained engagement one is likely to become more fluent in skills through practice. Though for people with handicaps this process may not be as sure and swift as with normally developing children, at the very least it is clear that unless some level of engagement is ongoing, the environment cannot shape and elaborate skills.

Finally, engagement fundamentally reflects whether an environment is humane. People have a right to live in an environment that is interesting and appropriate for them. Engagement reflects just that; it directly denotes that the environment offers activities and interactions that the individual finds reinforcing. One of the clearest and most basic indicators of an impoverished, unresponsive environment is the lack of activity by its inhabitants. people sitting passively with nothing to do, slouched or sprawled on furnishings and floors, idly milling about and engaged only in persistent stereotypies and periodic episodes of behavior problems—this is perhaps the ultimate image of an inhumane environment. These visions of early institutional environments can still be seen today. Though physical facilities may be attractive, habilitation plans well conceived, staff elaborately trained, and all other foundations of active treatment in place, a program cannot purport to be humane, educative, or acceptable if it does not promote active engagement in its clients. Though levels of engagement may vary across clients with differing characteristics, it is incumbent upon programs to investigate strategies that maximize engagement in each individual.

The benefits and importance of engagement articulated by Todd Risley and his Living Environment colleagues have served as a basis for reforming and reorganizing services for a wide variety of populations with special needs, ranging from infant, toddler, and preschool day care (O'Brien, Porterfield, Herbert-Jackson, & Risley, 1979; Twardosz, Cataldo, & Risley, 1974) to programs serving individuals with developmental disabilities (Risley & Favell, 1979). Measurements of engagement have been developed to track its variations across differing activities. The PLA Check, or planned activity check method (Risley & Cataldo, 1973), for example, consists of repeated instantaneous time samples in which the number of people present in an activity area is divided into the number of people engaged with that activity. The resulting percentage can reveal activities in which individuals are actually occupied and the time spent, as well as those services that are not having a functional effect because individuals are not engaged with them.

Such a measure, which may be used for a group or an individual, can then serve as a basis for reorganizing activities that have been found to have little or no engagement value. For instance, it is not uncommon to find low engagement during transitional periods from one activity to the next. As students move from classroom tasks to lunch, for example, some wait as others finish schoolwork, all wait while individual students wash their hands, and so on. These low-engagement periods, which reflect functional wastes of time, may be constructively filled by orchestrating routines such that children move individually from one activity to the next, rather than moving as a group and thus principally waiting for all to complete each step. This "activity zone" method of scheduling activities is one of many tactics utilized in the Living Environment programs by Risley and his colleagues to increase engagement and realize its attendant benefits (LeLaurin & Risley, 1972). This and many other strategies can similarly be employed in the design of services that optimize engagement and thus improve the educative, therapeutic, and humanitarian properties of environments (Favell, Favell, Riddle, & Risley, 1984).

In summary, measures of engagement are central to the definition of an acceptable treatment environment, for they directly reflect the functional impact of services through the behavior of individuals served. Engagement is the foundation on which functional habilitation, effective treatment, and humane living rests.

AN ACCEPTABLE TREATMENT ENVIRONMENT TEACHES AND MAINTAINS FUNCTIONAL SKILLS

There is virtually universal agreement that the acceptability of a setting or program must rest in large part on whether individuals learn skills that functionally improve their independence, enjoyment, and overall quality of life. Though there is agreement that the teaching of functional skills is central to the definition of an acceptable treatment environment, a number of points bear directly on how this dimension is measured, implemented, and interpreted.

When seeking to determine whether an environment has the mechanisms to teach each client functional skills, a variety of indicators are commonly reviewed. For example, a comprehensive written plan and evidence of an interdisciplinary planning process are typically considered essential elements in the delivery of habilitation services. Likewise, adequate documentation of progress in graphic and/or narrative form is a commonly accepted standard of quality. Although these are of clear value in developing and monitoring training programs, the means employed deserve careful analysis. It is commonly understood that written plans and progress notes do not assure that habilitative services are provided in a reliable fashion. Research and experience support the reality of inconsistent delivery of habilitative programs, despite the existence of written reports dictating and documenting their conduct (Repp & Barton, 1980). For example, the pattern of increased compliance to training and treatment prescriptions during monitoring surveys by funding agencies such as ICF-MR has been documented in a number of studies (Bible & Sneed, 1976; Reid, Parsons, Green, & Schepis, 1991).

Of equal concern is the inefficiency of these planning and monitoring processes (Jacobson, 1987). The many hours consumed in the development and documentation of training may actually result in a net reduction in actual training for clients as program staff invest substantial portions of their time to these efforts. A number of years ago, it was estimated that staff in one residential facility devoted 30% of their time to planning and paperwork. A given interdisciplinary team meeting typically included 20 staff members and consumed 2 hours (J. I. Riddle, 1978, personal communication). It was not known whether the cost of these processes was justified by benefits to clients.

Was the quality and consistency of programming and the client gains achieved worth the time and money invested? There was no formula to apply to the question or latitude to ask it. The standards and surveying practices that prevailed at the time focused heavily on the process of how plans were developed and documented; deviations in that process risked negative survey results and serious funding consequences. As the functional effects of these systems were increasingly questioned, standards and regulations were revised correspondingly. Currently, standards such as ICF-MR have de-emphasized the paper and planning process, focusing instead on observed evidence of training and demonstrable client progress.

Such a reorientation affords an opportunity to analyze experimentally alternative methods of planning, implementing, and monitoring training (Greene, Willis, Levy, & Bailey, 1978). These systems are as amenable to and worthy of empirical test as any other clinical or educational intervention. Measures of the functional impact of such processes as client evaluations, habilitation planning, and documentation and orchestration of training activities should include the cost of the process (i.e., the time invested in it) weighed against the tangible benefits to clients. Does a standardized client evaluation functionally alter the training goals and daily activities of that client? If so, what is the cost relative to the outcome achieved? Are there more efficient alternatives to the usual habilitative planning process? It should be possible to analyze the contribution of components of that process to assess their contribution to a quality product.

Similarly, it should be reasonably straightforward to investigate alternative means of devising the plan, in pursuit of methods that minimize time spent without compromising quality. Is a 2-hour interdisciplinary meeting necessary to devise a meaningful and manageable habilitation plan? Are there more time-efficient methods that can produce similar results? Such questions sound either obvious or heretical, but they must be asked if we are to find optimal means of service. Experimental analyses can be expected to shift the focus of definitions of acceptable treatment environments from untested processes and practices to those that have demonstrated efficacy in functionally benefiting clients.

An example of this empirically based evolution may be seen in the methods of training used to teach functional skills. In the past, the most common model of training involved specialized sessions in which a skill was taught in a controlled and contrived setting, often by a specialist in the domain being addressed. Thus, clients' programming days tended to be characterized by a series of discrete training sessions, often deliberately removed from ongoing activities. Although this model enabled documentation of training and was effective in teaching many skills, it had serious limitations. In particular, the skills taught under these conditions in some cases did not generalize or maintain well in the natural environment. Skills taught under sequestered circumstances were often not in evidence in the normal course of activities in which the skill would ordinarily be functional.

Though it is certainly possible to program for generalization and maintenance, it also became apparent that some skills were most efficiently and effectively taught in situ—that is, under natural conditions in which the skill should be appropriately displayed. Thus, incidental teaching strategies were developed to teach communication, self-care, and other adaptive skills in the context of individuals' everyday environments (Halle, 1987; Hart & Risley, 1974, 1975). This training is conducted within the setting that should naturally set the occasion for and reinforce the behavior and is focused on client-initiated engagement and interactions during which brief but frequent teaching interactions occur (McGee, Krantz, Mason, & McClannahan, 1983). This incidental approach to the training of skills is changing the standards and definition of appropriate education and habilitation. Documentation of discrete training sessions is increasingly not considered adequate evidence that training is being conducted. Greater emphasis is now placed on the demonstration of training in functional settings, times, and activities (Reid, Parsons, McCarn, et al., 1985; Schepis et al., 1982).

The shift in the definition of active treatment has altered the focus of methods used to evaluate its adequacy. The focus is now on evidence of frequent, positive interactions that include appropriate prompting and reinforcement procedures aimed toward increasing independence and use of skills in normal routines. The nature of the activities and materials is now examined more closely to ascertain whether they are functional and reinforcing, rather than arbitrarily selected and imposed on the individual (Favell & Cannon, 1977; Williams, Koegel, & Egel, 1981). This evolution in the methods of teaching skills serves as an important example of how the definition of acceptable treatment changes as the functional impact of practices is empirically tested.

Although certain methods of instruction are increasingly used to define an acceptable treatment environment, debate remains. For example, some contend that acceptable treatment consists solely of normalized methods. In this view, instructional strategies used with persons with developmental disabilities should match or closely resemble training methods used with nonhandicapped individuals. Normalized methods are associated with many advantages; they are less stigmatizing and may effectively teach skills and increase the probability of maintaining those skills in naturalized environments. For example, social praise may be a potent reinforcer in teaching adaptive behavior, and the fact that it is a socially normative reinforcer may greatly enhance the chances that skills will continue to be reinforced and thus maintained. Chapter 6, by Ron Van Houten and Ahmos Rolider, describes a variety of means by which natural conditions and contingencies may be used to promote behavior change effectively.

When normalized and natural consequences and educational methods are effective, they should of course be used in preference to more contrived and artificial procedures. In cases in which they are systematically sampled but found not to be sufficient, however, alternative means should be utilized. If edibles, tokens, and other contrived events are the only functional reinforcers identified for an individual, their use should not be prohibited for other reasons. In such situations, systematic efforts should be undertaken to establish more natural events as functional stimuli. Training efforts should be applied, for example, to pairing natural reinforcers (e.g., social approval) with the more contrived reinforcers that are currently functional. In a similar fashion, teacher prompts and other forms of externally imposed structure should be systematically replaced through familiar processes of fading and thinning, in which controlling conditions and contingencies are gradually changed.

The point is not to assume and remain content with contrived training procedures that may be unnecessary and may in fact impede a client's future progress. Instead, the point is to maintain a clear empirical and pragmatic referent for selecting and utilizing instructional strategies. A client's ongoing progress should not be sacrificed to others' values. As scientists and practitioners, we should assume neither that contrived procedures are the only vehicle for change nor that clients must respond to practices used with typical individuals. The challenge is to identify and analyze means of systematically teaching clients to learn with naturalized methods while not denying them effective education in the process.

Just as initial teaching efforts may require departures from wholly normalized practices, it may be necessary to maintain some level or type of specially designed therapeutic support in order to sustain improvement. Although it is desirable to aim training efforts toward environments and procedures that are as natural and normalized as possible, all such arrangements can only be justified if they are effective in maintaining improvement. For example, fading from highly structured caregiver-controlled conditions and contingencies to honor systems and other types of self-control and peer support programs may successfully maintain skills. In cases where progress deteriorates under less structured conditions, however, return to greater structure and external control is justified. Once again, the definition of an acceptable maintenance regime must rest on its functional properties in sustaining improvement, not on its normalized appearance or adherence to philosophical values. Though the degree of normalization should be extended as far as possible in the lives of each person with a handicap, all changes must be referenced against the habilitative and clinical rights of individuals served.

In summary, acceptable treatment environments are ones that teach and maintain functional skills. They are not defined solely by evidence of habilitation plans or other processes of planning, delivering, and monitoring training. The benefits of each dimension must be empirically tested and verified, validated by their functional effects in the acquisition and maintenance of skills in the natural environment.

An Acceptable Environment Ameliorates Behavior Problems

As with the development of functional skills, a defining dimension of an acceptable environment consists of its effectiveness in treating problem behavior. Problems such as self-injury and aggression are associated with substantial risks and often interfere with habilitative efforts and opportunities to live in less restrictive settings. For this reason, a primary focus is often placed on the methods and outcomes of treatment for such problems.

The acceptability of various methods of clinical intervention has been heavily debated in recent years (Harris & Handleman, 1990; Repp & Singh, 1990). One contingent advocates the sole use of positive treatment strategies, including reinforcement for alternative appropriate behavior, environmental alterations that set the occasion for desirable behavior, and benign behavioral consequences (e.g., verbal reprimands, brief interruption, or prompted redirection for problems). Proponents argue that such nonintrusive methods constitute the only ethical and acceptable means of treating these problems. Others contend that in addition to the procedures described above, severe cases of behavior problems may justify and require the use of behavioral consequences such as "room time out" or even contingent shock (see Chapter 14).

Resolution to the debate over acceptable methods will be aided by changes in both language and practice. First, the acceptability of a method is often based on a priori judgments of its restrictiveness, aversiveness, potential for harm and abuse, and conformance with social norms. Most standards and guidelines used in regulating treatment programs rank order techniques on these bases, allowing those considered most benign to be used routinely while requiring increased levels of due process, expertise, and monitoring for those considered most invasive. Some guidelines prohibit more invasive procedures altogether. The difficulty with these systems of defining acceptability lies in their use of categorical labels assigned to procedures without functional assessments of their actual properties in individual cases.

A procedure is typically labeled restrictive or nonrestrictive without defining the functional nature or extent of restriction that the technique actually imposes for an individual. Similarly, values of aversiveness, potential for harm and abuse, and social acceptability are assigned to techniques without reference to the realities of their application and effect. For example, verbal reprimanding is typically considered quite benign on most dimensions, and thus is viewed as an acceptable nonaversive consequence. In reality, whether or not a reprimand is aversive depends upon its definition and actual effects in an individual case.

The use of the term *aversive* often implies that it is synonymous with punishment. For an event to be functionally defined as a punisher, however, its presentation contingent upon a response must decrease the future probability of that response. Contingent reprimands may have that effect in an individual case (i.e., it may decrease behavior that it follows). Reprimands may have quite different functions, however, with other individuals or in other situations; it may be a neutral consequence (have no effect on behavior) or indeed be an effective reinforcer (increase behavior that it follows). If aversiveness is equated with the emotional reaction that a procedure evokes, reprimanding may have similar variable effects as a result of the individual's learning history. Reprimands may produce dismay, disinterest, or delight, depending upon whether they have been paired with punishment, neutral events, or positive reinforcement, respectively. In short, the effects of a procedure such as reprimanding are a function of its conditioning history and the parameters used in its application. It is not possible to determine this function on the basis of the appearance of the procedure; it must be demonstrated empirically (Van Houten, 1980).

Just as it is not possible to assign an arbitrary label of nonaversive to the procedure of verbal reprimanding, it is similarly not reasonable to assume that reprimands are benign on other dimensions. The procedure can clearly become abusive, drifting into denigrating and offensive diatribes. It can certainly be harmful. Many behavior problems (e.g., self-injury) are developed and maintained by the attention they produce; verbal reprimands constitute one form of attention and thus may similarly serve to reinforce harmful behavior. In these cases, a procedure that is "benign" in appearance may have extremely deleterious effects. Finally, social reprimanding is often viewed as socially acceptable in that it is widely employed in our culture. Many socially normalized practices including ridicule, ostracism, and reprimanding, however, must be questioned from both a humanitarian and a functional perspective.

A similar analysis of such categorical labels should be made of virtually every procedure. The acceptability of a procedure must be judged on the parameters of its application and on its functional properties in individual cases. For example, physical restraint can be punishing to some (Hamilton, Stephens, & Allen, 1967), but it can also be reinforcing, actually increasing the behavior upon which it is contingently applied (Favell, McGimsey, & Jones, 1978, 1981). Similarly, virtually any intervention can restrict freedom and access to opportunities to participate and develop. Such seemingly benign forms of time out as holding an individual's hands down or seating him or her a short distance from the group, if applied repeatedly and/or vigorously, can actually restrict access to activities for longer cumulative durations and to greater extents than versions of time out that are presently labeled more restrictive.

Just as any intervention can be aversive or restrictive; similarly, any procedure can be abusive or harmful. Virtually any procedure can be misapplied with unfortunate or even tragic results. Further, this potential for harm and abuse associated with any intervention must always be referenced against the harm and abuse that can result from lack of effective treatment. Behavior problems such as aggression and self-injury are themselves associated with stress, physical and psychological harm to oneself, and abuse from others and are equally associated with restrictions derived from practices (e.g., physical and chemical restraint) that are used to protect the individual.

In general, categorical and arbitrary labels do not contribute to functional definitions of acceptable treatment environments. These labels must be replaced by individually analyzed and defined procedures. Such a step is fundamental to holding programs and professionals accountable for using procedures that are functionally the least restrictive, and at the same time functionally the most effective, in individual cases (Van Houten et al., 1988).

Aside from labels placed on methods used to treat problems, a second issue bears on the definition of an acceptable treatment environment, in this case relating to measures of effective outcome. Though most would agree that a program must demonstrate successful amelioration of behavior problems, the demonstration of effects is now being critically analyzed. Research and practice in treatment of behavior problems has been appropriately criticized for its narrow focus on single targeted inappropriate behaviors. The reduction of a small number of inappropriate behaviors has traditionally defined a successful intervention. In current thought and practice, however, it is recognized that more expansive measures are required to assess the full benefits and limitations of treatment efforts. For example, in addition to measuring the rate of problem behavior, measures of main effects must be expanded to include methods of assessing changes in the severity and intensity of these problems. Without refined scales of measuring the severity of behavioral episodes, important clinical effects may be overlooked (Iwata, Pace, Kissel, Nan, & Farber, 1990).

Furthermore, the side effects of all interventions must be monitored as well. Though restrictive interventions are sometimes identified as uniquely causing negative side effects, in reality the use of these procedures has been associated with beneficial side effects as well (Newsom, Favell, & Rincover, 1983). At the same time, both positive and negative side effects have been correlated with positive interventions (Epstein, 1985). In short, the high likelihood of collateral changes in behavior associated with virtually any treatment strategy requires that methods of monitoring side effects be routinely incorporated into the evaluation of all treatments.

Third, the generality and durability of behavior change should be carefully monitored. Both the research literature and clinical practice have been characterized by relatively circumscribed and short-term evaluation of effects. In contrast, the goal of all treatment must be pervasive and durable improvement, that is, reductions in the rate and intensity of problems in all life settings and over extended periods. To that end, measurement systems capable of tracking behavioral improvement over extensive periods of time must be developed. This may require the use of different recording methods (e.g., reliable and valid rating scales) that are at once cost-efficient to employ and accurate in reflecting true behavioral change.

Finally, effectiveness of treatment must be measured and judged by the outcomes it produces in terms of functional changes in individuals' lives. The efficacy of treatment approaches and entire therapeutic environments must ultimately rest on whether behavioral improvements result in greater freedom, increased development, and enhanced quality of life (see Chapter 3). Such outcomes provide the most meaningful and legitimate method of evaluating whether means used are justified in terms of ends achieved. The use of invasive interventions can only be justified to the extent that they result in sufficiently improved outcomes (Lovaas & Favell, 1987). At the same time, positive interventions must be held to the same standard.

In short, acceptable treatments and environments of which they are a part must be defined ultimately by whether they positively affect a comprehensive array of measures of behavior change reflecting pervasive, durable improvement and whether these changes in turn result in measurable, meaningful life-style changes. The process of analyzing the adequacy with which an environment provides these means and achieves these ends is not served well by convenient (though unfounded) assumptions about methods, nor by narrow or shortsighted measures of success. Instead, the functional properties of a treatment approach must be analyzed in an individual case and its acceptability ultimately validated on the basis of not only the means employed, but also the outcomes it achieves for that individual.

AN ACCEPTABLE ENVIRONMENT IS THE LEAST RESTRICTIVE ALTERNATIVE

A major tenet appearing in many definitions of an acceptable environment refers to living in the least restrictive setting possible. In applying this doctrine, a placement continuum has evolved, with large segregated institutions and their associated practices typically considered the most restrictive, and community living with fully integrated work and educational opportunities typically viewed as the least restrictive. Along this continuum, varying residential, vocational, and educational arrangements are placed according to such variables as proximity to typical homes and individuals, location and nature of employment, and access to leisure activities commonly used by other members of the community.

It is relatively easy to define restrictiveness in physical terms, such as proximity to typical individuals or access to normalized activities. The true test, however, is whether a placement results in functionally fewer restrictions and functionally increased participation in these activities. Access and proximity do not define a least restrictive setting; that designation must be based on the actual behavior of the individual in that situation (e.g., whether the setting enables demonstrable increases in freedom of movement and engagement in reinforcing activities). In practice, restrictions typically attributed to institutional settings can be and are replicated in community arrangements. Lack of free access to the outdoors may be imposed by institutional inflexibility, but the prohibition has the same functional effect when imposed for reasons of neighborhood intolerance or proximity to a busy street. Similarly, access to community experiences is not enough; measurable differences in actual and successful participation in these activities must validate the claim of reduced restrictiveness. In short, the definition of restrictiveness must be based upon objective measures of each individual's behavior. Actual measures of restrictiveness must be substituted for those based upon assumptions and ideals (Van Houten et al., 1988).

AN ACCEPTABLE ENVIRONMENT IS A STABLE ENVIRONMENT

Of the many dimensions typically cited in the definition of an acceptable treatment environment, one of the most basic is often not explicitly addressed—its stability, that is, the degree to which its services and personnel provide clients with predictability and continuity in their lives. Like all human beings, people with challenging behaviors require and deserve consistency in their interactions and activities, a sense of stability in their daily routines, and order in their lives. Frequent changes in schedules, programs, caregivers, and peers are clear precipitators of problem behavior in many individuals with developmental disabilities. For some, even slight alterations in meal schedules or other expected events may provoke major outbursts. In addition to causing problems, constant change directly interferes with efforts to treat these clients. Effective treatment requires extraordinary degrees of consistency. If environmental arrangements, interactions, and contingencies are provided unreliably and unsystematically, little progress can be expected (Favell & Reid, 1988).

Despite the acknowledged importance of stability to the quality of a therapeutic environment, many programs evidence serious problems in this area. Staff absenteeism and turnover (withdrawal), perhaps the single most disruptive factor in providing stable services, is a chronic and widespread problem in most settings. What was thought to be an institutional problem was found to be equally troublesome in community programs (Zaharia & Baumeister, 1978). Though virtually everyone understands and acknowledges that caregiver withdrawal is an endemic and insidious problem, it continues unabated, viewed as an evil but immutable reality in our field. Although some research has been done with absenteeism, very little can be found in the area of turnover in human service settings. In actual experience, the most reliable variable affecting turnover appears to be the level of unemployment. When unemployment increases, turnover decreases; when the economy improves, human service staff leave to higher-paying and less demanding jobs.

Though staff withdrawal is a potent and pervasive problem, instability in therapeutic environments also occurs for other reasons. Chief among these is the premium placed on change itself. In habilitation plans, for example, emphasis is placed on teaching new skills and adding new dimensions of service. Though this is of unquestionable value, an equal emphasis should be placed on ensuring that previously acquired skills are maintained and that stable routines which clients have adjusted to and enjoy are not excessively disrupted. An opportunity to perform and practice a previously learned skill should be given as high a priority as learning a new one. The opportunity to relax to preferred music in the evening should similarly be honored, even as efforts are under way to teach new leisure skills.

The intent of this discussion is not to discourage efforts to improve services and skills. Instead, it is aimed toward highlighting the importance of stability in therapeutic environments. From that perspective, each factor that influences the continuity and predictability of clients' lives and programs should be critically scrutinized. We can no longer accept such "necessary" evils as staff turnover. Though advocating improved salary scales may seem naive and futile, there is no more important issue that can be addressed. Salaries aside, there are also many other ways of improving the quality of the work environment that can have important benefits for staff morale and performance, and thus for withdrawal. For example, ensuring that staff receive regular, positive feedback has been shown to be a powerful motivator, yet too often this is neglected by supervisors, who themselves too rarely receive positive support. Reorienting such practices can have effects on what is otherwise the most crippling intrusion on the quality of therapeutic environments. In a similar spirit, other factors, even those intended to improve services and skills, deserve careful analysis.

In assessing the adequacy of an environment or program, professional and funding credit should be placed on doing a manageable number of things well and unfailingly. "New and improved" practices and programs should remain the goal, but must be effected in such a way as not to influence negatively those aspects that are essential and in place.

AN ACCEPTABLE TREATMENT ENVIRONMENT IS A SAFE ENVIRONMENT

The acceptability of an environment very basically rests on whether individuals are safe within it. Individuals must be protected from physical and psychological harm, from injury resulting from behavior problems such as self-injury and aggression, from inappropriate access to activities and materials, and from treatments that improperly restrict freedoms or impose unnecessary stress, intrusion, and discomfort (Hannah, Christian, & Clark, 1981). The importance of safety transcends all other dimensions of program quality; without it, no other barometer of acceptability can be justified.

As clear as the mandate for safety may be, the issues surrounding it are complex. Safety from physical harm resulting from behavior problems can only be assured by the effective treatment of those problems. In attempts to remediate these problems, however, practitioners are constrained by a number of disparate forces. First, the clinical procedures available for use in treatment are not of guaranteed effectiveness. Even in the most competent hands and under the best of conditions, results of treatment are not predictable and rarely result in absolute amelioration of a problem. To this clinical imprecision is added strong ethical pressure to employ the least restrictive means of treating a problem. By this tenet, the more positive and benign methods of treatment should be attempted before resorting to more invasive and restrictive means.

The use of protective restraint (e.g., helmets to protect against head banging, and arm splints to reduce the likelihood of aggression against self or others) have been tightly restricted by current regulations, with pressure applied to discontinue their use quickly and permanently. These principles are reasonable and have properly challenged professionals to avoid unnecessary and excessive use of restrictive practices. Clinicians, however, are now faced with a double bind: attempting to treat problems with methods that may have less decisive clinical effects and that do not assure safety through means such as protective restraint, while being required to guarantee the safety of individuals against the harmful effects of problems.

Once again, this dilemma cannot be resolved by broadly framed policies or philosophies. Instead, practices to assure an individual's right to safety must be devised and analyzed in individual cases, with pragmatics taking precedence over philosophy. As the facts of an individual case are examined, realistic and imaginative solutions may be found. For example, when designing services around an individual, it often becomes apparent that changes in the design of the physical environment are required to assure safety and facilitate treatment. Collaboration between architects, designers, and behavior analysts can be expected to result in innovations in materials, furnishings, and other aspects of the physical environments in which people with challenging behaviors live. Far from the tile-and-terrazzo interiors of the past, living environments can be made both attractive and safe.

Just as new approaches to environmental design may be brought to bear in assuring safety, other practices within the environment must be evaluated as to their impact on safety. For example, shift staffing (which involves scheduling different staff for day, evening, and night duties) has been criticized as an institutionalized and nonnormative arrangement, and thus it is not allowed in some community programs. Certain behavior problems, however, require the constant vigilance of awake staff at all times. In such cases, the use of shift staffing seems a small compromise indeed if it allows an individual to live safely in a more integrated setting. If individuals instead are denied this opportunity because of their unique needs, our advocacy for full integration of people with challenging behaviors takes on a hallow and hypocritical tone.

In a similar spirit, other methods of protecting individuals must be individually analyzed. Protective devices such as helmets (to protect against head banging and to prevent pica) have in some cases been used for very prolonged periods as an alternative to treatment. This practice is now recognized as improper, and pressure is increasingly applied to eliminate chronic protective strategies. The appropriate emphasis on treating problems instead of preventing their occurrence through restraints and other restrictive means is well-founded. For example, many individuals who engage in pica respond well to treatment and thus can be freed from the helmets and other restraints that had been used to control the problem artificially (Mace & Knight, 1986). At the same time, it must be acknowledged that our therapeutic technology is imperfect, and clinicians cannot guarantee that even successful treatment will totally eliminate the risk of harm from this dangerous behavior.

To disallow the use of protective devices under all conditions places improper trust in the power of our technology and thus places individuals at risk. As an alternative to categorical prohibitions, a thorough analysis in an individual case may insist on sound treatment for problems such as pica while still allowing judicious use of protection. Methods of protection may be faded over time, but only to the extent that an individual's safety can be assured.

The protection of individuals extends beyond the realm of safety from physical harm. Acceptable treatment environments must provide safeguards to ensure that individuals' rights are protected. Human rights and peer review committees have been established to review and monitor programs for their adherence to legal and ethical standards, and for the appropriateness of the therapies that are employed. These mechanisms have been widely credited with controlling improper use of behavioral technology and holding professionals accountable for providing effective and acceptable treatment. Though in general these plaudits are deserved, it cannot be assumed that these systems work well in all cases. For example, in some instances the review process itself is so lengthy and cumbersome that it functionally becomes an impediment to providing treatment in a timely and efficacious manner. In other instances, these committees have improperly assumed the role of clinician, dictating practices and usurping professional judgement without assuming the responsibility and liability of the practitioner who is in fact responsible for treating the client (see Chapter 8).

A fine line is sometimes crossed between appropriately questioning the rationale and method of treatment and inappropriately requiring that a procedure be used or not used. Such drifts from the original intent and function of human rights and peer review committees may be relatively rare, but they highlight once again the need to analyze empirically the functional impact of all practices, in this case those of due process. At present, most standards and regulations require only that due process mechanisms be in place; the benefits of these procedures are assumed. In order to assure that these methods in fact promote acceptable and effective treatment, however, further analysis of these practices and decisions is needed.

AN ACCEPTABLE ENVIRONMENT IS ONE IN WHICH A CLIENT CHOOSES TO LIVE

Shifting the focus away from procedural definitions and toward measures of client behavior as the most fundamental and valid barometer of an acceptable treatment environment raises a final issue, notably that of client choice. In a very basic sense, an acceptable treatment environment may best be defined as one in which the client chooses to live. Expressed preference may be the ultimate index of the social validity of a setting and the practices within it. A number of issues are attendant, however, with the use of client choice as a basis for placement or as a means of defining the social acceptability of an environment.

First, methods of measuring preference are quite limited, especially for individuals who cannot verbalize their choices (Guess, Benson, & Siegel-Causey, 1985). On one hand, the task of measuring choice of foods and activities is relatively straightforward. In these cases, several items can be presented concurrently, and the percentage of times each is selected can be recorded. Such methods can be used in evaluating other aspects of a therapeutic setting, including preference for habilitative activities and reinforcement systems (Mithaug & Hanawalt, 1978; Parsons, Reid, Reynolds, & Bumgarner, 1990).

The challenge is more formidable when attempting to assess preference for one placement or environment relative to another. Though the logistics and measurement systems necessary to access choice between global variables such as living environments are difficult and at present limited, it is essential that such means be developed. Reliable and valid methods of enabling individuals to sample options and then to assess their preferences may provide important information in developing therapeutic services. The choice of particular caregivers, activities, and even living environments denotes that these are associated with some reinforcing valence that may be beneficial in teaching skills and treating problems. A task that is inherently nonreinforcing may both be more difficult to acquire and provoke behavior problems when presented. Changing that task to one that affords higher levels of reinforcement may increase its educative value and reduce the probability of problematic escape behavior. In the same fashion, assessing the reinforcing value of other aspects of the therapeutic environment (e.g., people, activities, and settings) may provide vital information in teaching skills and treating problems. Thus, asking a client's preference may enhance functional habilitation.

Aside from its therapeutic potential, client choice should clearly be included in any definition of an acceptable treatment environment. At present, social validation of procedures and settings is often based on broadly framed cultural norms and values that may be rigidly applied in treatment and placement decisions for persons with developmental disabilities. If we work for money, then people with developmental disabilities should only work for that version of "a token economy"; if many citizens live in neighborhoods, so should people with handicaps. Such pronouncements too often ignore the unique characteristics of an individual whose preferences and needs do not conform to a narrowly defined concept of social acceptability. Some of us elect to live in rural, sparsely populated settings, others in large cities. Living in an apartment is desirable to some, but isolating and demoralizing to others. We select our friends, our hobbies, our work, and the therapeutic treatments we receive. As with other citizens, the preferences of persons with developmental disabilities should be assessed and weighed seriously in decisions ranging from the selection of treatment techniques to living arrangements. Our own values cannot substitute for the development of means to access and act on their preferences.

Categorical assumptions regarding the need and desirability of institutional placement are wrong; assumptions regarding the need and desirability of neighborhood living are equally presumptuous. In the quest for an acceptable treatment environment, we too frequently substitute one set of imposed values for another. Instead, services should be developed around the individual, incorporating the unique preferences and needs of that person. The value of those services must be validated by demonstrable changes in the behavior of the individual, measured by his or her development of skills, reduction in aberrant behavior, and increased participation in reinforcing experiences. Analyzing the functional impact of an environment in individual cases may avoid arbitrary decisions about what is acceptable, decisions which may result in nonfunctional, even deleterious therapeutic efforts and environmental arrangements.

In summary, the acceptability of a treatment environment ultimately rests on the behavior of the individual within it. Explicit assessment of client behavior—including preferences, progress in development, and participation in reinforcing activities—needs to replace assumptions and arbitrary designations regarding what constitutes an acceptable treatment environment.

REFERENCES

Bible, G. H., & Sneed, T. J. (1976). Some effects of an accreditation survey on program completion at a state institution. *Mental Retardation, 14,* 14–15.

Bruinicks, R. H., Rotegard, L. L., Lakin, K. C., & Hill, B. K. (1987). Epidemiology of mental retardation and trends in residential services in the United States. In S. Landesman & P. Vietze (Eds.), *Living environments and mental retardation* (pp. 17–42). Washington, DC: American Association on Mental Retardation.

Christian, W. P., & Hannah, G. T. (1983). *Effective Management in Human Services.* Englewood Cliffs, NJ: Prentice-Hall.

Epstein, R. (1985). The positive side effects of reinforcement: A commentary on Balsam and Bondy (1983). *Journal of Applied Behavior Analysis, 18,* 71–78.

Favell, J. E., & Cannon, P. R. (1977). Evaluation of entertainment materials for severely retarded persons. *American Journal of Mental Deficiency, 81*(4), 367–361.

Favell, J. E., Favell, J. E., Riddle, J. I., & Risley, T. R. (1984). Promoting change in mental retardation facilities: Getting services from the paper to the people. In W. P. Christian, G. T. Hannah, & T. J. Glahn (Eds.), *Programming effective human services: Strategies for institutional change and client transition.* New York: Plenum.

Favell, J. E., McGimsey, J. F., & Jones, M. L. (1978). The use of physical restraint in the treatment of self-injury and as positive reinforcement. *Journal of Applied Behavior Analysis, 11,* 225–241.

Favell, J. E., McGimsey, J. F., & Jones, M. L. (1981). Physical restraint as positive reinforcement. *American Journal of Mental Deficiency, 85*(4), 425–432.

Favell, J. E., & Reid, D. H. (1988). Generalizing and maintaining improvement in problem behavior. In R. H. Horner, G. Dunlap, & R. L. Koegel (Eds.), *Generalization and maintenance: Lifestyle changes in applied settings.* Baltimore: Paul H. Brookes.

Greene, B. F., Willis, B. S., Levy, R., & Bailey, J. S. (1978). Measuring client gains from staff implemented programs. *Journal of Applied Behavior Analysis, 11,* 395–412.

Guess, D., Benson, H. A., & Siegel-Causey, E. (1985). Concepts and issues related to choice-making and autonomy among persons with severe disabilities. *Journal of the Association for Persons With Severe Handicaps, 10,* 79–86.

Halle, J. W. (1987). Teaching language in the natural environment: An analysis of spontaneity. *Journal of the Association for Persons With Severe Handicaps, 12,* 28–37.

Hamilton, J., Stephens, L., & Allen, P. (1967). Controlling aggressive and destructive behavior in severely retarded institutionalized residents. *American Journal of Mental Deficiency, 71,* 852–856.

Hannah, G. T., Christian, W. P., & Clark, H. B. (Eds.). (1981). *Preservation of client rights: A handbook for practitioners providing therapeutic, educational, and rehabilitative services.* New York: Free Press.

Harris, S. L., & Handleman, J. S. (Eds.). (1990). *Aversive and nonaversive interventions: Controlling life-threatening behavior by the developmentally disabled.* New York: Springer.

Hart, B., & Risley, T. R. (1974). Using preschool materials to modify the language of disadvantaged children. *Journal of Applied Behavior Analysis, 14,* 95–107.

Hart, B., & Risley, T. R. (1975). Incidental teaching of language in the preschool. *Journal of Applied Behavior Analysis, 8,* 411–420.

Holburn, C. S. (1990). Symposium overview: Our residential rules—have we gone too far? *Mental Retardation, 28,* 65–66.

Horner, R. D. (1980). The effects of an environmental "enrichment" program on the behavior of institutionalized profoundly retarded children. *Journal of Applied Behavior Analysis, 13,* 473–491.

Iwata, B. A., Pace, G. M., Kissel, R. C., Nan, P. A., & Farber, J. M. (1990). The Self-Injury Trauma (SIT) Scale: A method for quantifying surface tissue damage caused by self-injurious behavior. *Journal of Applied Behavior Analysis, 23,* 99–110.

Jacobson, J. W. (1987). Individual program plan goal content in developmental disabilities programs. *Mental Retardation, 25,* 157–164.

Koegel, R. C., O'Dell, M. C., & Koegel, L. K. (1987). A natural language teaching paradigm for non-verbal autistic children. *Journal of Autism and Developmental Disorders, 17,* 187–200.

Lattimore, J., Stephens, T. E., Favell, J. E., & Risley, T. R. (1984). Increasing direct care staff compliance to individualized physical therapy body positioning prescriptions: Prescriptive checklists. *Mental Retardation, 22,* 79–84.

LeLaurin, K., & Risley, T. R. (1972). The organization of day-care environments: "Zone" versus "man-to-man" staff assignments. *Journal of Applied Behavior Analysis, 5,* 225–232.

Lovaas, O. I., & Favell, J. E. (1987). Protection for clients undergoing aversive/restrictive interventions. *Education and Treatment of Children, 10*(4), 311–325.

Mace, F. C., & Knight, D. (1986). Functional analysis and treatment of severe pica. *Journal of Applied Behavior Analysis, 19,* 411–416.

McGee, G. G., Krantz, P. J., Mason, D., & McClannahan, L. E. (1983). A modified incidental-teaching procedure for autistic youth: Acquisition and generalization of receptive object labels. *Journal of Applied Behavior Analysis, 16*, 329–338.

Mithaug, D. E., & Hanawalt, D. A. (1978). The validation of procedures to assess prevocational task preferences in retarded adults. *Journal of Applied Behavior Analysis, 11*, 153– 162.

Newsom, C., Favell, J. E., & Rincover, A. (1983). The side effects of punishment. In S. Axelrod & J. Apsche (Eds.), *The effects of punishment on human behavior* (pp. 285–316). New York: Academic Press.

O'Brien, M., Porterfield, J., Herbert-Jackson, E., & Risley, T. R. (1979). *The Toddler Center: A practical guide to day care for one- and two-year olds*. Baltimore: University Park Press.

Parsons, M. B., Reid, D. H., Reynolds, J., & Bumgarner, M. (1990). Effects of chosen versus assigned jobs on the work performance of persons with severe handicaps. *Journal of Applied Behavior Analysis, 23*, 253–258.

Premack, D. (1959). Toward empirical behavior laws: I. Positive reinforcement. *Psychological Review, 66*, 219–233.

Reid, D. H., Parsons, M. B., Green, C. W., & Schepis, M. M. (1991). Evaluation of components of residential treatment by Medicaid ICI/MR surveys: A validity assessment. *Journal of Applied Behavior Analysis, 24*, 293–304.

Reid, D. H., Parsons, M. B., McCarn, J. M., Green, C. W., Phillips, J. F., & Schepis, M. M. (1985). Providing a more appropriate education for severely handicapped persons: Increasing and validating functional classroom tasks. *Journal of Applied Behavior Analysis, 18*, 289–301.

Repp, A. C., & Barton, L. E. (1980). Naturalistic observations of institutionalized retarded persons: A comparison of licensure decisions and behavioral observations. *Journal of Applied Behavior Analysis, 13*, 333–341.

Repp, A. C., & Singh, N. N. (Eds.), (1990). *Perspectives on the use of nonaversive and aversive interventions for persons with developmental disabilities*. Sycamore, IL: Sycamore.

Risley, T. R. (1990). *Treatment of severe behavior problems in persons with developmental disabilities*. Workshop presented at the annual convention of the Association for Advancement of Behavior Therapy.

Risley, T. R., & Cataldo, M. I. (1973). *Planned activity check: Materials for training observers*. Lawrence, KS: Center for Applied Behavior Analysis.

Risley, T. R., & Favell, J. E. (1979). Constructing a living environment in an institution. In L. A. Hamerlynck (Ed.), *Behavioral systems for the developmentally disabled: II. Institutional, clinic, and community environments*. (pp. 3–24). New York: Brunner/Mazel.

Schepis, M. M., Reid, D. H., Fitzgerald, J. R., Faw, G. D., van den Pol, R. A., & Welty, P. A. (1982). A program for increasing manual signing by autistic and profoundly retarded youth within the daily environment. *Journal of Applied Behavior Analysis, 15*, 363–379.

Sparr, M. P., & Smith, W. (1990). Regulating professional services in ICF's/MR: Remembering the past and looking to the future. *Mental Retardation, 28*, 95–99.

Steege, M. W., Wacker, D. P., Berg, W. K., Cigrand, K. K., & Cooper, L. J. (1989). The use of behavioral assessment to prescribe and evaluate treatments for severely handicapped children. *Journal of Applied Behavior Analysis, 22*, 23–33.

Twardosz, S., Cataldo, M. F., & Risley, T. R. (1974). Open environment design for infant and toddler day care. *Journal of Applied Behavior Analysis, 7*, 529–546.

Van Houten, R. (1980). Social validation: The evaluation of standards of competency for target behaviors. *Journal of Applied Behavior Analysis, 12*, 581–591.

Van Houten, R., Axelrod, S., Bailey, J. S., Favell, J. E., Foxx, R. M., Iwata, B. A., & Lovaas, I. (1988). The right to effective behavioral treatment. *Journal of Applied Behavior Analysis, 1988, 21*, 381–384.

Williams, J. A., Koegel, R. C., & Egel, A. L. (1981). Response-reinforcer relationships and improved learning in autistic children. *Journal of Applied Behavior Analysis, 14*, 53–60.

Zaharia, E. S., & Baumeister, A. A. (1978). Technician turnover and absenteeism in public residential facilities. *American Journal of Mental Deficiency, 82*, 580–593.

3

Building Functional Curricula for Students With Severe Intellectual Disabilities and Severe Problem Behaviors

ROBERT H. HORNER, JEFFERY R. SPRAGUE, AND K. BRIGID FLANNERY

People with severe intellectual disabilities who engage in dangerous behaviors present a major challenge. When building support plans (e.g., IEPs, IHPs) for these individuals, the severity of their harmful behaviors often overshadows all other support objectives. Recently, however, leaders in the field have encouraged a reevaluation of our strategies for delivering support (Touchette, 1989a; Wacker, 1989). We are encouraged to use functional analysis assessment procedures more prescriptively (Carr, Taylor, Carlson, & Robinson, 1989; Donnellan, LaVigna, Negri-Shoultz, & Fassbender, 1989; Durand & Crimmins, 1987; Favell, 1990; Iwata, Dorsey, Slifer, Bauman, & Richman, 1982; Mace et al., 1988; Meyer & Evans, 1989; Van Houten et al.,

ACKNOWLEDGMENTS. Preparation of this manuscript was supported in part by the U.S. Department of Education, Cooperative Agreement #G0087CO23488. The opinions expressed herein, however, do not necessarily reflect the position or policy of the U.S. Department of Education, and no official endorsement by the department should be inferred. The authors extend appreciation to Dr. Edward G. Carr, Dr. Richard W. Albin, and Dr. Robert E. O'Neill for their comments on earlier version of this chapter.

ROBERT H. HORNER, JEFFERY R. SPRAGUE, AND BRIGID FLANNERY • College of Education, University of Oregon, Eugene, Oregon 97403.

Behavior Analysis and Treatment, edited by R. Van Houten & S. Axelrod. Plenum Press, New York, 1993.

1988; Wacker et al., 1990) and to apply our technology of instruction in an effort to teach appropriate behaviors that achieve the behavioral function of the dangerous behaviors (Bailey & Pyles, 1989; Carr, 1988; Carr, Robinson, & Palumbo, 1990; Durand, 1990; Horner & Billingsley, 1988). This effort reflects a return to the roots of applied behavior analysis (Baer, Wolf, & Risley, 1968, 1987) and emphasizes that the *content* of instruction is an important concern for the reduction of problem behaviors. We are moving into an era in which durable, generalized behavior change is the standard for success, and where instructional technology will be viewed as among the most powerful approaches for reducing severe problem behavior.

This chapter addresses the role of instructional content (curriculum) in the reduction of problem behaviors, and it is based on two assumptions. The first assumption is that our task is not to discuss curriculum in general, but to meld curricular trends in the field with the unique curriculum needs of people who engage in severe problem behaviors. Typically these individuals are of school or adult age and have severe intellectual disabilities in addition to a history of dangerous behaviors. The second assumption is that curriculum development will need to be individualized; there will not be a specific curriculum for all people who perform problem behaviors. Although a case can be made that any curriculum should include certain communication skills (Lovaas, 1987), social skills (Calkins & Walker, 1990; Haring & Lovinger, 1989), pivotal learning skills (Koegel & Koegel, 1988), and so forth, there is no documentation of a skill sequence that uniquely avoids or remediates problem behaviors. Rather, each person will require unique curriculum content. The need is for an approach for building and revising curriculum content based on individual support needs.

Three important developments in the field are changing the way teachers and support staff build curricula. These developments are (a) a shift in the outcomes expected from behavioral support, from simple behavior reduction to broad change in the life-style of the person; (b) a recognition that although discrete behaviors (skills) are the unit of instruction, activities (skill clusters) are the unit of curriculum development; and (c) a recognition of the power of functional analysis assessment procedures for defining curriculum content. Together, these three developments provide dramatic opportunities for building curriculum content that is uniquely appropriate for an individual and is effective in both facilitating the development of new behaviors and reducing extreme problem behaviors.

EXPANDING THE OUTCOMES OF BEHAVIORAL SUPPORT

The outcomes expected from behavior programs are expanding, and this expansion has implications for the selection of instructional content. In the 1960s and 1970s, a challenge before the behavioral community was to document procedures for decreasing difficult, dangerous, and undesirable behaviors. The outcome measures for success were reductions in the frequency or rate of behaviors that were operationally defined and counted. In general, this challenge was met. Procedures were defined and validated for teaching new behaviors and reducing undesirable behaviors across a range of settings, people, and target behaviors (Alberto & Troutman, 1990; Carr et al., 1989; Cataldo, 1989; Kazdin, 1980; Matson & Taras, 1989; Wolery, Bailey, & Sugai, 1988). In the late 1980s, however, a growing number of individuals began to question the significance of these early gains (Guess, Helmstetter, Turnbull, & Knowlton, 1986; Meyer & Evans, 1989; Turnbull et al., 1986). The recent questioning includes an important "so what" message that should force the behavioral community to reexamine its roots. So what if George screams less than he did 6 weeks ago, if the rest of his life is still isolated, barren, and dysfunctional? The basic challenge is to show that the technology produces changes viewed as important for the overall life of the person, to go beyond demonstrations that behavior analysis works, and to show that it works to the advantage of people with disabilities (Sprague & Horner, 1991).

Behavioral Support in the Context of a Reasonable Life-Style

An acceptable support technology needs to result in people having reasonable life-styles. Though people will debate indefinitely the meaning of *life-style*, the point is that behavioral programming needs to affect what people do on a day-to-day basis: where they go, who they spend time with, and their access to friendships, as well as to work, recreation, learning, and living options that are valued by the individuals and society. Effective programming should affect the ability of a person to express and obtain preferences in his or her life. Wolf (1978) challenged us more than a decade ago to ensure that applied behavior analysis remains focused on socially important outcomes. The concerns he raised are of special importance when programs are developed for people with extreme behaviors. The reduction of severe self-injury or aggression is important; it is a necessary element of a behavior plan that will have life-style significance. The message of today, however, is that reduction of self-injury and aggression is a necessary but *insufficient* accomplishment if it occurs in a context of social isolation, physical segregation, and regimented activity patterns (Horner, 1990; Meyer & Evans, 1989; Turnbull et al., 1986).

This message has implications for our research focus, curriculum content, and intervention procedures. Behavior analysis is a field that is shaped by the selection of dependent variables (Baer, 1991; Horner, 1991); the current technology is a result of selecting frequency (rate) of undesirable variables as a guiding dependent variable. That approach has served us well. Now is not the time to discard what has been learned, or to reject the valuable work that has been conducted. Now is the time, however, to *add* the next level of standards that will give the technology increased validity. Future research and clinical work should include multiple dependent variables (Meyer, 1987; Meyer & Evans, 1989). In addition to measures of frequency, rate, and intensity, we should include measures that provide a broader index of how the person is living. Though this measurement technology is in its infancy (Bellamy, Newton, LeBaron & Horner, 1990; Emerson, 1985; Landesman, 1986; Newton et al., 1987; O'Brien, 1987; Schalock & Harper, 1982), some options include the following:

1. *Physical integration.* Measures should be included that indicate if a person is performing activities in his or her local community in a manner similar to nondisabled, same-age peers. Is the person shopping, traveling, working, and so on in the same places that nondisabled people live, work, learn, and play?

2. *Social integration.* Measures should be included that indicate if a person interacts regularly with others in his or her community. Does the person perform activities with people other than those with whom he or she lives or who are paid to provide support? Does the person have friends? Are there people who are considered important in his or her life? Does the person interact with his or her family?

3. *Variety.* Measures are needed that index the variety of different activities a person performs. Does the person engage in a very small number of activities and perform these over and over, or is there variety in the person's daily pattern of activities?

4. *Preference.* A difficult but important measure will be the index of choice or preference in a person's life (Dyer, Dunlap, & Winterling, 1990; O'Brien, 1987). To what extent does the person have the skills and learning history to define personal preferences, the assertiveness skills to express those preferences, and daily activity patterns that reflect them?

5. *Social Roles.* Measures that are of special value for adults with severe disabilities may focus on the social and professional roles a person maintains (O'Brien, 1987). Does a person participate in activities that serve typically valued roles, such as renter, home owner, employee, employer, community volunteer, and so forth (Berkman & Meyer, 1988)?

The variables listed above typically are not measures included in behavior management programs. They are, however, the kind of measures that should accompany frequency and rate data if we are to show that programs designed to reduce difficult behaviors also improve the quality of life led by people receiving support. Figure 1 provides an example of one format in which traditional measures of problem behaviors are integrated with broader indices of life-style. The data came from a residential support program in Oregon that provides assistance to individuals with severe intellectual disabilities. These individuals moved to the community after being selected by

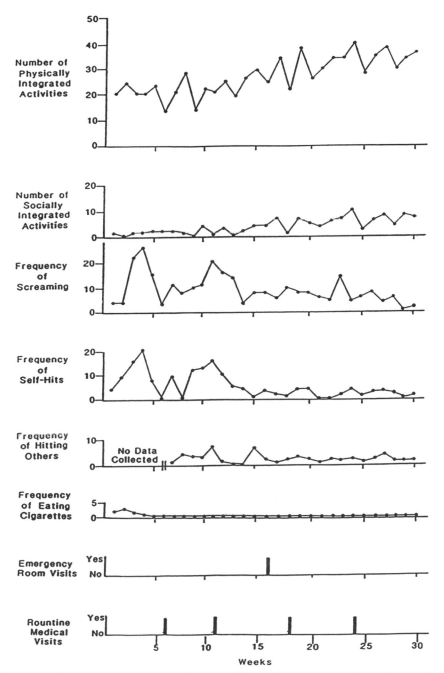

FIGURE 1. The frequency of integrated activites (physical integration and social integration), problem behaviors (screaming, self-hits, hitting others, eating cigarettes), and medical visits (emergency visits, routine doctor visits) per week across 30 weeks of support for one adult with severe intellectual disabilities and a history of severe problem behaviors.

institution staff as among a group of 20 people with the most extreme challenging (i.e., dangerous) behaviors in the institution.

The results in Figure 1 are clinical data for one person collected over 30 weeks by residential staff who monitored targeted behaviors on a 24-hour basis. The purpose of the figure is to show an example in which reductions in problem behaviors were assessed simultaneously with life-style measures such as the number of activities performed in the community (physical integration) and the number of activities performed with people other than housemates or people who were paid to provide support (social integration). The data in Figure 1 do not document experimental control and are not offered in a research format. They indicate, however, that simultaneous with a reduction in screaming, hitting oneself, hitting others, and eating cigarette butts, the frequency of physically and socially integrated activities increased. No causal relationship among these measures is implied, but the combined message from these multiple indices is more compelling than if any one or two measures were presented alone.

Implications of Life-Style Measures for Curriculum Development

Expanding the outcome measures for individuals with severe problem behaviors has two important curriculum implications: (a) addition of broad environmental variables to program plans, and (b) expansion of the range of interventions proposed. Because support plans are evaluated for their influence on the life-style of the students, a need exists to include more focus on the setting, activities, and social contact in the curriculum. It is no longer enough to indicate simply *what* the student is to learn; the curriculum should also indicate *where* and *with whom* behaviors are expected to occur. The expanded outcomes required of support plans will force curriculum developers to attend to the context in which behavior occurs as well as the topography, rate, and intensity of the behavior.

A second implication of the expanded outcomes is the need for more comprehensive support plans. For many students, simple solutions will not produce dramatic outcomes. A student who is 16 years old, lives in a barren environment, and hits his head whenever he is approached by staff may not experience the types of life-style changes desired simply by modifying his schedule of reinforcement. Although the power of effective reinforcement is well documented, we anticipate that the use of life-style outcomes will result in support plans that simultaneously incorporate changes in the physical structure of a living (work/school) setting, changes in social options, changes in instructional goals, and changes in medical support, as well as changes in the consequences for behavior. As the array of outcomes expands, so will the array of procedures used to deliver support. The net result will be support plans that are more comprehensive and include simultaneous manipulation of many variables (Evans & Meyer, 1987; Voeltz & Evans, 1983).

It is not enough to change an isolated behavior if that change is not related to how a person lives. For the teacher or staff person designing the curriculum for an individual, this means assessing how the content of instruction and behavior support plans affects how the individual will work, play, learn, make friends, and be part of his or her ongoing community life. This approach to curriculum development is related to the second major change in curriculum theory: a shift from skills to activities as the unit of curriculum development.

MOVING FROM SKILLS-BASED CURRICULA TO ACTIVITY-BASED CURRICULA

A curriculum defines the content of instruction. Skills are the content that have guided curriculum development during the past 20 years. Skills are the core of language, math, and reading programs. We teach people how to perform certain skills (behaviors) more often, and to perform other skills (behaviors) less often. Typically, skills are selected for inclusion in a curriculum because they are perceived as important prerequisites for future development, or because they are a set of behaviors typically performed by others in our society (Brown, Branston, Baumgart, et al., 1979; Brown, Branston, Hamre-Neitupski, et al., 1979; Ferguson & Wilcox, 1987; Wilcox & Bellamy, 1987).

An alternative approach to curriculum development is based on two concepts: (a) build the curriculum around the *functions* or accomplishments of behavior, not the specific skills, and (b) sequence the curriculum content so the full cluster or set of behaviors needed to achieve a desired function is taught as a unit (i.e., teach the learner to achieve the outcome, not just perform a skill). This approach has its roots in the mandate from Brown and his colleagues that students need to meet the "criterion of ultimate functioning" (Brown, Neitupski, & Hamre-Neitupski, 1976)—that is, that students should be able to perform a newly acquired behavior to the criterion demanded by the natural environment. The behavior should occur in the full range of appropriate situations encountered in typical daily routines, should not occur in inappropriate situations, and should be performed in a way that produces the natural "function" in these natural situations (e.g., is effective in obtaining natural reinforcers; Baer, 1982; Baer & Wolf, 1970; Horner, Bellamy, & Colvin, 1984; Horner, Dunlap, & Koegel, 1988; Sailor et al., 1989; Stokes & Baer, 1977).

A growing group of authors (Falvey, 1986; Ferguson & Wilcox, 1987; Ford et al., 1989; Guess et al., 1986; Neel & Billingsley, 1989; Sailor et al., 1989; Wilcox & Bellamy, 1987) have recently presented similar variations of an approach to curriculum development that meets Brown's challenge. It is based on activities (also labeled "tasks," "routines," or "skill clusters") as the unit of analysis, rather than skills. An activity is a sequence of behaviors that, if performed in the natural environment, will produce a socially important outcome (Wilcox & Bellamy, 1987). Activities define the cluster or set of behaviors that are needed to produce a functional effect. Some of the skills may be taught, some may be performed with the help of prosthetics and alternative performance strategies, and some may be avoided altogether through creative sequencing or external assistance.

Activities are the units of behavior that nondisabled people typically use in describing their own behavior: Allen shopped for groceries, Amy visited a friend, Paul went to the gym and played basketball. The importance of defining activities is that they focus curricular attention on the social outcome of behavior. The objective of instruction for students with severe disabilities should not be to teach students to behave exactly like their nondisabled peers, but to *achieve the same outcomes* that are achieved by the latter. Activities focus on socially important outcomes and allow substantial discretion in the chains of behavior used to achieve those outcomes.

Traditional curricula are developed by defining the discrepancy between what typical people do and what the student with disabilities does (e.g., John is 5 years old, nondisabled, and ties his shoes; therefore, we need to teach Allen, who is 7 years old, and severely disabled, how to tie his shoes). An activity-based curriculum is designed by defining the accomplishments (Gilbert, 1978) that typical people achieve and assessing the discrepancy between those accomplishments and those of the student with severe disabilities. For example, John puts his shoes on by himself; it happens that he does this by lacing them up and tying the laces. Allen may be able to attain the same accomplishment (i.e., putting on his shoes as part of getting dressed) by learning to tie laces, wearing loafers, wearing shoes with velcro fasteners or using a prosthetic that holds his shoe while he inserts his foot. The shift to activities as the unit of curriculum development is a shift from skills to accomplishments as the foundation for curriculum analysis.

An activities-based approach to curriculum development avoids two errors. First, it avoids the assumption that one student needs to learn exactly the same behaviors as other students. The student may need to achieve the same functions, but how he or she does that may be unique for each learner. The second error is teaching individual skills in isolation. An activities-based curriculum assumes that the learner must achieve the desired effect, not just perform an isolated skill. For example, the skill of street crossing would never be taught in isolation; a person learning to cross streets would always perform the behavior in the context of an activity (e.g., going shopping, going to the park, visiting a friend).

The shift to activities-based curricula is very consistent with behavioral theory. With an activities-based approach, behaviors are taught in a functional context (i.e., are followed by natural stimuli that are presumed reinforcers). In addition, the emphasis on function over topography of responding is consistent with a response-class analysis of adaptive behavior (Johnston & Pennypacker, 1980; see Chapter 10).

Curriculum Content Should Focus on Immediate Effects

Among the most important implications of a functional approach to curriculum is the expectation that a curriculum should have an *immediate* effect on the person's life. The content of a curriculum should be logically related to overall patterns of where individuals go, what they do, and with whom they spend time. Curricula can be restricted if the focus is only on preparing the learner for future events and ignores (or undervalues) the immediate impact of the skills to be learned. A typical rationale for curriculum content is that the skills taught in the curriculum are building blocks that the student will need either later in life or in more complex tasks (Haring & Bricker, 1976). This rationale led to the creation of skill sequences that were designed to provide the "prerequisite" skills needed for participation in typical community contexts (Brown et al., 1976; Guess & Helmstetter, 1986; Wilcox & Bellamy, 1982). The "prerequisite" logic works well for math, reading, and language (Lovaas, 1987; Schiefelbusch, 1978); for example, there are prerequisite skills that should be mastered before presenting multiplication (e.g., Engelmann & Carnine, 1982).

The logic of skills sequences, however, is less clear for students with moderate, severe, or profound intellectual disabilities. You do not need to learn to identify colors before you learn to dress yourself, do your own laundry, or hold a job. In fact, the logic behind teaching prerequisite skills may serve as a trap for many students with severe disabilities. By failing to acquire so-called prerequisite skills, students are denied access to events that would have a significant positive impact on their immediate lives. A curriculum logic that assumes a student must be able to count before he or she goes into real work settings can result in a 19-year-old student studying preschool number skills when supported employment at a local bakery would have a more dramatic impact on his or her life (Ferguson & Wilcox, 1987; Ford et al., 1989; McDonnell & Horner, 1985; Snell, 1987; Wilcox & Bellamy, 1982).

Curriculum Content Should Be Socially and Behaviorally Functional

The importance of making curriculum content functional is generally accepted (Brown, Branston, Baumgart, et al., 1979; Brown, Branston, Hamre-Neitupski, et al., 1979; Falvey, 1986; Wilcox & Bellamy, 1987). For students with disabilities who engage in severe problem behaviors, however, the way in which *functional* is defined may need expansion. Brown and his colleagues have determined that an activity is functional if a nondisabled person would need to perform the activity if the student with disabilities did not. This is an excellent criterion for assessing the extent to which a behavior is socially functional. From a behavior analytic perspective, however, a functional response is one that increases the probability of reinforcement (positive or negative). Although both standards are valid, it is important to acknowledge the shift in perspective used to assess functionality. An activity is socially functional if it produces an outcome valued by society; it is behaviorally functional if it produces an outcome valued by the individual. For students with severe problem behaviors, it may be important to build a curriculum that meets *both* of these standards of functionality.

Curriculum Content Should Be Locally Referenced

A curriculum is functional for an individual only if it is referenced to the specific stimuli, opportunities, and outcomes available in the environment where the person behaves. This requires special attention to the demands of the local community. No two communities are alike; being a participating member of the community of Philadelphia, Pennsylvania, is entirely different than it is in tiny Sweet Home, Oregon. A person's curriculum should include things that are relevant in the community in which he or she spends time—the community at large, the residential community, the work or school community, and so forth. The activities included, as well as the criteria of performance, should be determined by the demands of that community.

The focus of the curriculum becomes one of teaching enough so that the learner is competent locally rather than teaching a prescribed set of generic skills that will result in competence across all environments. The curriculum should be more specific to the individual and the community in which he or she lives. In the past, the same set of skills were learned by all persons. This may have included making a bed, identifying the foods in each of the four food groups, and crossing all types of streets. Yet in Mary's home, for example, it may be acceptable to just pull the sheets and covers to the top of the bed. She does not need to make the bed and tuck in the covers. Similarly, John may not need to learn to cross all types of streets, just those he will encounter in his normal daily routines. The content of instruction is based on individual needs and makes the curriculum (a) more likely to influence the student's life-style, (b) less likely to teach irrelevant behavior, and (c) more likely to teach behavior that will be maintained by natural consequences.

Curriculum Content Should Be Peer Referenced

Curriculum content should be guided by the activity patterns of same-aged peers (Brown, et al., 1976; Wilcox & Bellamy, 1987). This will facilitate interactions between the person with disabilities and her or his nondisabled peers (Falvey, 1986). Storey, Stern, and Parker (1990) found that the perceptions of a person's capabilities are influenced by the types of activities in which the person participates. Typical community members viewed adolescents with severe disabilities as more competent and more likely to assume adult roles if they watched slides of the students performing the same activities similar to their nondisabled peers than when they watched slides of these same students performing activities within a juvenile context (e.g., golfing with plastic clubs and balls versus golfing with regular equipment on a regulation course). The use of age-appropriate materials and activities as the content for curriculum will decrease social misperceptions (Brown, Branston, Hamre-Neitupski, et al., 1979).

FUNCTIONAL ANALYSIS ASSESSMENT AND CURRICULUM DEVELOPMENT

Functional analysis assessment is a process for determining the reinforcers maintaining a behavior and the stimulus conditions that set the occasion for the behavior. Traditionally, there has been only one process for conducting a functional analysis. That process is to monitor a target behavior over time and to manipulate antecedent stimuli and response consequences systematically to determine the features of the environment that reliably predict and maintain the behavior (Iwata, 1989; Iwata, Dorsey, et al., 1982). The use of single-subject research designs (Barlow & Hersen, 1984) allows documentation of a functional relationship between the behavior and events in the environment. The power of this process is the precision and experimental rigor that it allows. The disadvantages are the time required to complete the analysis, the high experimental expertise required of the clinicians, and the difficulty in identifying the range of different variables that may be affecting the behavior (especially those that are *not* temporally proximal to the target behavior).

In response to the needs of clinicians, there have been many recent efforts to expand the array of strategies used to conduct functional analysis assessments (Lennox & Miltenberger, 1989; Romanczyk, 1989). Two additions to the assessment strategy of environmental manipulations are interviews with people who know (and work or live with) the individual with disabilities (Durand & Crimmins, 1987; O'Neill, Horner, Albin, Storey, & Sprague, 1990; Touchette, 1989b; Willis, LaVigna, & Donnellan, 1989) and systematic observations in clinical settings (Iwata, Wong, Reardon, Dorsey, & Lau, 1982; Miltenberger & Fuqua, 1985; Miltenberger & Veltum, 1988; Touchette, Mac-Donald, & Langer, 1985). In both cases, attention is given to defining conditions in which problem behaviors are most and least likely. The attempt is to identify patterns of antecedent and consequent events associated with the problem behaviors. Although these interviews and clinical observations do not meet the rigorous standards of functional analysis manipulations (Iwata,

Pace, Kalsher, Cowdery, & Cataldo, 1990), they have been useful in defining settings, people, places, situations, demands, and reinforcers associated with difficult behaviors (Durand, 1990).

The three strategies for obtaining assessment information (interview, observation, and manipulation) are increasing the number of behavior support plans developed from hypotheses concerning the function(s) of a problem behavior (Carr et al., 1990; Carr et al., 1989). A major assumption in the field is that we will be able to develop more effective (and less intrusive) behavioral programs if we have information about the antecedent and consequent events associated with a behavior. For example, a teacher or clinician who designs a support plan for a person who engages in severe head hitting may develop a different plan if all that is known is that the person hits his head, versus knowing that head hitting is restricted to only three times during the day, that difficult demands are made during each of these times (and at no other times), and that the person is able to avoid the demands when he hits his head.

Functional analysis assessment information has relevance for many elements of behavioral programming (Carr et al., 1990; Favell, 1990; Koegel & Koegel, 1988). We will focus on the significant implications of this assessment information for curriculum development.

Problem Behaviors as Skill Deficits

Teaching new skills is among the most powerful behavior management strategies we have. If a clinician can determine the function of a problem behavior, and if a socially desirable and functionally equivalent behavior can be identified and taught, there is reason to believe that the problem behavior will decrease and the alternative behavior will maintain and generalize (Carr, 1988; Carr et al., 1990; Cataldo, Ward, Russo, Riordan, & Bennett, 1986; Durand, 1987; Favell & Reid, 1988; LaVigna & Donnellan, 1986; Meyer & Evans, 1989). In effect, the new desirable behavior will compete with, and thereby reduce, the problem behavior (see Chapter 10; Repp, Singh, Olinger, & Olsen, 1990; Sasso & Reimers, 1988; Wacker et al., 1990). The logic of teaching new behaviors as a strategy for decreasing undesirable behaviors transforms functional analysis from a behavior management procedure to a procedure with direct curriculum implications. The message is that dangerous and undesirable behavior may serve as a direct guide to defining the most important skills (activities) that should be taught.

Examples of the impact that functional analysis assessment is having on curricular decisions are documented in a growing research literature (Carr et al., 1990; Repp, Felce, & Barton, 1988; Wacker, 1989). Horner and Budd (1985) worked with a 9-year-old boy who grabbed and screamed during instruction. An informal functional assessment suggested that the problem behaviors were maintained by access to desired objects such as toys and food. Rather than developing an intervention based upon a negative consequence for grabbing and screaming, the authors used this assessment hypothesis to change the curriculum for this boy to include instruction on communication skills (ASL signs) for requesting the desired objects. When the communication skills were taught in the natural context, the boy shifted from grabbing and screaming to formal communication. The frequency of grabbing and screaming decreased to near-zero levels as long as the formal communication was effective in achieving access to the objects.

Similarly, Carr and Durand have provided a series of studies documenting the use of functional analysis to guide curricular decisions (Carr & Durand, 1985a, b; Durand & Crimmins, 1987). Durand and Carr (1987) examined the function of stereotyped behavior with four children. Through direct observations, they hypothesized that stereotypy during instruction was maintained by escape from the instructional sessions where teachers presented tasks that were difficult (e.g., resulted in errors). When time out followed an instance of stereotypy, the rate of stereotypy during instruction increased. The authors concluded that stereotypic behavior was used to avoid difficult tasks. An alternative, functionally equivalent behavior would be to ask for help from the teacher. Based on this hypothesis, Durand and Carr taught students to ask for help when they encountered a task that was difficult. The result was that as asking increased, the rate of stereotypic behaviors decreased. Once again, the functional analysis was used to direct the clinicians to a skill that needed to be taught.

Using functional analysis results to teach new skills may also improve the generalized outcomes of instruction. Durand (1984) reported an impressive analysis with 12 youths who were assessed as using aggressive and resistive behaviors to avoid difficult tasks. Half of these students received training in communication skills that they could use to request teacher assistance when faced with difficult instructional demands; the other half received a time-out program to decrease their aggression. All 12 students decreased their levels of problem behavior during instruction. The difference between the two groups appeared when they were presented with novel teachers. Students who had been in the time-out program responded to the new teacher by reverting to the original levels of aggression and resistance. The students who had been trained to use communication behaviors to avoid difficult situations continued to use communication rather than aggression when faced with a novel teacher. The implications of this analysis hold great promise as a foundation for building a technology of generalized response reduction (Favell & Reid, 1988).

The Role of Response Efficiency

A recent supplement has been offered to the recommendations that functional analysis assessment be used to select training objectives. The addition is the critical role that *response efficiency* plays in the selection of functionally equivalent training objectives. Response efficiency refers to (a) the physical effort required to perform a behavior (e.g., it may be more effortful to throw objects and hit the teacher than to use a simple manual sign), (b) the schedule of reinforcement (e.g., an extremely self-injurious behavior may only need to be performed once to get teacher attention, whereas a more benign behavior may need to be performed many times before the same outcome is achieved), and (c) the latency between delivery of the Sd (discriminative Stimulus) and delivery of the reinforcer (e.g., a communication response that takes 10 seconds to perform and results in the teacher saying, "OK, you may take a break in a minute," may be less efficient than a short, aggressive response that results in immediate escape from an undesirable task).

Response efficiency is an important curricular variable when selecting instructional objectives. Recent research has documented the critical role of response efficiency (Day & Horner, 1990). Horner, Sprague, O'Brien, and Heathfield (1990) used a functional analysis manipulation to document that the hitting and property destruction of a 14-year-old boy with moderate mental retardation was maintained by escape from difficult instructional tasks (e.g., tasks in which he got 33% or fewer trials correct). When the student received extra teacher assistance during difficult tasks, he did not engage in aggression. The authors taught the student two behaviors for requesting teacher assistance. One procedure involved using a small communicator on which the student typed out the message "Help, please." This was a difficult response chain for this student, partly because of his mild cerebral palsy. A second, more efficient, strategy was to press one button on the same communicator. That button was programmed to produce the same "Help, please" response.

Systematic manipulations of treatment conditions documented that the student learned both communication strategies. When he was only given access to the hard skill of typing out "help, please," he was more likely to use aggression than to use the communication alternative. When he learned that a single button push produced teacher assistance, however, the rate of aggression plummeted. The more efficient communication behavior effectively replaced aggression. The onerous spelling response was less efficient than aggression, and it did not replace aggression even though it generated the same functional effect (escape from a difficult learning trial). The central message for clinicians is that the efficiency of both the problem behavior and the desirable alternative needs to be assessed when using functional analysis to guide curriculum decisions.

Focusing on the function of severe problem behaviors is an exciting development that holds much promise for clinical success. Functional analysis procedures can assist in the development of more effective and efficient support plans. It should be noted, however, that functional analysis is not a panacea. We do not believe functional analysis assessment will define the support programs for behaviors maintained by variables such as endogenous opiates, homeostatic imbalance, or hormonal abnormalities. Nor do we believe that functional analysis assessment will preclude the need for all reductive procedures (Wacker et al., 1990). We do, however, believe that the information from functional analysis assessment will lead to hypothesis-based interventions that are more comprehensive, more effective, and generally less intrusive than interventions developed without such information (Carr et al., 1990).

MODIFYING INSTRUCTIONAL STIMULI THAT ARE DISCRIMINATIVE FOR PROBLEM BEHAVIOR

An effective functional analysis defines not only the stimuli that maintain a problem behavior, but the stimuli that set the occasion for the behavior (O'Neill et al., 1990; Touchette et al., 1985; Willis et al., 1989). Given an instructional context in which high rates of aggression or self-injury are occurring, the functional analysis results should be useful in addressing several curricular questions.

1. *Consider changing the curriculum content.* The first question is whether the task is functional for the learner. Is the outcome of the task sufficiently reinforcing that it could be expected to maintain the skill once the student has met the training criterion? If the functional analysis data suggest that the student is attempting to avoid instruction and there are no data to support that the skill (activity) is reinforcing, then consideration should be given to changing the focus of instruction (i.e., changing the activity).

2. *Consider removing discriminative stimuli for problem behavior.* If the functional analysis suggests that the task is appropriate but that it includes stimuli that are discriminative for problem behavior, the curricular decision may be to remove the instructional stimuli that occasion the problem behavior. Albin, O'Brien, and Horner (1990) present an analysis in which a high school–age woman performed an escalating sequence of problem behaviors when her teacher used a harsh voice to remind her of classroom rules. When low levels of problem behavior were ignored and the harsh reminders were eliminated, the rate and intensity of problem behaviors dropped dramatically. The functional analysis had been effective in identifying a stimulus that was associated with problem behaviors. When the teachers removed that stimulus (harsh reminder), the likelihood of the problem behaviors decreased.

3. *Consider adding extra teacher assistance.* If the specific stimuli that occasion the problem behavior cannot be identified or cannot be manipulated, additional teacher assistance may reduce the problem behaviors. As mentioned earlier, several studies have shown that the addition of staff

prompts with difficult tasks has been effective at reducing escape behaviors (Carr & Durand, 1985a; Horner, et al., 1990). It may be that students who have a history of instructional failure treat errors, and error corrections, as functional punishers. When extra teacher assistance is provided and errors are reduced, the student is more likely to work on a hard task without problem behavior.

4. *Consider interspersing easy tasks.* If the functional analysis suggests that problem behaviors are associated with task difficulty, one curricular decision may be to add known, easy tasks to each session of instruction on the difficult task (Dunlap, 1984; Dunlap & Koegel, 1980; Dunlap & Plienis, 1988; Engelmann & Carnine, 1982; Engelmann & Colvin, 1983; Neef, Iwata, & Page, 1980). Dunlap (1984) and Winterling, Dunlap, and O'Neill (1987) have shown that when a functional analysis assessment indicates that task difficulty is related to problem behavior, the addition of such "maintenance tasks" can both increase acquisition of the new skills and decrease the rate of problem behaviors. Maintenance tasks are behaviors that the learner has already acquired to criterion. They are interspersed after every one to five trials of the difficult task. The learner receives a mixture of known, easy trials and more difficult, new trials. The result is much higher levels of responding to the difficult trials, better acquisition, and less problem behavior.

This basic strategy has been modified slightly and reported in several recent analyses of "interspersed requests" (Horner, Day, Sprague, O'Brien, & Heathfield, 1991; Mace et al., 1988; Singer, Singer, & Horner, 1987). In each of these studies a series of short, easy requests were delivered as part of instruction with students whose aggressive and self-injurious behavior was maintained by avoiding instruction on difficult tasks. The teacher would present three to five requests that (a) required less than 3 seconds to complete, (b) had a very high probability of being performed correctly, (c) were followed by praise, (d) were delivered in rapid succession, and (e) were presented immediately before presentation of a trial on the difficult task. In each study, a functional analysis documented that the problem behavior of the learner was maintained by escape from the difficult task. When the interspersed request strategy was employed, aggressive and self-injurious behavior was reduced or eliminated, and the students attempted to complete the difficult tasks more often.

Taken together, the above considerations point to an array of important curricular decisions that teachers can make in response to students who perform problem behaviors during instruction. Functional analysis assessment is an effective procedure for assessing whether the skills (activities) in the curriculum are functional for the learner and whether specific stimuli in the instructional presentation are associated with the problem behavior. If these stimuli can be isolated, often they can be eliminated without hindering the instructional process. The message is that an effective functional analysis offers considerable information for determining the stimuli presented during instruction.

Selecting Functional Reinforcers

Among the most significant challenges for teachers of students with severe intellectual disabilities is the identification of functional reinforcers. Functional analysis assessment procedures have been suggested as one approach for addressing this curricular need. Recently, Mark Durand and his colleagues have proposed using functional assessment of problem behaviors as a guide for defining reinforcers that can be used to build adaptive behavior (Durand, 1987, 1988, 1990; Durand, Crimmins, Caulfield, & Taylor, 1989). The basic idea is that if a specific consequence can function to maintain a problem behavior, it should also be effective at building and maintaining an adaptive behavior. This approach is consistent with the central theme of functional equivalence training (Carr, 1988), but it has special value for those learners who have few identified reinforcers and high levels of problem behavior.

In a recent innovative analysis, Durand et al., (1989) examined the disruptive and aggressive behavior of six students during instruction. The assessment suggested that the problem behavior of some students was maintained by escape from the learning situation, whereas the problem behavior of other students was maintained by attention from the teaching staff. All of the students received instructional sessions in which enthusiastic teacher praise was delivered for working on the task. In addition, all students received sessions in which the teacher turned away (time out from teacher) when the student performed well on the task. The results indicated that the students who were hypothesized to work for teacher attention performed very well during the praise condition and exhibited high levels of disruptive behavior during the sessions when the teacher turned away. Conversely, the students who were viewed as working to escape the instructional setting did well during the sessions when the teacher turned away and were very disruptive during the sessions when their task performance was followed by praise. The study demonstrated that the information from a functional analysis assessment can be useful in tailoring the reinforcers used during instruction. Even events typically viewed as punishers (e.g., the teacher turning away) may function as powerful reinforcers for some students.

Curricular Issues in the Assessment and Design of Setting Events

Functional analysis assessment also holds promise for guiding the manipulation of more generic features of a setting—the physical surroundings, proximity to others, schedule, meals, sleep cycles, and so forth. The field of behavior analysis traditionally has placed an emphasis on measuring individual events that are present immediately before and after a behavior occurs (Alberto & Troutman, 1990; Kazdin, 1977; Sulzer & Mayer, 1972). Researchers and clinicians now are beginning to emphasize the role of proximally distant stimuli in affecting problem behavior (Colvin & Sugai, 1989; Leigland, 1984; Meyer & Evans, 1989; Wahler & Fox, 1981). There is growing evidence that a number of problem behaviors are associated with multiple discriminative stimuli (Gardner, Cole, Davidson, & Karan, 1986; Patterson, 1982). Though there is some debate about the technical appropriateness of the term (see Michael, 1982), a number of studies refer to these temporally distant stimuli as *setting events*.

Setting events are stimuli that interact with existing discriminative stimuli to produce momentary changes in existing stimulus-response relationships (Bijou & Baer, 1961; Kantor, 1959; Leigland, 1984; Michael, 1982). The setting-events literature for persons with severe disabilities focuses on describing the relationships between specific setting features and stereotypical behaviors (Brusca, Nieminen, Carter, & Repp, 1989; Favell, 1990; Horner, 1980), self-injurious behaviors (Schroeder et al., 1982), rumination (Lazar & Rucker, 1984), and aggression (Gardner et al., 1986). Each of these studies has demonstrated a relationship between setting events and the behaviors of concern. Some of the events that have been identified with serious behavior events include illness or pain, schedule changes, noise level, irregular sleep patterns, and serious disruptions (i.e., a fight at home before coming to school or work).

Although it has been difficult to arrange systematic manipulation of setting factors for functional analysis, successful measurement strategies include completing checklists of identified events (Colvin & Sugai, 1989; Gardner et al., 1986; Patterson, 1982), filling simple matrices of behaviors and events by time period (O'Neill et al., 1990; Touchette et al., 1985), and direct observation of the effects of such environmental features as type or materials or density of staff interaction (Horner, 1980; Repp et al., 1988). Logistical issues affecting the assessment of specific setting factors also extend to the development of curricular interventions. Certain setting modifications, such as including more materials to interact with (Horner, 1980) or changing the schedule of food intake (Lazar & Rucker, 1984), are relatively clear-cut and easy to implement. Attempting to decrease the frequency of fighting or disruption at home may be more difficult to modify (Patterson, 1982).

Summary

As behavior analysis is shaping the technology of support for people with severe problem behaviors, so people with severe problem behaviors are shaping the development of applied behavior analysis. This is true especially in the area of curriculum development. The successes of the past three decades have brought us a new set of challenges. Frequency of problem behaviors has served us well as a guiding dependent variable, yet it is time to expand our outcome variables to include valued indices of a quality life-style. The addition of these life-style variables will challenge both our measurement and intervention technologies. We must show not only that interventions make a difference, but that they make a difference across all hours of the day, for many days, in many settings, with many different materials, and many different people. The ante has risen.

To meet this challenge, we need curricula that are both behaviorally and socially functional, curricula that are based not only on a social logic but on a behavioral logic that predicts that the outcome of performing an activity will be reinforcing for the learner. This has led to a shift from isolated sequences of skills as the basis of curriculum development to a focus on clusters of skills, or activities, that result in functional outcomes. Among the most basic implications is that students with problem behavior should receive support in those settings where they can (a) live reasonable life-styles, (b) learn new skills, and (c) use those new skills to achieve functional outcomes. Said differently, if we implement the above curriculum logic, we should take our technology to students in their typical homes, schools, communities, and workplaces. Problem behaviors should guide how we provide support, not force removal of the student from the mainstream of society. This shift will have major implications for all students with disabilities, but especially for those students who perform severe problem behaviors in instructional contexts. Teachers now face the task of ensuring that the content and context of instruction are behaviorally functional for the learner.

REFERENCES

Alberto, P., & Troutman, A. (1990). *Applied behavior analysis for teachers: Influencing student performance* (3rd ed.). Columbus, OH: Charles E. Merrill.

Albin, R. W., O'Brien, M., & Horner, R. H. (1990). *A case study analysis of an escalating sequence of problem behaviors.* Manuscript submitted for publication.

Baer, D. M. (1982). The imposition of structure on behavior and the demolition of behavioral structures. In D. J. Bernstein (Ed.), *Response structure and organization: 1981 Nebraska symposium on motivation* (pp. 217–254).

Baer, D. M. (1991). The future of applied behavior analysis for people with severe disabilities: Commentary II. In L. Meyer, C. Peck, & L. Brown (Eds.), *Critical issues in the lives of people with severe disabilities* (pp. 613–615). Baltimore: Paul H. Brookes.

Baer, D. M. & Wolf, M. M. (1970). The entry into natural communities of reinforcement. In R. Ulrich, T. Stachnik, & J. Mabry (Eds.), *Control of human behavior* (pp. 319–324). Glenview, IL: Scott, Foresman.

Baer, D. M., Wolf, M. M., & Risley, T. R. (1968). Some current dimensions of applied behavior analysis. *Journal of Applied Behavior Analysis, 1,* 91–97.

Baer, D. M., Wolf, M. M., & Risley, T. R. (1987). Some still current dimensions of applied behavior analysis. *Journal of Applied Behavior Analysis, 20,* 313–327.

Bailey, J. S., & Pyles, D. A. M. (1989). Behavioral diagnostics. In E. Cipani (Ed.), *The treatment of severe behavior disorders: Behavior analysis approaches* (pp. 85–107). Washington, DC: American Association of Mental Retardation.

Barlow, E., & Hersen, M. (1984). *Single case experimental designs: Strategies for studying behavior change*. New York: Pergamon.

Bellamy, G. T., Newton, J. S., LeBaron, N., & Horner, R. H. (1990). Quality of life and lifestyle outcomes: A challenge for residential programs. In R. L. Schalock (Ed.), *Quality of life: Perspectives and issues* (pp. 127–137). Washington, DC: American Association on Mental Deficiency.

Berkman, K. A., & Meyer, L. H. (1988). Alternative strategies and multiple outcomes in the remediation of severe self-injury: Going all out nonaversively. *Journal of the Association for Persons With Severe Handicaps, 13*, 76–86.

Bijou, S. W., & Baer, D. M. (1961). *Child development I: A systematic and empirical theory*. Englewood Cliffs, NJ: Prentice-Hall.

Brown, L., Branston, M. B., Baumgart, D., Vincent, L., Falvey, M., & Schroeder, J. (1979). Using the characteristics of current and subsequent least restrictive environments as factors in the development of curricular content for severely handicapped students. *Journal of the Association for Persons With Severe Handicaps, 4*, 407–424.

Brown, L., Branston, M. B., Hamre-Neitupski, S., Pumpian, I., Certo, N., & Greunwald, L. A. (1979). A strategy for developing chronological age appropriate and functional curricular content for severely handicapped adolescents and young adults. *Journal of Special Education, 13*, 81–90.

Brown, L., Neitupski, J., & Hamre-Neitupski, S. (1976). The criterion of ultimate functioning. In M. A. Thomas (Ed.), *Hey, don't forget about me*. Reston, VA: Council for Exceptional Children.

Brusca, R. M., Nieminen, G. S., Carter, R., & Repp, A. C. (1989). The relationship of staff contact and activity to the stereotypy of children with multiple disabilities. *Journal of the Association for Persons With Severe Handicaps, 14*, 127–136.

Calkins, C. F., & Walker, H. M. (1990). *Social competence for workers with developmental disabilities*. Baltimore: Paul H. Brookes.

Carr, E. G. (1988). Functional equivalence as a means of response generalization. In R. H. Horner, G. Dunlap, & R. L. Koegel (Eds.), *Generalization and maintenance: Life-style changes in applied settings* (pp. 221–241). Baltimore: Paul H. Brookes.

Carr, E. G., & Durand, V. M. (1985a). Reducing behavior problems through functional communication training. *Journal of Applied Behavior Analysis, 18*, 111–126.

Carr, E. G., & Durand, V. M. (1985b). The social-communicative basis of severe behavior problems in children. In S. Reiss & R. Bootzin (Eds.), *Theoretical issues in behavior therapy* (pp. 219–254). New York: Academic Press.

Carr, E. G., Robinson, S., & Palumbo, L. W. (1990). The wrong issue: Aversive versus nonaversive treatment. The right issue: Functional versus nonfunctional treatment. In A. Repp & N. Singh (Eds.), *Perspectives on the use of nonaversive and aversive interventions for persons with developmental disabilities* (pp 361–379). DeKalb, IL: Sycamore.

Carr, E. G., Taylor, J. C., Carlson, J. I., & Robinson, S. (1989). Reinforcement and stimulus-based treatments for severe behavior problems in developmental disabilities. In U. S. Department of Health and Human Services *Treatment of destructive behaviors in persons with developmental disabilities* (pp. 173–229). Washington, DC: National Institutes of Health.

Cataldo, M. F. (1989). The effects of punishment and other behavior reducing procedures on the destructive behaviors of persons with developmental disabilities. In *Treatment of destructive behaviors in persons with developmental disabilities*. Washington, DC: National Institutes of Health.

Cataldo, M. F., Ward, E. M., Russo, D. C., Riordan, M., & Bennett, D. (1986). Compliance and correlated behavior in children: Effects of contingent and noncontingent reinforcement. *Analysis and Intervention in Developmental Disabilities, 6*, 264–282.

Colvin, G., & Sugai, G. (1989). *Managing escalating behavior.* Eugene, OR: Behavior Associates.

Day, M., & Horner, R. H. (1990, March). *Response efficiency and deceleration of problem behaviors via functional equivalence training.* Presentation at the 1990 Northern California Association for Behavior Analysis, San Francisco, CA.

Donnellan, A., LaVigna, G. W., Negri-Shoultz, N. & Fassbender, L. L. (1989). *Progress without punishment: Effective approaches for learners with behavior problems.* New York: Teachers College Press.

Dunlap, G. (1984). The influence of task variation and maintenance tasks on the learning and affect of autistic children. *Journal of Experimental Child Psychology, 37,* 41–64.

Dunlap, G., & Koegel, R. L. (1980). Motivating autistic children through stimulus variation. *Journal of Applied Behavior Analysis, 13,* 619–627.

Dunlap, G., & Plienis, A. L. (1988). Generalization and maintenance of unsupervised responding via remote contingencies. In R. H. Horner, G. Dunlap, & R. L. Koegel (Eds.), *Generalization and maintenance: Lifestyle changes in applied settings.* Baltimore: Paul H. Brookes.

Durand, V. M. (1984). *Attention-getting problem behavior: Analysis and intervention.* Unpublished doctoral dissertation, State University of New York, Stony Brook.

Durand, V. M. (1987). Look homeward angel: A call to return to our functional roots. *Behavior Analyst, 10,* 299–302.

Durand, V. M. (1988). *Functional reinforcer assessment: II. An evaluation of multiple influences.* Manuscript submitted for publication.

Durand, V. M. (1990). *Severe behavior problems: A functional communication training approach.* New York: Guilford.

Durand, V. M., & Carr, E. G. (1987). Social influences on self-stimulatory behavior: Analysis and treatment application. *Journal of Applied Behavior Analysis, 20,* 119–132.

Durand, V. M., & Crimmins, D. B. (1987). Assessment and treatment of psychotic speech in an autistic child. *Journal of Autism and Developmental Disorders, 17,* 17–28.

Durand, V. M., Crimmins, D. B., Caulfield, M., & Taylor, J. (1989). Reinforcer assessment: I. Using problem behavior to select reinforcers. *Journal of the Association for Persons With Severe Handicaps, 14,* 113–126.

Dyer, K., Dunlap, G., & Winterling, V. (1990). The effects of choice-making on the problem behaviors of students with severe handicaps. *Journal of Applied Behavior Analysis, 23,* 515–524.

Emerson, E. B. (1985). Evaluating the impact of deinstitutionalization in the lives of mentally retarded people. *American Journal of Mental Deficiency, 90,* 277–288.

Engelmann, S., & Carnine, D. (1982). *Theory of instruction: Principles and applications.* New York: Irvington.

Engelmann, S., & Colvin, G. (1983). *Generalized compliance training: A direct-instruction program for managing severe behavior problems.* Austin, TX: Pro-Ed.

Evans, I. M., & Meyer, L. H. (1987). Moving to educational validity: A reply to Test, Spooner, and Cooke. *Journal of the Association for Persons With Severe Handicaps, 12,* 103–106.

Falvey, M. A. (1986). *Community based curriculum.* Baltimore: Paul H. Brookes.

Favell, J. E. (1990). Issues in the use of nonaversive and aversive interventions. In S. L. Harris & J. S. Hendleman (Eds.), *Life-threatening behavior: Aversive versus nonaversive intervention* (pp. 36–56). New Brunswick, NJ: Rutgers University Press.

Favell, J. E., & Reid, D. H. (1988). Generalizing and maintaining improvement in problem behavior. In R. H. Horner, G. Dunlap, & R. L. Koegel (Eds.), *Generalization and maintenance: Life-style changes in applied settings* (pp. 171–196). Baltimore: Paul H. Brookes.

Ferguson, D., & Wilcox, B. (1987). *The elementary/secondary system: Supportive education for students with severe handicaps. Module 1: The activity-based IEP.* Eugene: Specialized Training Program, University of Oregon.

Ford, A., Schnorr, R., Meyer, L., Davern, L., Black, M. S., & Dempsey, P. (Eds.). (1989). *The Syracuse community-referenced curriculum guide for students with moderate and severe disabilities.* Baltimore: Paul H. Brookes.

Gardner, W. I., Cole, C. L., Davidson, D. P., & Karan, O. C. (1986). Reducing aggression in individuals with developmental disabilities: An expanded stimulus control, assessment, and intervention model. *Education and Training of the Mentally Retarded, 21,* 3–12.

Gilbert, T. F. (1978). *Human competence: Engineering worthy performance.* New York: McGraw-Hill.

Guess, D., & Helmstetter, E. (1986). Skill cluster instruction and the individualized curriculum sequencing model. In R. H. Horner, L. H. Meyer, & H. D. Fredericks (Eds.), *Education of learners with severe handicaps* (pp. 221–248). Baltimore: Paul H. Brookes.

Guess, D., Helmstetter, E., Turnbull, H. R., & Knowlton, S. (1986). *Use of aversive procedures with persons who are disabled: An historical review and critical analysis.* Seattle: Association for Persons With Severe Handicaps.

Haring, N. G., & Bricker, D. (1976). Overview of comprehensive services for the severely profoundly handicapped. In N. G. Haring & L. J. Brown (Eds.), *Teaching the severely handicapped, vol. 1* (pp. 2–16). New York: Grune & Stratton.

Haring, T. G., & Lovinger, L. (1989). Promoting social interaction through teaching generalized play initiation responses to preschool children with autism. *Journal of the Association for Persons With Severe Handicaps, 14,* 58–67.

Horner, R. D. (1980). The effects of an environment "enrichment" program on the behavior of institutionalized profoundly retarded children. *Journal of Applied Behavior Analysis, 13,* 473–491.

Horner, R. H. (1990). Ideology, technology and typical community settings: The use of severe aversive stimuli. *American Journal on Mental Retardation, 95*(2), 166–168.

Horner, R. H. (1991). The future of applied behavior analysis for people with severe disabilities: Commentary I. In L. Meyer, C. Peck, & L. Brown (Eds.), *Critical issues in the lives of people with severe disabilities* (pp 607–611). Baltimore: Paul H. Brookes.

Horner, R. H., Bellamy, G. T., & Colvin, G. T. (1984). Responding in the presence of nontrained stimuli: Implications of generalization error patterns. *Journal of the Association for Persons With Severe Handicaps, 9,* 287–296.

Horner, R. H., & Billingsley, F. F. (1988). The effect of competing behavior on the generalization and maintenance of adaptive behavior in applied settings. In R. H. Horner, G. Dunlap, & R. L. Koegel (Eds.), *Generalization and maintenance: Life-style changes in applied settings* (pp. 197–220). Baltimore: Paul H. Brookes.

Horner, R. H., & Budd, C. M. (1985). Teaching manual sign language to a nonverbal student: Generalization of sign use and collateral reduction of maladaptive behavior. *Education and Training of the Mentally Retarded, 20,* 39–47.

Horner, R. H., Day, M., Sprague, J. R., O'Brien, M., & Heathfield, L. T. (1991). Interspersed requests: A nonaversive procedure for decreasing aggression and self-injury during instruction. *Journal of Applied Behavior Analysis, 24*(2), 265–278.

Horner, R. H., Dunlap, G., & Koegel, R. L. (1988). *Generalization and maintenance: Life-style changes in applied settings.* Baltimore: Paul H. Brookes.

Horner, R. H., Sprague, J. R., O'Brien, M., & Heathfield, L. T. (1990). The role of response efficiency in the reduction of problem behaviors through functional equivalence training: A case study. *Journal of the Association for Persons With Severe Handicaps, 15*(2), 91–97.

Iwata, B. A. (1989, May). Discussant comments. In D. Wacker (Chair), *Functional analysis of severe problem behaviors: Recent applications and novel approaches.* Symposium presented at the 5th annual conference of the Association for Behavior Analysis, Milwaukee, WI.

Iwata, B. A., Dorsey, M. F., Slifer, K. J., Bauman, K. E., & Richman, G. S. (1982). Toward a functional analysis of self-injury. *Analysis and Intervention in Developmental Disabilities, 2,* 3–20.

Iwata, B. A., Pace, G. M., Kalsher, M. J., Cowdery, G. E., & Cataldo, M. F. (1990). Experimental analysis and extinction of self-injurious escape behavior. *Journal of Applied Behavior Analysis, 23,* 11–27.

Iwata, B. A., Wong, S. E., Reardon, M. M., Dorsey, M. F., & Lau, M. M. (1982). Assessment and training of clinical interviewing skills: Analogue analysis and field replication. *Journal of Applied Behavior Analysis, 15,* 191–204.

Johnston, J. M., & Pennypacker, H. S. (1980). *Strategies and tactics of human behavioral research.* Hillsdale, NJ: Lawrence Erlbaum.

Kantor, J. R. (1959). *Interbehavioral psychology.* Granville, OH: Principia.

Kazdin, A. E. (1977). Assessing the clinical or implied importance of behavior change through social validation *Behavior Modification, 1,* 427–452.

Kazdin, A. E. (1980). *Behavior modification in applied settings* (2nd ed.). Homewood, IL: Dorsey.

Koegel, R. L. & Koegel, L. (1988). Generalized responsivity and pivotal behaviors. In R. H. Horner, G. Dunlap, & R. L. Koegel (Eds.), *Generalization and maintenance: Life-style changes in applied settings,* (pp. 41–66). Baltimore: Paul H. Brookes.

Landesman, S. (1986). Quality of life and personal life satisfaction: Definition and measurement issues. *Mental Retardation, 24,* 141–143.

LaVigna, G. W., & Donnellan, A. M. (1986). *Alternatives to punishment: Solving behavior? problems with nonaversive strategies.* New York: Irvington.

Lazar, J. B., & Rucker, W. L. (1984, November). *The effectiveness of manipulating setting factors on the ruminative behavior of a boy with profound retardation.* Paper presented at the annual conference of the Association for Persons With Severe Handicaps, Chicago.

Leigland, S. (1984). On "setting events" and related concepts. *Behavior Analyst, 7,* 41–45.

Lennox, D. B., & Miltenberger, R. G. (1989). Conducting a functional assessment of problem behavior in applied settings. *Journal of the Association for Persons With Severe Handicaps, 14,* 304–311.

Lovaas, O. I. (1987). Behavioral treatment and normal educational and intellectual functioning in young autistic children. *Journal of Consulting and Clinical Psychology, 55,* 3–9.

Mace, F. C., Hock, M. L., Lalli, J. S., West, B. J., Belfiore, P., Pinter, E., & Brown, D. F. (1988). Behavioral momentum in the treatment of noncompliance. *Journal of Applied Behavior Analysis, 21,* 123–141.

Matson, J. L., & Taras, M. E. (1989). A 20 year review of punishment and alternative methods to treat problem behaviors in developmentally delayed persons. *Research in Developmental Disabilities, 10,* 85–104.

McDonnell, J. J., & Horner, R. H. (1985). Effects of in vivo versus simulation-plus-in vivo training on the acquisition and generalization of grocery item selection by high school students with severe handicaps. *Analysis and Intervention in Developmental Disabilities, 5,* 323–343.

Meyer, L. M (1987). *Program quality indicators (POI): A checklist of most promising practices in educational programs for students with severe disabilities.* Seattle, WA: Association for Persons With Severe Handicaps.

Meyer, L. M., & Evans, I. M. (1989). *Nonaversive intervention for behavior problems: A manual for home and community.* Baltimore: Paul H. Brookes.

Michael, J. L. (1982). Distinguishing between discriminative and motivational functions of stimuli. *Journal of the Experimental Analysis of Behavior, 37,* 149–155.

Miltenberger, R. G., & Fuqua, R. W. (1985). Evaluation of a training manual for the acquisition of behavioral assessment interviewing skills. *Journal of Applied Behavior Analysis, 18,* 323–328.

Miltenberger, R. G., & Veltum, L. (1988). Evaluation of an instructions and modeling procedure for training behavioral assessment interviewing. *Journal of Behavior Therapy and Experimental Psychiatry, 19,* 31–41.

Neef, N. A., Iwata, B. A., & Page, T. J. (1980). The effects of interspersal training versus high density reinforcement on spelling acquisition and retention. *Journal of Applied Behavior Analysis, 13,* 153–158.

Neel, R. S., & Billingsley, F. F. (1989). *Impact: A functional curriculum handbook for students with moderate to severe disabilities.* Baltimore: Paul H. Brookes.

Newton, J. S., Bellamy, G. T., Horner, R. H., Boles, S. M., LeBaron, N. M., & Bennett, A. (1987). Using the Activities Catalog in residential programs for individuals with severe disabilities. In B. Wilcox & G. T. Bellamy, *A comprehensive guide to the Activities Catalog: An alternative curriculum for youth and adults with severe disabilities* (pp. 125–149). Baltimore: Paul H. Brookes.

O'Brien, J. (1987). A guide to lifestyle planning: Using the Activities Catalog to integrate services and natural support systems. In B. Wilcox and G. T. Bellamy (Eds.), *A comprehensive guide to the Activities Catalog:* (pp. 175–189). Baltimore: Paul H. Brookes.

O'Neill, R. E., Horner, R. H., Albin, R. W., Storey, K., & Sprague, J. R. (1990). *Functional analysis: A practical assessment guide*. Sycamore, IL: Sycamore.

Patterson, G. R. (1982). *Coercive family process*. Eugene, OR: Castalia.

Repp, A. C., Felce, D., & Barton, L. E. (1988). Basing the treatment of stereotypic and self-injurious behaviors on hypotheses of their causes. *Journal of Applied Behavior Analysis, 21*, 281–289.

Repp, A. C., Singh, N. N., Olinger, E., & Olsen, D. (1990). A review of the use of functional analysis to test causes of self-injurious behavior: Rationale, current status, and future directions. *Journal of Mental Deficiency Research, 34*, 95–105.

Romanczyk, R. G. (1989). *Self-injurious behavior: Etiology and treatment*. New York: Plenum.

Sailor, W., Anderson, J. L., Halvorsen, A. T., Doering, K., Filler, J., & Goetz, L. (1989). *The comprehensive local school: Regular education for all students with disabilities*. Baltimore: Paul H. Brookes.

Sasso, G. M., & Reimers, T. M. (1988). Assessing the functional properties of behavior: Implications and applications for the classroom. *Focus on Autistic Behavior, 3*, 1–15.

Schalock, R. L., & Harper, R. S. (1982). Skill acquisition and client movement indices: Implementing cost-effective analysis in rehabilitation programs. *Evaluation and Program Planning, 5*, 223–231.

Schiefelbusch, R. L. (1978). *Bases of language intervention*. Baltimore: Paul H. Brookes.

Schroeder, S. R., Kanoy, J. R., Mulick, J. A., Rojahn, J., Thios, S. J., Stephens, M., & Hawk, B. (1982). The effects of the environment on programs for self-injurious behavior. In J. H. Hollis & C. E. Meyers (Eds.), *Life threatening behavior: Analysis and intervention* (pp. 105–159). Washington, DC: American Association on Mental Deficiency.

Singer, G. H. S., Singer, J., & Horner, R. H. (1987). Using pretask requests to increase the probability of compliance for students with severe disabilities. *Journal of the Association for Persons With Severe Handicaps, 12*, 287–291.

Snell, M. E. (Ed.). (1987). *Systematic instruction of persons with severe handicaps*. Columbus, OH: Charles E. Merrill.

Sprague, J. R., & Horner, R. H. (1991). Determining the acceptability of behavior support plans. In M. Wang, H. Wahlberg, & M. Reynolds (Eds.), *Handbook of special education* (pp. 125–142). Oxford, London: Pergamon Press.

Stokes, T. F., & Baer, D. M. (1977). An implicit technology of generalization. *Journal of Applied Behavior Analysis, 10*, 349–367.

Storey, K., Stern, R., & Parker, R. (1990). A comparison of attitudes towards typical recreational activities versus the Special Olympics. *Education and Training in Mental Retardation 25*(1), 94–99.

Sulzer, B., & Mayer, G. R. (1972). *Behavior modification procedures for school personnel*. New York: Holt, Rinehart and Winston.

Touchette, P. E. (1989a) Humane, permanent elimination of destructive behavior via analysis and manipulation of stimulus control. In U. S. Department of Health and Human Services *Treatment of destructive behaviors in persons with developmental disabilities* (pp. 73–75). Washington, DC: National Institutes of Health.

Touchette, P. E. (1989b). *A stimulus control model for the elimination of severe maladaptive behavior*. Paper presented at the NIDRR National Conference on Data-Based Strategies for Behavior Management in Community Settings, Santa Barbara, CA.

Touchette, P. E., MacDonald, R. F., & Langer, S. N. (1985). A scatter plot for identifying stimulus control of problem behavior. *Journal of Applied Behavior Analysis, 18*, 343–351.

Turnbull, H. R., Guess, D., Backus, L. M., Barber, P. A., Fiedler, C. R., Helmstetter, E., & Summers, J. A. (1986). A model for analyzing the moral aspects of special education and behavioral interventions: The moral aspects of aversive procedures. In P. R. Dokecki & R. M. Zaner (Eds.), *Ethics of dealing with persons with severe handicaps* (pp. 167–210). Baltimore: Paul H. Brookes.

Van Houten, R., Axelrod, S., Bailey, J. S., Favell, J. E., Foxx, R. M., Iwata, B. A., & Lovaas, O. I. (1988). The right to effective behavioral treatment. *Behavior Analyst, 11*(2), 111–114.

Voeltz, L. M., & Evans, I. M. (1983). Educational validity: Procedures to evaluate outcomes in programs for severely handicapped learners. *Journal of the Association of the Severely Handicapped, 8*(1), 3–15.

Wacker, D. P. (1989). Further evaluation of functional communication training: An analysis of active treatment components. In U. S. Department of Health and Human Services *Treatment of destructive behaviors in persons with developmental disabilities* (pp. 70–72). Washington, DC: National Institutes of Health.

Wacker, D. P., Steege, M. W., Northup, J., Sasso, G., Berg, W., Reimers, T., Cooper, L., Cigrand, K., & Donn, L. (1990). A component analysis of functional communication training across three topographies of severe behavior problems. *Journal of Applied Behavior Analysis, 23*, 417–429.

Wahler, R. G., & Fox, J. J. (1981). Setting events in applied behavior analysis: Toward a conceptual and methodological expansion. *Journal of Applied Behavior Analysis, 14*, 327–338.

Wilcox, B. W., & Bellamy, G. T. (1982). *Design of high school programs for students with severe handicaps*. Baltimore: Paul H. Brookes.

Wilcox, B. W., & Bellamy, G. T. (1987). *A comprehensive guide to the activities catalog*. Baltimore: Paul H. Brookes.

Willis, T. J., LaVigna, G. W., & Donnellan, A. M. (1989). *Behavior assessment guide*. Los Angeles: Institute for Applied Behavior Analysis.

Winterling, V., Dunlap, G., & O'Neill, R. (1987). The influence of task variation on the aberrant behavior of autistic students. *Education and Treatment of Children, 10*, 105–119.

Wolery, M., Bailey, D. B., & Sugai, G. M. (1988). Structuring the environment for effective teaching. In M. Wolery, D. B. Bailey, & G. M. Sugai *Effective teaching: Principles and procedures of applied behavior analysis with exceptional students*, (pp. 187–213). Boston: Allyn and Bacon.

Wolf, M. M. (1978). Social validity: The case for subjective measurement, or how applied behavior analysis is finding its heart. *Journal of Applied Behavior Analysis, 11*, 203–214.

II

The Role of Behavioral Assessment in Providing Quality Care

4

Functional Analysis and Treatment of Aberrant Behavior

F. Charles Mace, Joseph S. Lalli, Elizabeth Pinter Lalli, and Michael C. Shea

Introduction

The field of applied behavior analysis has developed an impressive technology for reducing the myriad aberrant behaviors engaged in by individuals with developmental disabilities. Most interventions apply basic behavioral principles (e.g., positive and negative reinforcement, punishment, and stimulus control) to discourage aberrant responses and promote adaptive behavior. In pursuit of an effective technology, the field has focused on the development and refinement of intervention procedures that produce large, durable, and general changes in socially meaningful behaviors (Baer, Wolf, & Risley, 1968; Stokes & Baer, 1977).

Although technological advances have been responsible for improving the lives of persons with handicaps (Bailey, Shook, Iwata, Reid, & Repp, 1986), many behavior analysts consider the emphasis on technology to detract from the field's scientific advancement (e.g., Dietz, 1978, 1982; Hayes,

ACKNOWLEDGMENTS. This chapter was originally published in *Research in Developmental Disabilities*, 1991, 12, 155–180 and is reprinted here with permission from Pergamon Press.

F. Charles Mace and Joseph S. Lalli • Department of Pediatrics, University of Pennsylvania School of Medicine, Philadelphia, Pennsylvania 19104. Elizabeth Pinter Lalli • Council Rock School District, Langhorne, Pennsylvania 18940. Michael C. Shea • Graduate School of Applied and Professional Psychology, Rutgers University, Piscataway, New Jersey 08855.

Behavior Analysis and Treatment, edited by R. Van Houten & S. Axelrod. Plenum Press, New York, 1993.

Rincover, & Solnick, 1980; Johnston & Pennypacker, 1980; Michael, 1980; Pierce & Epling, 1980). The trend in applied behavioral research has been toward development and evaluation of intervention procedures without analyzing the variables responsible for aberrant behavior (Hayes et al., 1980; Pierce & Epling, 1980). For example, interventions such as token economies, time out, and overcorrection are typically implemented without assessing the variables that maintain the aberrant target behavior. These techniques are effective to the extent that they successfully compete with reinforcement contingencies that support maladaptive behavior. When therapeutic effects are not achieved, however, few guidelines exist for selecting an alternative intervention. An analytic approach not only promotes the discovery of unique contingencies but encourages application of laboratory-derived findings to better understand and alter problem behavior.

In recent years, various methodologies have evolved to analyze and treat a wide range of problem behaviors, including self-injury, aggression, pica, disruption, reluctant and bizarre speech, and stereotypy. Our goal here is to review this emerging literature and discuss (a) the general classes of variables found to control aberrant behavior, (b) the specific methods used to analyze behavior-environment interactions, and (c) a comprehensive model for conducting functional analysis and treatment of aberrant behavior.

General Classes of Controlling Variables

Several investigators have examined the functional relationship between various environmental conditions and aberrant behavior. Generally, these variables have been found to influence maladaptive behavior via positive or negative reinforcement contingencies, or to facilitate discrimination of known or unknown reinforcement contingencies. The following is a summary of the major research findings in different classes. Although some of these studies restrict their investigation to the functional analysis of aberrant behavior, many applied the results of the analysis to develop effective interventions.

Attention

Ayllon and Michael (1959) provided one of the first empirical demonstrations of the influence of attention on aberrant behavior. An informal analysis suggested that the psychotic speech of a psychiatric inpatient was positively reinforced by attention from nursing staff. When nurses stopped replying to the subject's statements, the rate of aberrant comments dropped sharply. In a similar vein, Budd, Green, and Baer (1976) trained a parent of a child with developmental disabilities to withhold attention contiguous to disruptive behavior and noncompliance, on the assumption that the parent's attention reinforced the maladaptive behaviors. The mother learned to avoid repeating instructions and to wait at least 5 seconds after disruptive behavior occurred before interacting with her child. Both tactics resulted in substantial reductions in the child's disruptive behavior; however, a brief time-out procedure was added to withholding attention in order to achieve a complete remediation of the problem. Finally, Hunt, Alwell, and Goetz (1988) taught three students with severe disabilities to initiate conversations independently in order to obtain the peer and staff attention produced by the students' inappropriate social behaviors.

Formal experimental analyses have confirmed attention's capacity to reinforce positively a wide range of aberrant responses. Thomas, Becker, and Armstrong (1968) were among the first to verify experimentally that disapproving comments contingent on inappropriate comments can increase the rate of aberrant responding. The authors had a classroom teacher vary the number of disapproving comments in reference to students' disruptive behavior during successive experimental phases. Disruptions occurred consistently more often when teacher disapproval was high. Mace, Page, Ivancic, and O'Brien (1986) similarly found aggressive and disruptive behavior in children with mental retardation to be a function of therapists' social disapproval of their behavior. Therapists reacted to aberrant behavior with comments such as, "Stop that, Joel, you know you shouldn't throw toys" on a continuous reinforcement schedule that was later thinned to a variable ratio schedule. All three subjects in the study emitted high rates of disruptive or aggressive behavior under these contingencies. These findings prompted the authors to select interventions that minimized attention for aberrant behavior such as ignoring, response blocking (for aggression), and time out.

Iwata, Dorsey, Slifer, Bauman, and Richman (1982) developed a comprehensive pretreatment assessment protocol to analyze the relationship between self-injurious behavior and various positive and negative reinforcement contingencies. One assessment condition involved the presentation of social disapproval contingent on self-injury. Iwata and his colleagues found contingent disapproving comments to be a primary motivator of self-injury for some subjects and one of multiple motivating factors for other individuals. Finally, forms of attention other than social disapproval have been shown also to reinforce maladaptive behavior. For example, Anderson, Dancis, and Alpert (1978) compared the effects of noncontingent attention versus attention contingent on the self-injurious behavior of subjects with Lesch-Nyhan Syndrome. Contingent attention occurred in the form of quick intervention to prevent self-injurious responses, followed by reassuring statements and stroking the child. Self-injury occurred at extremely high rates during the contingent attention condition. This finding is important because Lesch-Nyhan Syndrome is a gene-linked disorder that is invariably associated with specific topographies of self-injury (i.e., mouth and lip biting). The study provides evidence that even behavior elicited by biological conditions may be controlled by social influences.

Sensory and Perceptual Consequences

Certain types of aberrant behavior may also be positively reinforced by the automatic sensory or perceptual consequences that the maladaptive response produces. Research has implicated sensory or perceptual consequences as maintaining variables for stereotypy, self-injury, and pica. Lovaas, Newsom, and Hickman (1987) provided a comprehensive theoretical formulation of the role of sensory or perceptual reinforcement in the genesis and maintenance of repetitive, stereotyped behaviors. Briefly, Lovaas et al. considered stereotypy as a class of learned, operant behaviors that result automatically in internal or external stimulation with powerful reinforcing properties. Several studies have demonstrated that visual, auditory, tactile, and kinesthetic stimuli can reinforce nonstereotyped behavior in animals and in normal and handicapped humans (see Lovaas et al., 1987, for a complete review).

Evidence for these stimuli maintaining stereotyped behavior in humans comes from two types of investigations. First, Wolery (1978) tested the hypothesis that sensory stimulation from repetitive motor movements can function as a positive reinforcer by imitating the sensory stimulation of various stereotyped topographies. Patting the leg of one subject and rubbing the arm of another to simulate stimulation derived from stereotypy was found to function as a positive reinforcer. Wolery, Kirk, and Gast (1985) similarly found contingent opportunities to engage in stereotypy effective in teaching autistic children new classroom behaviors. The second method of testing the sensory-consequences hypothesis relies on inferring the existence of a positive reinforcement process on the basis of observing behavior consistent with extinction. Rincover and his colleagues reduced stereotyped movements by masking the auditory, visual, or proprioceptive consequences resulting from such behavior (Rincover, Cook, Peoples, & Packard, 1979; Rincover, Newsom, & Carr, 1979). For example, a small vibrator attached to the back of a child's hand masked the proprioceptive stimulation produced by finger and arm waving, resulting in marked reductions in stereotypic behavior (i.e., sensory extinction). Similar reductions were reported for repetitive plate spinning by carpeting a tabletop as a means of minimizing auditory consequences of the behavior.

The role of sensory consequences in maintaining self-injury and pica has also been investigated. One theory of the etiology of self-injury is that such individuals have defective pain mechanisms that permit them to engage in self-injurious forms of stereotypy for sensory stimulation or possibly to produce addictive levels of endogenous opiates (Cataldo & Harris, 1982). Given this etiology, researchers have reasoned that sensory extinction procedures or provision of alternate sensory activities should suppress self-injury. Rincover and Devany (1982) illustrated sensory extinction using subjects whose self-injury appeared relatively unaffected by social influences and, therefore, was possibly maintained by sensory reinforcement. Head banging was sharply reduced with a padded helmet for one child and padding the floor and walls for another subject. A third child's face scratching was eliminated by covering his hands with thin rubber gloves. Similar treatment success was reported by Favell, McGimsey, and Schell (1982) by providing subjects with profound mental retardation sensory alternatives to self-injury. Enriching the environment with toys and prompting and reinforcing toy play resulted in reduced self-injury and increased manipulation of toys. Interestingly, the topography of toy manipulation corresponded to the senses stimulated by self-injury (e.g., eye poking was replaced by waving toys in front of the eyes).

Favell et al. (1982) also applied this principle to substitute a noninjurious form of gustatory reinforcement for pica. The availability of popcorn and toys, as well as providing popcorn contingent on toy holding, produced substantial reductions in ingestion of inedible objects. Steege, Wacker, Berg, Cigrand, and Cooper (1989) provided an individual with severe multiple disabilities an alternative method to produce reinforcing stimuli through the activation of a microswitch. The microswitch was connected to previously identified reinforcing stimuli (e.g., radio, fan), and its use was prompted by the individual's classroom teacher. Increased use of the microswitch was accompanied by a decrease in the frequency of self-injurious behaviors. Finally, Durand (1982) observed decreases in an individual's self-injury when a small, cylindrical vibrator (which produced an indirect form of sensory stimulation) was attached to the individual's hand.

Access to Materials or Activities

Aberrant behavior may also be positively reinforced by access to materials or activities that an individual's adaptive repertoire produces less effectively or efficiently. Examples include the child who picks up a toy while shopping and throws a tantrum until his or her parent purchases it; the aggressive, bullylike behavior of a child that permits him or her to monopolize preferred toys and games; and the adult whose somatic complaints result in reinforcing medical examinations. Some evidence for the validity of this hypothesis comes from a study by Patterson, Littman, and Bricker (1967), who found a clear association between the aggressive behavior of nursery-school children and their victims relinquishing toys or other materials. Recent support has been provided by Day, Rea, Schussler, Larsen, and Johnson (1988) and Durand and Kishi (1987). In each of these investigations, the authors conducted pretreatment assessments to identify the environmental events associated with their respective participants' self-injury. Findings from the pretreatment assessments indicated that access to preferred items maintained three of the eight participants' problem behaviors.

Escape-Avoidance of Aversive Demand Conditions

Several studies have shown that aberrant behavior can be maintained by escape or avoidance of aversive stimuli. When presented with certain situations, an individual may engage in one or more maladaptive responses because these behaviors result in (a) complete avoidance of aversive stimuli, (b) delay in the presentation of aversive stimuli, (c) attenuation of the strength of the aversive stimuli, or (d) alleviation of aversive conditions. When aberrant behavior has any of the above functions, it is maintained, at least in part, by negative reinforcement (Skinner, 1969).

Several studies have employed rigorous experimental methods to establish the escape-avoidance motivations of many aberrant behaviors. One strategy has been to assess maladaptive behavior in the presence or absence of task-related demands. Using this research paradigm, demands are conceptualized as discriminative stimuli for aberrant behavior that effect the attenuation or alleviation of the aversive properties of the demand. If problem behavior is more prevalent under demand conditions, it is inferred that the aberrant responses are motivated by escape or avoidance contingencies. Carr, Newsom, and Binkoff (1980) employed this methodology with two highly aggressive boys with mental retardation and autism. Demand conditions for one child consisted of a requirement to remain seated in a chair throughout the experimental session, whereas the second subject was prompted through a buttoning task. No-demand conditions were unstructured with no instructions and minimal interaction. Aggressive responses occurred at high rates, and almost exclusively during demand sessions. Interestingly, when a safety signal was provided indicating that demands would be discontinued, the aggressive behavior of both subjects dropped sharply. Carr and Newsom (1985) used similar methods to determine that tantrum behaviors of developmentally disabled students were demand related. Tasks for the demand conditions were taken from the students' classroom curriculum and consisted of various nonverbal and verbal imitation tasks and simple questions to describe pictures depicting an action sequence. Results for all three students were almost identical to those of the Carr et al. (1980) study, including the impact of the signal indicating termination of demands.

A second method of investigating the validity of the escape-avoidance hypothesis involves manipulation of the consequences for aberrant behavior during task-related demands. Researchers have examined directly the escape-avoidance function of aberrant behavior by arranging experimentally for maladaptive responses to be followed by either periods of escape from demands or a delay in the onset of demands. In the third experiment of the Carr et al. (1980) study, the experimenters applied a negative reinforcement contingency to the subject's aggressive behavior. On an intermittent, fixed-ratio schedule that was progressively thinned, aggression resulted in a 1-minute period without demands, after which time demands resumed.

Aggression was alternately strengthened and weakened when this contingency was applied to aggressive acts and nonaggressive behaviors, respectively.

Escape or time-out periods from task-related demands have also been found to negatively reinforce self-injury (Iwata et al., 1982), stereotypy (Durand & Carr, 1987), reluctant speech (Mace & West, 1986), psychotic speech (Durand & Crimmins, 1987), and aggression and disruption (Mace et al., 1986). Tasks used in these studies were functional and nonfunctional academics and escape contingencies were applied on a rich schedule of reinforcement (in some cases a CRF schedule). Mace, Browder, and Lin (1987) found that stereotypy occurred at higher rates when the behavior delayed the onset of demands. Prompts to participate in a table game were provided only when the subject was not engaged in repetitive motor behaviors. Thus, the student could avoid instructions to participate in the game by engaging in stereotypy. When the experimenters did not allow stereotypy to produce this effect (i.e., prompts to engage in the task were presented on a VT 60-s [variable-time 60-second] schedule), stereotypic acts occurred less often.

A third source of evidence for the escape-avoidance motivations of some aberrant behavior comes from research showing a functional relationship between task difficulty and maladaptive responding. Investigators have reasoned that increases in task difficulty should produce corresponding increases in aberrant behavior if the function of the response class is to attenuate or alleviate demands. Similarly, shifts from easy to difficult tasks contingent on aberrant behavior should punish the maladaptive response. Several dimensions of task difficulty have been varied to test this hypothesis. Among the first investigations was by Sailor, Guess, Rutherford, and Baer (1968), who assessed tantrums during four task conditions that varied according to difficulty. A girl with severe mental retardation was presented with a vocal imitation task using word or phrase lists that were graded by length (i.e., 20 versus 14) and complexity (e.g., "dog" versus "stepping over cardboard boxes"). When the experimenters alternated from easy to difficult lists and from difficult to easy lists contingent on tantrums, aberrant behavior decreased and increased, respectively, demonstrating that the more difficult tasks functioned as aversive stimuli.

Weeks and Gaylord-Ross (1981) found self-injury to occur at higher rates when subjects were given difficult versus easy figure-discrimination tasks. Easy discriminations contrasted figures of different shapes, sizes, and colors, whereas difficult discriminations involved comparisons of black and white reversed forms. Similar effects on the disruptive behavior of students with learning problems were reported by Center, Deitz, and Kaufman (1982); aberrant responses occurred at high rates when students were given math problems beyond their achievement level. In the same vein, stereotyped movements have been found to be a function of increasing the number of leisure task components (Mace et al., 1987) and increasing the complexity of receptive labeling tasks beyond the child's skill level (Durand & Carr, 1987).

A final dimension of task difficulty that has been studied is the subject's familiarity or reinforcement history with a particular task. Holding the number of task components and complexity generally constant, Mace et al. (1987) reported higher levels of stereotypy when a student with multiple handicaps was presented with novel tasks (i.e., tasks with which he had no known reinforcement history) than when asked to perform familiar tasks for which he had developed skills. Finally, Gaylord-Ross, Weeks, and Lipner (1980) demonstrated that the effects reported above may depend on the presence or absence of other variables. These researchers found increases in self-injury during demand conditions to depend on a combination of task type (e.g., sorting colored buttons) and the experimenter requests during the task. Thus, demand conditions may occasion aberrant behavior only when specific stimuli combine to produce an aversive situation that may motivate escape-avoidance behavior.

Interventions derived from an analysis of demand conditions have taken a variety of forms. First, some investigators have reduced maladaptive behavior by removing the escape-avoidance function of the response. Procedures that do not permit or minimize attenuation or alleviation of task demands can result in extinction of the aberrant behavior (Catania, 1984). Carr et al. (1980) illustrated this approach by confining a child to a chair with a seat belt for 1-hour sessions. Previous data indicated that the boy's aggression was maintained by escape from the chair; when escape was no longer permitted, aggressive behavior ceased. Guiding compliance with task demands can also serve to remove the function of aberrant behavior. Mace et al. (1987) eliminated escape-motivated stereotypy using a prompt hierarchy that culminated with manual guidance. Extinction of aberrant behavior during tasks calling for responses that cannot be guided (e.g., vocal behavior) may be achieved by consistently presenting the task until compliance occurs (see Mace & West, 1986, in the treatment of reluctant speech and Repp, Felce, & Barton, 1988, in the treatment of SIB, self-injurious behavior).

A second approach to intervention with escape or avoidance-motivated behavior has been to reduce the aversiveness of the demand and thereby reduce the incentive for aberrant behavior. Carr et al. (1980), Carr and Newsom (1985), and Steege et al. (1989) achieved this by introducing strong positive reinforcers for task-related behaviors that resulted in elimination of aggressive and tantrumous behavior. One explanation may be that positive reinforcement for task-related behaviors exceeded the negative reinforcement of escape-avoidance. Alternatively, the aversiveness of demands may be reduced by eliminating opportunities for error, thus increasing reinforcement for task responses. Weeks and Gaylord-Ross (1981) eliminated self-injury related to difficult discrimination tasks using an errorless learning procedure. A difficult two-choice discrimination was made easy by beginning with maximally different options and gradually fading the stimuli toward the target stimuli over numerous trials. Finally, a series of studies by Carr and Durand and their associates demonstrated the therapeutic value of training an adaptive response to produce the same or similar function as that produced by the aberrant behavior. If the substitute adaptive response can effect greater reinforcement or be performed with less effort than the aberrant behavior, and if reinforcement for the aberrant behavior can be minimized, the client should eventually respond predominantly on the reinforcement schedule for the adaptive behavior in order to maximize his or her reinforcement (Myerson & Hale, 1984).

In one experiment from the Carr et al. (1980) study, negatively reinforced aggression was reduced sharply by permitting escape from demands contingent on finger tapping rather than aggression. This contingency also resulted in very high rates of finger tapping. Carr and Durand (1985) applied the same rationale to select adaptive replacements for misbehavior. Interventions were based on an analysis that showed aggression, tantrums, and self-injury occurred most often under conditions of low adult attention and high task demands. Thus, children with severe disabilities were taught socially appropriate methods to solicit adult attention and to request assistance during tasks as a means of effecting a class of reinforcers similar to that produced by the maladaptive behavior. A similar tact was taken by Durand and Carr (1987) and Durand and Kishi (1987) by teaching subjects to say "Help me" following incorrect responses to task-related requests. In both cases, the rate of aberrant behavior declined when the adaptive substitute was trained and reinforcement for aberrant behavior was minimal. Finally, Koegel, Dyer, and Bell (1987) used simulated conditions to observe autistic children's play activities in order to identify child-preferred activities and associated levels of social avoidance behavior. Once identified, child-preferred activities were utilized to decrease the children's social avoidance behaviors.

Antecedent and Concurrent Stimuli

Numerous investigations have assessed the relationship between aberrant behavior and stimuli presented antecedent to or concurrent with it. Unlike the studies reviewed above, the focus of these investigations is on identifying events that set the occasion for maladaptive behavior rather than on the consequences that maintain it. This tactic may be especially useful for behaviors that are maintained by consequences that are not directly observable or amenable to manipulation (e.g., sensory or perceptual consequences). Although such research has been useful in designing effective interventions, it has contributed less to the field's understanding of the function of aberrant behavior. First, behavior analysts recognize that behavior is a function of the consequences it produces (Skinner, 1953). Antecedent and concurrent stimuli are generally believed to influence behavior by being discriminative of the specific consequences that follow a particular response. Thus, the power of antecedent and concurrent stimuli to occasion behavior is linked directly to the effect a behavior has on the environment. To understand these effects is the principle goal of the science of behavior. Secondly, most research of this kind has not analyzed the specific function of antecedent or concurrent stimuli. For example, it is not clear whether these stimuli function as (a) discriminative stimuli, (b) a chain of discriminative stimuli, (c) setting events (Wahler & Fox, 1981), (d) establishing operations (Michael, 1982), or (e) elements in an unknown operant process. These mechanisms should be the focus of future research on controlling antecedent and concurrent stimuli.

The following studies illustrate the functional analysis of aberrant behavior and antecedent or concurrent stimuli. First, enriching the environment with leisure, educational, or social stimuli has been found to decrease rates of aberrant behavior and increase the incidence of adaptive responses. For example, several researchers have reported that the availability of toys and/or social interaction was associated with less stereotypy, self-injury, disruption, or pica in individuals with developmental disabilities (e.g., Berkson & Mason, 1963: Favell et al., 1982; Horner, 1980; Mosely, Faust, & Reardon, 1970). One plausible explanation for this effect is that the enriched environment provides discriminative stimuli and reinforcement for adaptive behaviors that effectively compete with maladaptive responses (Favell et al., 1982). In a second example, Matheny (1968) found that teacher use of tacts and mands differentially affected the echolalia of autistic children. When presented with tacts, echoic behavior increased, whereas teacher mands were associated with lower levels of echolalia and more frequent nonechoic vocalizations. Third, a number of studies have shown that increasing the pace of instructions can reduce a variety of disruptive classroom behaviors (e.g., Carnine, 1976). Again, this effect may be attributable to an increased rate of discriminative stimuli and reinforcement for adaptive behavior that results in a corresponding decrease in maladaptive responses.

A fourth type of research evaluates the effects of continuous and noncontingent stimuli on aberrant behavior. For example, Mace, Yankanich, and West (1989) measured the stereotypic behavior of a child with severe mental retardation under four different conditions: (a) no music (classroom), (b) music (classroom), (c) music with headphones (classroom), and (d) a quiet room. The quiet room and music-with-headphones conditions were associated with very low levels of stereotypy, which suggested to the authors that stereotypy may have been a response to aversive classroom noise that was not present in these two conditions. Finally, Mace and Knight (1986) conducted a two-phase analysis of the effects of different levels of social interaction with staff and protective equipment on severe pica. The analysis showed that increased social interaction with staff and no protective equipment were associated with the lowest levels of pica. These findings prompted the design of an intervention that combined these variables to produce large reductions in the aberrant response.

TOWARD A COMPREHENSIVE FUNCTIONAL ANALYSIS METHODOLOGY

A variety of methodologies have been used to analyze the relationship between aberrant behavior and its controlling variables. Some have focused on a descriptive analysis of behavior under natural conditions (e.g., Bijou, Peterson, & Ault, 1968). Others have emphasized the experimental analysis of aberrant behavior under controlled laboratory conditions (Iwata, et al. 1982). Further, most approaches have either proposed or demonstrated the value of linking the results of descriptive or experimental analysis with the design of interventions that interfere with the environment's capacity to evoke aberrant behavior.

Recently, some researchers have evaluated an indirect method for analyzing the relationship between environmental events and individuals' aberrant behaviors. The Functional Analysis Interview (O'Neill, Horner, Albin, Storey, & Sprague, 1989) is a set of questions directed to the relevant service provider related to the problem behaviors and their associated environmental conditions and events. The function of the interview is to provide the clinician with preliminary information to help structure the direct observation data collection procedures. The Motivation Assessment Scale (MAS; Durand & Crimmins, 1988) is a questionnaire developed to assess the hypothesized function of problem behavior. Informants are instructed to rate the likelihood of a target behavior occurring in different antecedent conditions. Obtained data are then analyzed in order to identify the hypothesized maintaining variables.

Preliminary investigations suggest that these assessment methods may provide the clinician with useful information regarding a problem behavior and its controlling variables. It should be noted, however, that indirect assessment methods such as these instruments rely on the service provider's retrospective accounts of behavior or verbal representations of behavior that occurred previously, and thus are not formal analyses. Therefore, the utility of these instruments may be as an adjunct to more formal functional analyses, as suggested by their respective authors.

In the following sections, we propose a comprehensive methodology for analyzing and treating aberrant behavior. The proposed sequence attempts to integrate proven functional analysis methods to provide clinicians and researchers with specific guidelines for conducting a multistage analysis and intervention. These phases discussed below include (a) a descriptive analysis of natural conditions; (b) formulation of hypotheses of functional relation-ships; (c) an experimental analysis under analogue conditions; (d) interven-tion development, implementation, and evaluation; and (e) maintenance and generalization of intervention effects.

Descriptive Analysis of Natural Conditions

The overwhelming majority of studies reviewed in the first part of this chapter employed experimental methods to identify functional relationships between behavior and the environment. That is, experimenters manipulated the variables under investigation during conditions that controlled extraneous variables in order to isolate the effects of the independent variable(s). Typ-ically, experimental conditions were designed to be analogues of the subjects' natural environment (e.g., Carr et al., 1980; Iwata et al., 1982; Mace et al., 1986). For most investigations, however, the rationale for studying specific reinforcement contingencies or occasioning stimuli was based on either prior research, informal observations, or care provider reports of behavior-environment interactions. Rarely have formal functional analyses been based on empirical data showing a relationship between an individual's aberrant behavior and events antecedent and subsequent to such behavior under natural circumstances.

Having an empirical basis for formulating and testing hypotheses of functional relationships is important for at least two reasons. First, for many subjects, aberrant behavior is a high-probability response. Exposing a re-sponse that is likely to occur to a reinforcement contingency may result in that response coming under control of the contingency. It may be risky, though, to assume that a contingency that controls a response under experimental conditions is the same contingency that maintains the behavior in the natural environment. Such an assumption would have greater validity if aberrant behavior and certain antecedent and subsequent events were observed to covary naturally in the subject's home, school, or work setting. Second, interventions based on a functional analysis are likely to be effective to the extent that the contingencies/stimuli in the analogue conditions parallel those in the subject's natural environment. For example, a functional analysis of analogue conditions may identify social disapproval as a positive reinforcer for self-injury and suggest that attention be withheld to extinguish the response (e.g., Carr, 1977). If social disapproval does not occur contingent on self-injury in the natural environment and the behavior is controlled by other unidentified contingencies, however, withholding attention is not likely to reduce the aberrant behavior.

Several methodologies have been proposed for collecting descriptive data on the natural covariation among behaviors and between behaviors and environmental events. For example, Vyse, Mulick, and Thayer (1984) used an interval recording procedure (partial interval and momentary time sampling) to assess behavior-behavior relationships for several child behaviors in the classroom. Correlational analyses showed that some aberrant behaviors covaried in clusters both within and between children. Patterson (1969), Wahler (1975), and Strain and Ezzell (1978), among others, employed complex observational codes to identify interrelationships among behaviors and behavioral sequences as well as between behaviors and specific settings and situational events. Similar observational methods have proven useful to identify natural covariation among behaviors of medical personnel and patient responses in a pediatric intensive care unit (Cataldo, Bessman, Parker, Pearson, & Rogers, 1979), eating behaviors and concurrent activities of obese and nonobese children (Epstein, Parker, McCoy, & McGee, 1976), and beer consumption of college students in bars and group size and the size of the container in which beer is purchased (Geller, Russ, & Altomari, 1986).

The methodology we have adopted to conduct a descriptive analysis of aberrant behavior is based largely on the work of Bijou and his colleagues (Bijou et al., 1968; Bijou, Peterson, Harris, Allen, & Johnston, 1969). The procedures begin with unstructured observations of the subject in his or her natural setting en route to objective specification of response classes and events that may occur antecedent and subsequent to the aberrant responses. Typically, this results in the identification of three to five categories each of antecedent events, response topographies, and subsequent events. Categories within each of the three classes may be as refined as necessary to identify response classes and their maintaining variables. For instance, antecedent events can be as global as instruction, noninstruction, and social interaction, or as refined as eye contact, proximity of others, and type of comment from others (statement, question, reprimand, praise, etc).

Data on antecedents, responses, and subsequents are collected by two independent observers for purposes of establishing interobserver agreement. Observations are conducted in the subject's natural setting during 15- to 60-minute sessions, depending on the amount of time required to obtain representative samples. A 10-second partial-interval recording procedure is used to record concurrently aberrant behaviors and their antecedent and subsequent events (see Figure 1). Because all events are potential antecedents, categories in this column are recorded continuously throughout the observation session. Aberrant responses are recorded when they occur, and events that follow these behaviors within two 10-second intervals (or up to 30 seconds) are recorded as subsequent events that may be sufficiently contiguous to the aberrant behavior to reinforce it. Both antecedent and subsequent events are recorded as *environmental events* on the data sheet in Figure 1, and aberrant responses are recorded as *responses*. As with all intrasubject research, sessions are conducted until clear patterns are apparent in the data.

These descriptive data can be graphed in a multielement fashion to depict variability over time. We have found it useful to graph the data as

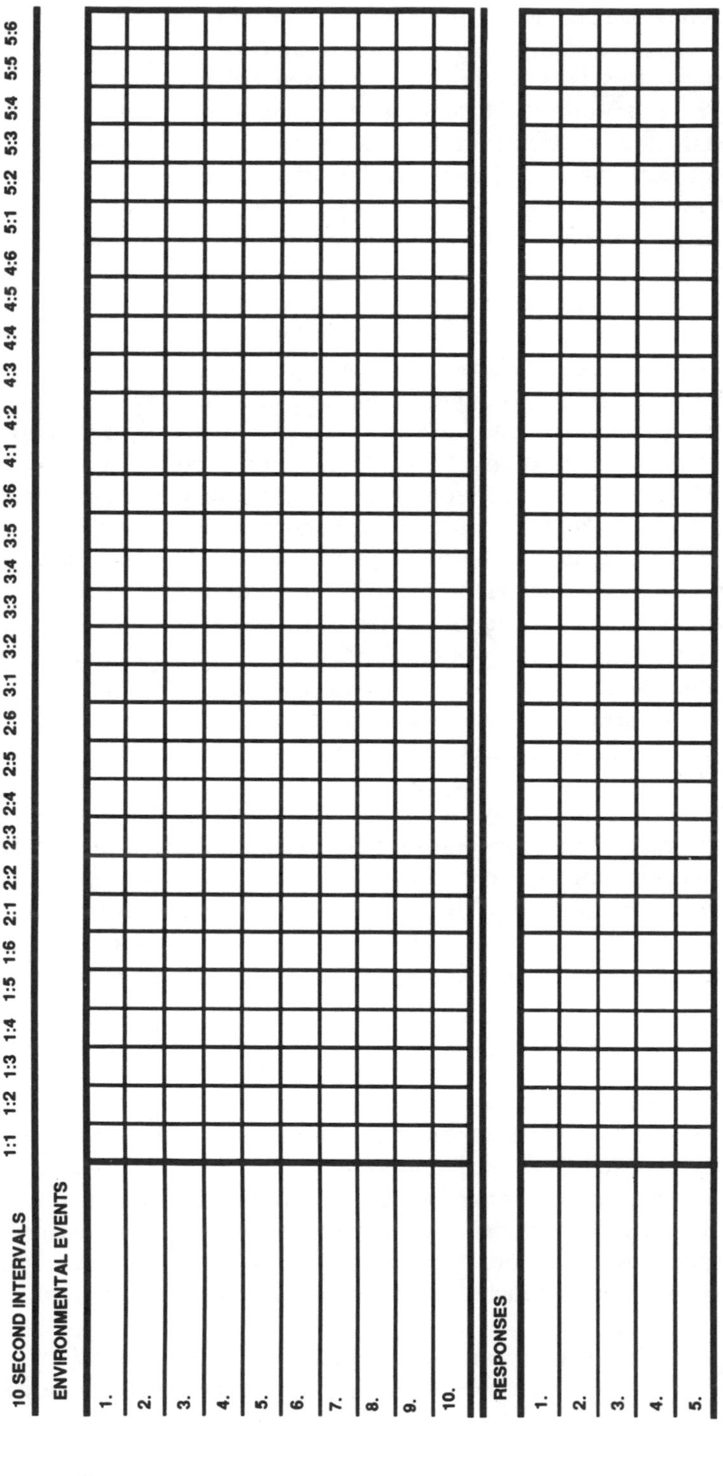

FIGURE 1. Descriptive analysis data sheet used to record concurrent occurrences of environmental events and target responses. This form is designed for continuous 10-second partial interval recording.

estimates of conditional probabilities (see Bijou et al., 1968, 1969). For example, it is possible to estimate the power of each antecedent event to evoke or occasion the aberrant response class (i.e., given an antecedent event, the probability of observing a contiguous aberrant response). In this regard, session data are expressed as the percentage of intervals scored for a given antecedent event that are followed (within two intervals) by an aberrant response. Antecedents that are followed frequently by aberrant behavior may be discriminative stimuli for the maladaptive responses. It is also helpful to express the descriptive data as the percentage of aberrant responses that are followed by each subsequent event (i.e., given an aberrant response, the probability of observing a given contiguous subsequent event). These data identify events that naturally follow the aberrant behavior and may occur as a consequence of the response. In addition, expressing these data in a time series provides a rough estimate of how intermittently a subsequent event is linked to aberrant behavior (e.g., 20% of aggressive incidents followed by social disapproval is suggestive of a VR-5 schedule of reinforcement).

Hypotheses of Functional Relationships

The major purpose of a descriptive analysis is to provide an empirical basis for the formulation of hypotheses of possible functional relationships between aberrant behavior and environmental variables (Bijou et al., 1968, 1969; Kohler & Greenwood, 1986; Wahler, 1975). A successful descriptive analysis demonstrates the natural covariation between maladaptive behavior and contiguous antecedent and subsequent events. It is important to emphasize, however, that descriptive data are only suggestive of functional relationships. Experimental methods are necessary to verify the functional relationships that were suggested by the descriptive data (Bijou et al., 1968).

Specific hypotheses of functional relationships may be formulated by careful examination of the descriptive data. For example, Baskett and Johnson (1982) conducted repeated observations of unstructured parent-child and child-sibling interactions in the home during 45-minute periods. Several adaptive and maladaptive child behaviors were recorded, along with parent and sibling reactions to these behaviors. The authors found that child disruptive behaviors such as whining, demanding, and noncompliance were frequently followed by both positive and negative reactions from their parents. This covariation under natural conditions suggested that parent attention (in a variety of forms) may positively reinforce the child's disruptive behavior. In a similar investigation, Atwater and Morris (1988) conducted naturalistic observations of preschool teachers' instructions and children's compliance over the course of three consecutive school semesters. Data were collected on the form and frequency of teachers' instructions, teachers' positive and negative feedback, and the students' compliance to instructions. The descriptive analysis data suggested that the children's compliance was directly related to the context of an instruction (e.g., large group, small group, preacademic, nonpreacademic, transition), but not to its form (e.g., instructions, questions, declaratives).

Other response-event or event-response covariations may lead to different hypotheses. For example, aberrant behavior may appear to be motivated by escape or avoidance contingencies when it occurs frequently during task-related demands, when demands are increased, or when there is a disparity between client skill and the requirements of a particular task (Carr, 1977; Durand, 1982). A similar hypothesis may be plausible if task demands are alleviated or attenuated intermittently subsequent to aberrant responses. On the other hand, sensory or perceptual consequences may be implicated as maintaining variables when behaviors such as stereotypy, pica, or self-injury occur at high rates in austere environments (e.g., Finney, Russo, & Cataldo, 1982; Iwata et al., 1982), when specific sensory consequences of aberrant behavior occur consistently (e.g., Rincover, Cook, et al., 1979), or when such potentially aversive environmental stimuli as novel settings (Davenport & Berkson, 1963) or unpleasant visual or auditory stimuli (Forehand & Baumeister, 1970) are introduced.

The examples above are only samples of the multitude of hypotheses that can be derived from inspection of descriptive data. The hypotheses selected for a particular investigation will depend on the type and pattern of descriptive data collected and the researcher's knowledge of the literature and behavior analysis.

Experimental Analysis Under Analogue Conditions

The first step in conducting an experimental analysis of aberrant behavior is to design experimental conditions to test the hypotheses derived from the descriptive analysis. The variables controlling aberrant behavior are experimentally analyzed by performing one or more well-controlled experiments under conditions that are analogues of the subject's natural environment. Results are more likely to generalize to the subject's natural environment to the extent that natural and analogue conditions overlap. In an experimental analysis, the researcher defines specific independent variables and presents them to the subject at times and under conditions determined by the experimenter. The goal is to direct the interaction between behavior and the environment and to isolate the factors responsible for the occurrence of aberrant behavior (Johnston & Pennypacker, 1980).

A cardinal rule in any experimental analysis is to hold constant or eliminate as many extraneous variables as possible in the experimental setting and, to the extent feasible, to vary one factor at a time in each experimental condition. Thus, if the consequences of an aberrant behavior are being studied, antecedent conditions such as the experimenter, instructions, and materials should be held constant while the events planned as consequences of the maladaptive behavior are varied in different experimental conditions. For example, to test the hypothesis of positive reinforcement of aggression via contingent social disapproval, an experimenter might design one condition in which an adult and the subject are seated in a playroom together with a variety of toys. The adult's attention could be focused on some task other than the child (e.g., magazine reading); however, contingent on aggressive behavior, the adult would provide disapproving comments to the child on some intermittent schedule. This experimental condition could be contrasted with one in which the setting and adult remain constant, but adult attention is available for appropriate play responses and social disapproval is withheld (see Mace et al., 1986). Higher rates of aggression in the former condition would suggest strongly that aggressive acts were positively reinforced by disapproving adult attention.

Alternatively, an analysis of the effects of different antecedent or concurrent events on aberrant behavior would vary these stimuli across experimental conditions while holding constant the planned consequences for maladaptive behavior. For instance, Durand and Carr (1987) studied the escape-avoidance motivations of stereotypy by varying the difficulty level of academic tasks across different experimental sessions. In order to isolate the effects of these antecedent stimuli, the experimenters uniformly ignored stereotyped behaviors across conditions while task difficulty was varied. Levels of stereotypy were higher when subjects were presented with more difficult tasks, suggesting to the authors that repetitive movements may function as escape responses for some individuals.

Researchers have employed diverse methods of varying experimental conditions to test single or multiple hypotheses. Carr et al. (1980) and Carr and Newsom (1985) varied a single factor in many of their experiments. Aberrant behaviors assessed as task-related demands were alternately presented and withdrawn across different experimental phases. Iwata et al. (1982) developed a preintervention assessment protocol to test multiple hypotheses regarding the function of self-injury. All subjects were exposed to three experimental conditions and one control condition designed to test the following hypotheses: (a) Self-injury is positively reinforced by social disapproval, (b) self-injury is negatively reinforced by escape or avoidance of demands, and (c) sensory or biochemical consequences of self-injury maintain the response. Another strategy has been to analyze the effects of different dimensions or levels of single or multiple variables. For example, Mace and Knight (1986) conducted two separate preintervention analyses to determine the effects that different levels of social interaction and protective equipment had on a subject's pica. One analysis compared frequent, limited, and no social interaction, whereas the other analysis compared a helmet with face shield, helmet without face shield, and no protective equipment. Finally, several researchers have conducted follow-up analyses subsequent to an initial assessment to clarify unresolved issues. This approach resulted in better understanding of and more effective interventions for self-injury (Pace, Ivancic, Edwards, Iwata, & Page, 1985), stereotypy (Durand & Carr, 1987; Mace et al., 1987), and aggression (Carr et al., 1980; Mace et al., 1986).

Presenting analogue conditions to subjects in the context of an intrasubject experimental design permits valid conclusions to be drawn regarding the effects the various conditions have on the target aberrant behavior. Two general types of experimental designs have been used for this purpose. Withdrawal or reversal designs have generally been used to compare two experimental conditions. A different experimental condition is in effect in each phase; conditions are alternated in a sequence of phases as a pattern of stable responding is achieved in each phase. Within-subject replication of experimental conditions and their effects permits scientifically valid conclusions to be drawn (see Carr et al., 1980; Carr & Newsom, 1985; Durand & Carr, 1987, for examples). The second tactic has been to present experimental conditions to subjects in the context of a multielement or alternating-treatments design. In this approach, subjects are typically presented with the experimental conditions in a random or counterbalanced order each day of the analysis. It is reasonable to conclude that conditions that result in high levels of aberrant behavior contain variables that have functional control of the aberrant response (see Iwata et al., 1982; Mace et al., 1987; Mace et al., 1986; Thomas et al., 1968, for examples). We should note that the multielement design is not the best choice when the experimental conditions cannot be made discriminable for a particular subject.

Intervention Development, Implementation, and Evaluation

The applied value of preintervention descriptive and experimental analyses of aberrant behavior is their contribution to intervention development. The results of the descriptive and experimental studies can provide specific information about how the environment controls each subject's maladaptive behavior. Analysis of the consequences produced by aberrant responses can identify positive and/or negative reinforcement contingencies that maintain the problem behavior. Likewise, an analysis of antecedent and/or concurrent stimuli contiguous to aberrant responses can help define the persons, materials, situations, or interactions that increase or decrease the probability that an individual will engage in maladaptive activities.

Understanding the interface between an individual and his or her environment that results in aberrant behavior can have clear implications for the design of effective intervention procedures. The general strategy is to alter the environment so as to minimize the reinforcement for aberrant behavior and, whenever possible, provide reinforcement for adaptive responses to compete with maladaptive behavior. When the functional analysis identifies specific reinforcement contingencies operating to maintain behavior. A logical intervention tactic is extinction. Extinction of behavior maintained by positive reinforcement involves discontinuing the presentation of the positive reinforcer contingent on the aberrant response (Skinner, 1969). This tactic was illustrated by Ayllon and Michael (1959) by having nursing staff ignore bizarre speech (i.e., withhold indulging comments) and Mace et al. (1986) when experimenters ignored (i.e., discontinued social disapproval) and blocked aggressive responses. By contrast, extinction in a negative reinforcement process consists of discontinuing the contingent relationship between aberrant behavior and the delay, attenuation, or alleviation of aversive stimuli (Catania, 1984). Thus, extinction procedures would prevent the aberrant behavior from resulting in escape or avoidance of task-related demands (see Carr et al., 1980; Carr & Newsom, 1985; Mace et al., 1987).

When maladaptive behavior is shown to correlate with certain antecedent or concurrent stimuli, intervention often entails minimizing the presentation of these stimuli in the subject's environment. For example, studies showing increased disruptive behavior from students when they are presented with difficult academic tasks have achieved reduction in aberrant behavior by reducing task difficulty (Center et al., 1982), eliminating errors via errorless learning procedures (Weeks & Gaylord-Ross, 1981), and altering the pace of instruction to encourage academic responses (Carnine, 1976). When stimuli that are discriminative for aberrant behavior cannot be minimized or eliminated from the subject's environment, however, an alternative may be to provide a new reinforcement history with these stimuli that will weaken their discriminative control of the maladaptive behavior. For example, Mace and West (1986) found that a child engaged consistently in mute behavior in response to his teacher's queries. When the teacher was trained to persist with her questions despite the student's mute behavior and praise the vocal responses when they occurred, the subject spoke reliably in the teacher's presence.

Extinction and alteration of antecedent or concurrent stimuli are likely to be most effective when combined with procedures to prompt and reinforce adaptive behavior. A familiar strategy is to employ a prompt hierarchy to occasion an adaptive academic, vocational, or social response that is then reinforced on a rich schedule (e.g., Cuvo, Leaf, & Borakove, 1978). The rationale for this procedure is rooted largely in Hernstein's matching law (1961): If the rate of reinforcement for the adaptive target response exceeds that for the aberrant class of behaviors, adaptive responding should increase, whereas rates of aberrant behavior should decrease (see Myerson & Hale, 1984, for a discussion of applications of the matching law). Carr and Durand (1985), Durand and Carr (1987), Durand and Kishi (1987), and Day et al. (1988) illustrated an innovative variation of this strategy that directly links preintervention analysis with teaching procedures for adaptive behavior. In each of the studies, an experimental analysis indicated that a variety of aberrant behaviors were maintained by either escape-avoidance or demands for adult attention. Thus, these researchers trained subjects to emit an adaptive response that would serve a function similar to their maladaptive behavior. Aberrant behaviors decreased when children were taught to demand adult attention or "help" vocally following task errors.

A distinct advantage of designing interventions on the basis of a preintervention analysis is that treatments are often positive in nature and include few (if any) aversive components. This is attributable largely to the focus on identifying and interrupting reinforcement contingencies that maintain maladaptive behavior patterns. It is important to note, however, that the methodology is not a panacea for eliminating the therapeutic use of aversive contingencies to reduce severe maladaptive behavior. For very difficult (i.e., highly aggressive or self-injurious) clients, enduring lengthy and sometimes incomplete extinction processes may be a less compassionate and less therapeutic alternative than combining extinction and differential reinforcement procedures with effective punishment techniques.

Maintenance and Generalization of Intervention Effects

An experimental analysis of aberrant behavior is, to one degree or another, only an analogue of the subject's natural environment. Yet the methodological requirements for controlled measurement and manipulation of variables may yield findings that do not generalize to the natural setting. Differences between the experimental and natural settings along the dimensions of personnel, materials, times, procedures, and extraneous influences (e.g., peers, illness, novel events) may account for a failure to generalize (Kohler & Greenwood, 1986; Stokes & Baer, 1977). This final phase of functional analysis and intervention has been largely overlooked by researchers at this point in the evolution of the methodology. It would seem, though, that this phase is critical to the long range success of the methodology in applied settings.

SUMMARY AND DIRECTIONS FOR FUTURE RESEARCH

This chapter reviewed conceptual and empirical literature describing a behavior analytic approach to functionally analyzing and treating a wide variety of aberrant behaviors. Functional analysis research has identified several general classes of variables that control problem behavior. Maladaptive responses may be positively reinforced by contingent attention, access to materials or activities, or the sensory and perceptual consequences produced by the aberrant response. Alternatively, behaviors that produce escape or avoidance of aversive conditions (especially task-related demands) may be maintained by negative reinforcement. Finally, analysis of antecedent and concurrent events can identify variables that predict differential rates of aberrant responding. Both approaches—analysis of antecedent/concurrent stimuli and of consequent events—can lead to the development of effective interventions by interrupting reinforcement contingencies that may maintain aberrant behavior. We also described a comprehensive, multistage functional analysis methodology for maladaptive behavior. Its components included (a) a descriptive analysis of natural conditions; (b) formation of hypotheses of functional relationships; (c) experimental analysis of analogue conditions; (d) intervention development, implementation, and evaluation; and (e) maintenance and generalization of intervention effects.

As functional analysis research gains momentum, there are several areas that hold promise for future investigation. First, including the descriptive analysis phase and the maintenance and generalization phase will strengthen our understanding of the genesis and persistence of aberrant behavior and enhance the applied value of the functional analysis methodology. Much more research is needed to understand how the natural environment fosters aberrant behavior and impedes progress in remediating it. Second, virtually all applications of the functional analysis methodology have been with high-rate responses, yet many serious behavior problems occur only a few times per day, per month, or per year. Clearly, a methodology for analyzing low-rate behaviors is needed. Third, additional applications of the analysis of antecedent and concurrent events may prove useful in identifying environmental predictors of low-rate behaviors, responses maintained by extremely thin schedules of reinforcement, and behaviors that by nature or convention are maintained by reinforcers that the researcher may not be able to observe or manipulate directly (e.g., peer influences, physiological events, sexual relations). Finally, there are obvious benefits to extending the functional analysis methodology to the study of adaptive social, vocational, and academic behaviors. Such research might identify natural conditions that promote the development and maintenance of adaptive behavior, which in turn may have clear implications for designing more therapeutic and educational environments.

REFERENCES

Anderson, L., Dancis, J., & Alpert, M. (1978). Behavioral contingencies and self-mutilation in Lesch-Nyhan disease. *Journal of Consulting and Clinical Psychology, 46,* 529–536.

Atwater, J. B., & Morris, E. K. (1988). Teacher's instructions and children's compliance in preschool classrooms: A descriptive analysis. *Journal of Applied Behavior Analysis, 21,* 157–167.

Ayllon, T., & Michael, J. (1959). The psychiatric nurse as a behavioral engineer. *Journal of the Experimental Analysis of Behavior, 2,* 323–334.

Baer, D. M., Wolf, M. M., & Risley, T. R. (1968). Some current dimensions of applied behavior analysis. *Journal of Applied Behavior Analysis, 1,* 91–97.

Bailey, J. S., Shook, H., Iwata, B., Reid, D., & Repp, A. (1986). *Journal of Applied Behavior Analysis Reprint Series on Developmental Disabilities. 1968–1985*. Lawrence, KS: Society for Experimental Analysis of Behavior.

Baskett, L. M., & Johnson, S. M. (1982). The young child's interactions with parents versus siblings: A behavioral analysis. *Child Development, 53,* 643–650.

Berkson, G., & Mason, W. A. (1963). Stereotyped movements of mental defectives: IV. The effects of toys and the character of tacts. *American Journal of Mental Deficiency, 68,* 511–524.

Bijou, S. W., Peterson, R. F., & Ault, M. H. (1968). A method to integrate descriptive and experimental field studies at the level of data and empirical concepts. *Journal of Applied Behavior Analysis, 1,* 175–191.

Bijou, S. W., Peterson, R. F., Harris, F. R., Allen, K. E., & Johnson, M. S. (1969). Methodology for experimental studies of young children in natural settings. *Psychological Record, 19,* 177–210.

Budd, K. S., Green, D. R., & Baer, D. M. (1976). An analysis of multiple misplaced parental social contingencies. *Journal of Applied Behavior Analysis, 9,* 459–470.

Carnine, D. W. (1976). Effects of two teacher-presentation rates on the off-task behavior, answering correctly, and participation. *Journal of Applied Behavior Analysis, 9,* 199–206.

Carr, E. G. (1977). The motivation of self-injurious behavior: A review of some hypotheses. *Psychological Bulletin, 84,* 800–816.

Carr, E. G., & Durand, M. (1985). Reducing behavior problems through functional communication training. *Journal of Applied Behavior Analysis, 18,* 111–126.

Carr, E. G., & Newsom, C. (1985). Demand-related tantrums. *Behavior Modification, 9,* 403–426.

Carr, E. G., Newsom, C., & Binkoff, J. (1980). Escape as a factor in the aggressive behavior of two retarded children. *Journal of Applied Behavior Analysis, 13,* 101–117.

Cataldo, M. F., Bessman, C. A., Parker, L. H., Pearson, J., & Rogers, M. C. (1979). Behavioral assessment for pediatric intensive care units. *Journal of Applied Behavior Analysis, 12,* 83–97.

Cataldo, M. F., & Harris, J. (1982). The biological basis for self-injury in the mentally retarded. *Analysis and Intervention in Developmental Disabilities, 2,* 21–39.

Catania, A. C. (1984). *Learning* (2nd ed.). Englewood Cliffs, NJ: Prentice-Hall.

Center, D. B., Deitz, S. M., & Kaufman, M. (1982). Student ability, task difficulty, and inappropriate classroom behavior. *Behavior Modification, 6,* 355–374.

Cuvo, A. J., Leaf, R. B., & Borakove, L. S. (1978). Teaching janitorial skills to the mentally retarded: Acquisition, generalization and maintenance. *Journal of Applied Behavior Analysis, 11,* 345–355.

Day, R. M., Rea, J. A., Schussler, N. G., Larsen, S. E., & Johnson, W. L. (1988). A functionally based approach to the treatment of self-injurious behavior. *Behavior Modification, 12,* 565–589.

Davenport, R. K., & Berkson, G. (1963). Stereotyped movements of mental defectives: II. Effects of novel objects. *American Journal of Mental Deficiency, 67,* 879–882.

Dietz, S. M. (1978). Current status of applied behavior analysis. *American Psychologist, 33,* 805–814.

Dietz, S. M. (1982). Defining applied behavior analysis: An historical analogy. *Behavior Analyst, 5,* 53–64.

Durand, V. M. (1982). Analysis and intervention of self-injurious behavior. *Journal of the Association for the Severely Handicapped, 7,* 44–53.

Durand, V. M., & Carr, E. G. (1987). Social influences on "self-stimulatory" behavior: Analysis and treatment application. *Journal of Applied Behavior Analysis, 20,* 119–132.

Durand, V. M., & Crimmins, D. B. (1987). Assessment and treatment of psychotic speech in an autistic child. *Journal of Autism and Developmental Disorders, 17,* 17–28.

Durand, V. M., & Crimmins, D. B. (1988). Identifying variables maintaining self-injurious behavior. *Journal of Autism and Developmental Disorders, 18,* 99–117.

Durand, V. M., & Kishi, G. (1987). Reducing severe behavior problems among persons with dual sensory impairments: An evaluation of a technical assistance model. *Journal of the Association for the Persons With Severe Handicaps, 12,* 2–10.

Epstein, L. H., Parker, L., McCoy, J. F., & McGee, G. (1976). Descriptive analysis of eating regulation in obese and nonobese children. *Journal of Applied Behavior Analysis, 9*, 407–415.

Finney, J., Russo, D., & Cataldo, M. (1982). Reduction of pica in young children with lead poisoning. *Journal of Pediatric Psychology, 7*, 197–207.

Favell, J. E., McGimsey, J. F., & Schell, R. M. (1982). Treatment of self-injury by providing alternate sensory activities. *Analysis and Intervention in Developmental Disabilities, 2*, 83–104.

Forehand, R., & Baumeister, A. A. (1970). The effect of auditory and visual stimulation of stereotyped rocking behavior and general activity of severe retardates. *Journal of Clinical Psychology, 26*, 426–429.

Gaylord-Ross, R., Weeks, M., & Lipner, C. (1980). An analysis of antecedent, response, and consequence events in the treatment of self-injurious behavior. *Education and Training of the Mentally Retarded, 15*, 35–42.

Geller, E. S., Russ, N. W., & Altomari, M. G. (1986). Naturalistic observations of beer drinking among college students. *Journal of Applied Behavior Analysis, 19*, 391–396.

Hayes, S. C., Rincover, A., & Solnick, J. V. (1980). The technical drift of applied behavior analysis. *Journal of Applied Behavior Analysis, 13*, 275–285.

Herrnstein, R. J. (1961). Relative and absolute strength of response as a function of reinforcement. *Journal of the Experimental Analysis of Behavior, 4*, 267–272.

Horner, R. D. (1980). The effects of an environmental "enrichment" program on the behavior of institutionalized profoundly retarded children. *Journal of Applied Behavior Analysis, 13*, 473–491.

Hunt, P., Alwell, M., & Goetz, L. (1988). Acquisition of conversation skills and the reduction of inappropriate social interaction behaviors. *Journal of the Association for the Severely Handicapped, 7*, 44–53.

Iwata, B., Dorsey, M., Slifer, K., Bauman, K., & Richman, G. (1982). Toward a functional analysis of self-injury. *Analysis and Intervention in Developmental Disabilities, 2*, 3–20.

Johnston, J. M., & Pennypacker, H. (1980). *Strategies and tactics of human behavioral research.* Hillsdale, NJ: Lawrence Erlbaum.

Koegel, R. L., Dyer, K., & Bell, L. K. (1987). The influence of child-preferred activities on autistic children's social behavior. *Journal of Applied Behavior Analysis, 20*, 243–252.

Kohler, F. W., & Greenwood, C. R. (1986). Toward a technology of generalization: The identification of natural contingencies of reinforcement. *Behavior Analyst, 9*, 19–26.

Lovaas, I., Newsom, C., & Hickman, C. (1987). Self-stimulatory behavior and perceptual reinforcement. *Journal of Applied Behavior Analysis, 20*, 45–68.

Mace, F. C., Browder, D., & Lin, Y. (1987). Analysis of demand conditions associated with stereotypy. *Journal of Behavior Therapy and Experimental Psychiatry, 18*, 25–31.

Mace, F. C., & Knight, D. (1986). Functional analysis and treatment of severe pica. *Journal of Applied Behavior Analysis, 19*, 411–416.

Mace, F. C., Page, T. J., Ivancic, M. T., & O'Brien, S. (1986). Analysis of environmental determinants of aggression and disruption in mentally retarded children. *Applied Research in Mental Retardation, 7*, 203–221.

Mace, F. C., & West, B. (1986). Analysis of demand conditions associated with reluctant speech. *Journal of Behavior Therapy and Experimental Psychiatry, 17*, 285–294.

Mace, F. C., Yankanich, M. A., & West, B. (1989). Toward a methodology of experimental analysis and treatment of aberrant classroom behaviors. *Special Services in the School, 4*, 71–88.

Matheny, A. P. (1968). Pathological echoic responses in a child: Effect of environment mand and tact control. *Journal of Experimental Child Psychology, 6*, 624–631.

Michael, J. (1980). Flight from behavior analysis. *Behavior Analyst, 3*, 1–22.

Michael, J. (1982). Distinguishing between discriminative and motivational functions of stimuli. *Journal of the Experimental Analysis of Behavior, 37*, 149–155.

Mosely, A., Faust, M., & Reardon, D. M. (1970). Effects of social and nonsocial stimuli on the stereotyped behaviors of retarded children. *American Journal of Mental Deficiency, 74,* 809–811.

Myerson, J., & Hale, S. (1984). Practical implications of the matching law. *Journal of Applied Behavior Analysis, 17,* 367–380.

O'Neill, R. E., Horner, R. H., Albin, R. W., Storey, K., & Sprague, J. R. (1989). The functional analysis interview. In R. H. Horner, J. L. Anderson, E. G. Carr, G. Dunlap, R. L. Koegel, & W. Sailor (Eds.), *Functional analysis: A practical assessment guide* (pp. 10–23). Eugene: University of Oregon Press.

Pace, G. M., Ivancic, M. T., Edwards, G. L., Iwata, B., & Page, T. J. (1985). Assessment of stimulus preference and reinforcer value with profoundly retarded individuals. *Journal of Applied Behavior Analysis, 18,* 249–255.

Patterson, G. R. (1969). Behavioral intervention procedures in the classroom and in the home. In A. E. Bergin & S. L. Garfield (Eds.), *Handbook of psychotherapy and behavior change.* New York: John Wiley.

Patterson, G. R., Littman, R. A., & Bricker, W. (1967). Assertive behavior in children: A step toward a theory of aggression. *Monographs of the Society for Research in Child Development, 32*(5, Whole No. 113).

Pierce, W. D., & Epling, W. F. (1980). What happened to analysis in applied behavior analysis? *Behavior Analyst, 3,* 1–9.

Repp, A. C., Felce, D., & Barton, L. E. (1988). Basing the treatment of stereotypic and self-injurious behaviors on hypotheses of their causes. *Journal of Applied Behavior Analysis, 21,* 281–289.

Rincover, A., Cook, R., Peoples, A., & Packard, D. (1979). Sensory extinction and sensory reinforcement principles for programming multiple adaptive behavior change. *Journal of Applied Behavior Analysis, 12,* 221–233.

Rincover, A., & Devany, J. (1982). The application of sensory extinction procedures to self-injury. *Analysis and Intervention in Developmental Disabilities, 2,* 67–81.

Rincover, A., Newsom, C. D., & Carr, E. G. (1979). Use of sensory extinction procedures in the treatment of compulsive-like behavior of developmentally disabled children. *Journal of Consulting and Clinical Psychology, 47,* 695–701.

Sailor, W., Guess, D., Rutherford, G., & Baer, D. M. (1968). Control of tantrum behavior by operant techniques during experimental verbal training. *Journal of Applied Behavior Analysis, 1,* 237–243.

Skinner, B. F. (1953). *Science and human behavior.* New York: Macmillan.

Skinner, B. F. (1969). *Contingencies of reinforcement: A theoretical analysis.* Englewood Cliffs, NJ: Prentice-Hall.

Steege, M. W., Wacker, D. P., Berg, W. K., Cigrand, K. K., & Cooper, L. J. (1989). The use of behavioral assessment to prescribe and evaluate treatments for severely handicapped children. *Journal of Applied Behavior Analysis, 22,* 23–33.

Stokes, T. F., & Baer, D. M. (1977). An implicit technology of generalization. *Journal of Applied Behavior Analysis, 10,* 349–367.

Strain, P. S., & Ezzelle, D. (1978). The sequence and distribution of behaviorally disordered adolescents' disruptive/inappropriate behaviors. *Behavior Modification, 2,* 403–425.

Thomas, D. R., Becker, W. C., & Armstrong, M. (1968). Production and elimination of disruptive classroom behavior by systematically varying teachers' behavior. *Journal of Applied Behavior Analysis, 1,* 35–45.

Vyse, S., Mulick, J. A., & Thayer, B. M. (1984). An ecobehavioral assessment of a special educational classroom. *Applied Research in Mental Retardation, 5,* 395–408.

Wahler, R. G. (1975). Some structural aspects of deviant child behavior. *Journal of Applied Behavior Analysis, 8,* 27–42.

Wahler, R. G., & Fox, R. M. (1981). Setting events in applied behavior analysis: Towards a conceptual and methodological expansion. *Journal of Applied Behavior Analysis, 14,* 327–338.

Weeks, M., & Gaylord-Ross, R. (1981). Task difficulty and aberrant behavior in severely handicapped students. *Journal of Applied Behavior Analysis, 14,* 449–463.

Wolery, M. R. (1978). Self-stimulatory behavior as a basis for devising reinforcers. *AAESPH Review, 3,* 23–29.

Wolery, M. R., Kirk, K., & Gast, L. (1985). Stereotypic behavior as a reinforcer: Effects and side effects. *Journal of Autism and Developmental Disorders, 15,* 149–161.

5

Treatment Classification and Selection Based on Behavioral Function

BRIAN A. IWATA, TIMOTHY R. VOLLMER, JENNIFER R. ZARCONE, AND TERESA A. RODGERS

INTRODUCTION

Results from more than 25 years of research on behavioral approaches to the treatment of self-injury, aggression, and related disorders in developmentally disabled individuals indicate that these problems are learned behaviors and can be reduced significantly using interventions derived from operant conditioning principles. A consistent finding has been that behavior disorders are responsive to treatment across an extremely wide range of procedural variation. Because so many options are available in a given clinical situation, issues related to treatment selection have become increasingly important in recent years, and a number of decision-making models have been proposed. Yet the question of how best to proceed when attempting to reduce a serious behavior problem has been difficult to answer and is often the subject of controversy. Some treatments are viewed as more effective, intrusive, or costly than others, and there has been disagreement over the relative "ranking" of treatments based on these factors. The ultimate criteria used in making treatment decisions should take into account scientific, ethical, and economic factors, as well as consumer preference (e.g., see the extensive

BRIAN A. IWATA, TIMOTHY R. VOLLMER, JENNIFER R. ZARCONE, AND TERESA A. RODGERS • Psychology Department, University of Florida, Gainesville, Florida 32611.

Behavior Analysis and Treatment, edited by R. Van Houten & S. Axelrod. Plenum Press, New York, 1993.

discussion of these factors in Repp & Singh, 1990). Much of the current controversy, however, arises from more basic misconceptions about the characteristics of treatment procedures and the behavior disorders they are designed to eliminate, resulting in either arbitrary or erroneous classification.

Of the many refinements seen in assessment and treatment research over the past decade, two are particularly relevant to treatment classification and selection. First, assessment research has evolved from having a primary focus on target-response measurement to the identification of variables that are correlated with—or that may actually exert functional control over—the occurrence of behavior disorders. Second, questions posed in treatment research have extended beyond the typical focus on *which* treatments work to include *why* (i.e., according to what principles) treatments work. The recent integration of methods and findings from these areas of research has led to the emergence of what is becoming known as the *functional analysis model* of assessment and treatment. The model has profound implications for treatment classification and selection because it suggests a general strategy for predicting which interventions are likely to be effective (and, conversely, which are likely to be ineffective) prior to actual implementation.

In this chapter, we will review several treatment models and their limitations, which are best understood following a brief discussion of the learned (functional) characteristics of behavior disorders. We will then describe an approach to treatment based on the functional analysis of behavior and will outline specific interventions consistent with each behavioral function. Our goal here is to provide a general framework for treatment classification. It is not our intent to provide detailed instructions on procedural implementation (as in a clinical manual) or to provide a comprehensive review of research on the effects of a given intervention.

THE FUNCTIONAL CHARACTERISTICS OF BEHAVIOR DISORDERS

There is strong evidence that behavior disorders have a significant learned component. For many years, support for this view came from two sources: (a) the assumed generality of basic research on operant conditioning, which showed repeatedly that many forms of behavior can be shaped and maintained through reinforcement; and (b) retrospective interpretation of clinical data. If treatment results showed that it was possible to "unlearn" a behavior problem, one might reasonably assume that the problem was "learned" in the first place. How this learning actually occurred in individuals who exhibited severe behavior disorders was of incidental interest, even though its relevance to treatment was proposed a number of years ago (e.g., Bachman, 1972; Carr, 1977). At that time, there appeared to be a general consensus that therapeutic contingencies could be implemented with little regard to factors initially responsible for the development and maintenance of aberrant behavior.

Because of the lack of consistent success found with every behavioral treatment, including punishment, there has been renewed interest in the direct examination of conditions that produce behavior disorders. Several learning-based interpretations have evolved, and although there is considerable overlap among them, differences exist at the level of both interpretation (i.e., specification of controlling variables) and description (nomenclature). The present account of behavioral function offers the following advantages: (a) It classifies function according to basic principle (contingency) rather than lay interpretation, which reduces confusion and promotes integration of theory with both basic and applied research; (b) it provides a relatively complete account of the major determinants of operant behavior while invoking a small number of key variables; and (c) it therefore should be generalizable across different topographies of learned behavior disorders.

The proposed functional classes include the two types of contingencies (positive versus negative reinforcement) responsible for behavioral development and two sources of stimulus delivery/removal (socially mediated versus automatic). A brief description of these four functional classes is presented here; a more extensive review can be found in Iwata, Vollmer, and Zarcone (1990). Identification of the specific reinforcer delivered or removed (e.g., attention, food, activities), although important from the standpoint of treatment development, is neither critical nor even beneficial for the purpose of classification, for two reasons. First, an analysis of behavior disorders based on specific maintaining stimuli will never be complete until all reinforcers are identified. Second, specific reinforcers historically have been extremely idiosyncratic, so that the same event could serve as either positive or negative reinforcement.

Socially Mediated Positive Reinforcement

Disruptive behaviors reliably produce a response from those in the immediate vicinity. Screaming children must be checked for injury, injured children require medical attention, and those injuring others must be stopped. In each of these examples, attention and perhaps additional events are delivered by another person (hence the term *social*) contingent on the occurrence of behavior and may serve as positive reinforcement. The effects of social reinforcement on self-injurious behavior (SIB) were demonstrated a number of years ago by Lovaas and Simmons (1969); more recently, it has been shown that aggression and disruption can be maintained in a similar manner (Mace, Page, Ivancic, & O'Brien, 1986). One might expect these unavoidable or inadvertent consequences to promote the development of behavior disorders when an individual has limited ability to attract attention through other means, or when the environment is relatively unresponsive to more benign forms of getting attention. These risk factors—behavioral and environmental deficit—probably account for observed correlations between a problem such as SIB and both degree of retardation (Griffin, Williams, Stark, Altmeyer, & Mason, 1984) and restricted living environment (Borthwick, Meyers, & Eyman, 1981).

Automatic-Positive Reinforcement

Some behaviors, rather than being reinforced by consequences that others deliver, directly produce stimulation that serves as positive reinforcement. Over the years, these behaviors have been called *mannerisms* and *stereotypy*, which describe topographical characteristics but do not refer to any controlling variable. Another frequently used term, *self-stimulation*, does refer to process but is a lay interpretation of the source of reinforcement. A more accurate description would be that these positive reinforcers are produced *automatically* by the behavior (Skinner, 1969). Appetitive behaviors maintained directly by primary reinforcement (e.g., food seeking) are examples of automatic reinforcement, as are some higher forms of creativity (e.g., playing a musical instrument). Although specific accounts of the source of reinforcement for behavior disorders have ranged form perceptual stimulation in autistic individuals (Lovaas, Newsom, & Hickman, 1987) to endogenous opioids as one maintaining factor for SIB (Cataldo & Harris, 1982), the common feature of this contingency is that responding produces reinforcement independent of the action of others.

Socially Mediated Negative Reinforcement

In addition to—or instead of—receiving attention for disruptive behavior, some individuals experience cessation of ongoing activity. They are removed from class, sent home from the workshop, not required to complete their chores, or even placed in "time out" following episodes of SIB, aggression, or property destruction. Events that are removed, attenuated, or prevented by others contingent on the occurrence of behavior problems may strengthen these problems through the process of negative reinforcement (Iwata, 1987). As is the case with behavior disorders maintained by social-positive reinforcement, developmentally disabled individuals may be at greater risk for the strengthening of inappropriate "avoidance" or "escape" behavior because of both behavioral and environmental limitations. Severe behavioral deficits often require intensive remediation, and slower response acquisition during training may lead to reinforcement reduction as well as continued presentation of difficult tasks, which can be terminated only through extreme behavior.

Automatic-Negative Reinforcement

Response-contingent termination of ongoing events need not be arranged by others. Instead, some behaviors can directly and automatically disrupt or terminate ongoing stimulation. Common examples include scratching the skin at the site of an insect bite or rubbing the jaw when experiencing a toothache. In most individuals, these behaviors eventually give way to more adaptive alternatives, such as applying antiseptic to the bite or calling the dentist to arrange an appointment. Many developmentally disabled individuals have not learned these latter behaviors and are left with their own means of terminating "aversive states" associated with physical pain or discomfort. Thus, scratching may occur whenever there is localized irritation to the skin; it may later persist as a result of the additional irritation it produces. This source of reinforcement may account for observed correlations between specific medical conditions and SIB. For example, one form of SIB—head banging—has been associated with ear infections in children (DeLissovoy, 1963). It is important to note that the initial source of stimulation (e.g., headache, skin condition) does not cause the behavior to occur through a reflexive or other biological mechanism; rather, the presence of stimulation allows its termination through responding to serve as negative reinforcement. Ear infections do not produce head banging, but they may arrange a condition in which head banging is reinforced when it otherwise would not be.

Implications

Assuming that the above account is an accurate description of the contingencies that develop and maintain most behavior disorders, our ability to identify the relevant contingency on an individual basis will serve a number of purposes. First, it will identify the conditions that promote the initial development of behavior disorders (e.g., deprivation from attention, in the case of behavior maintained by social-positive reinforcement). Second, it will indicate the source of reinforcement (e.g., attention contingent on inappropriate behavior) that should be eliminated through extinction. Third, it will suggest a general contingency, as well as specific reinforcing events, that should form the basis for treatment (e.g., differential reinforcement of alternative behavior using attention). Fourth, it should indicate which approaches to treatment are either irrelevant or perhaps even countertherapeutic (e.g., "sensory" extinction). Finally, by matching behavioral function to the active components (functions) of treatment, it should be possible to classify, develop, and select behavioral interventions based on the functions of behavior for which they are effective. Before describing how such a classification system would operate, the alternatives will be reviewed.

APPROACHES TO TREATMENT CLASSIFICATION AND SELECTION

Arbitrary Selection

The least sophisticated method of selecting treatment procedures consists of adopting a more or less uniform approach to behavior management based on some arbitrary criterion (e.g., organizational regulation, apparent ease of administration). Examples of this approach include the use of "response blocking" following all observed instances of SIB, environmental repair (perhaps a variant of overcorrection) for all destructive behavior, restraint or time out for aggressive behavior, restriction of privileges for running away, or differential reinforcement of other behavior (DRO) for all of these undesirable activities. Both the rationale for using this approach and the expected results are poor, because no specific form of treatment has been shown to be sufficiently effective for general application (i.e., across behavior disorders, maintaining contingencies, and situations).

Classification by Procedural Description (Treatment Topography)

Most textbook authors organize behavior reduction techniques according to contingency or function (e.g., extinction, differential reinforcement, time out, response cost, punishment), which can accommodate a wide range of procedural or topographical variation. For example, treatment procedures containing a time-out contingency have been implemented through ignoring the inappropriate behavior (Nelson & Rutherford, 1983), contingent observation (Porterfield, Herbert-Jackson, & Risley, 1976), discriminative arrangements such as the time-out ribbon (Foxx & Shapiro, 1978), facial screening (Lutzker, 1978), movement suppression (Rolider & Van Houten, 1985), restraint (Edwards, 1974), and the use of time-out rooms (Harris, Ersner-Hershfield, Kaffashan, & Romanczyk, 1974). Because many therapeutic procedures can be derived from a given contingency, consistent implementation requires precise description. Thus, general contingency descriptions found in texts usually give way to more detailed procedural descriptions in most administrative and treatment manuals, which place emphasis on the topographical aspects of intervention (e.g., Florida Department of Health and Rehabilitative Services, 1989; Ontario Ministry of Community and Social Services, 1987).

This approach to treatment classification results in a well-defined system of techniques specifying the acceptable "boundaries" for a given intervention, which can be extremely useful in developing staff training and quality control programs. Classification based on procedural rather than functional description, however, also results in treatment programs whose behavioral effects are difficult to predict because the actions of the therapist, although perhaps adequately described, entail the use of unidentified or unknown contingencies. An example of this limitation can be seen in procedural definitions of extinction, which have fostered a popular misconception among some practitioners that extinction is defined as "ignoring the behavior" (LaVigna & Donnellan, 1986, p. 50). The function of extinction is to eliminate reinforcement for an undesirable behavior. "Ignoring" and variations thereof limit the *delivery* of certain consequences for behavior (social-positive reinforcement). To the extent that delivery of these social consequences does not reinforce the behavior (e.g., the behavior is automatically reinforced), the procedural form of "extinction" based on ignoring will not be effective treatment. Worse yet, to the extent that removal of social interaction serves as negative reinforcement, ignoring the behavior by terminating social interaction would be countertherapeutic.

Selection Based on the Least Restrictive Alternative

Treatment classification by procedure does not dictate any particular method for selecting one intervention over another. It does, however, provide a convenient basis for applying additional criteria to the selection process. One important historical criterion within the field of developmental disabilities is the philosophy of the "least restrictive alternative" (Evans & Meyer, 1985). Consistent with the general practice in medicine favoring low- over high-risk interventions, the criterion of least restrictive alternative dictates severe limitation on, if not complete prohibition of, interventions that pose risk for injury, pain, discomfort, humiliation, or social stigmatization. Emphasis is placed on interventions consistent with "normalized" functioning typical of that seen in nonhandicapped individuals; in other words, treatments should be selected based on whether or not they would be freely chosen by nonhandicapped individuals. In principle, this approach to treatment selection is ideal because it allows consumers to exercise choice. In reality, however, methods used to define "restrictiveness" almost never involve real choice exercised by actual consumers of service.

A number of surveys have been conducted in an attempt to establish social acceptability ratings for behavioral interventions (see O'Brien & Karsh, 1990, for a review). The general paradigm involves providing raters (college students, parents, therapists, etc.) with brief descriptions of client, problem, and treatment options. Although the results of these surveys are easily summarized as procedural hierarchies based on degree of "acceptability," interpretation of the data is extremely difficult because it is not clear how well raters understand the nature of the problem, the exact procedures being evaluated, the relative risks associated with both problem and procedure, or the relative effectiveness of different procedures. In fact, Axelrod (1990) and Mulick and Kedesdy (1988) have provided compelling arguments suggesting that acceptability evaluations even by professionals often are based on erroneous assumptions about effectiveness, intrusiveness, risk, and normalcy.

For example, in every survey or administrative manual we have examined, differential reinforcement is considered the least restrictive of all behavior reduction procedures. This is based on the fact that reinforcement delivery for the nonoccurrence of the target behavior or for the occurrence of an alternative is viewed as a friendly interaction between therapist and client, whereas the nondelivery of reinforcement for the occurrence of the target behavior is essentially an "unobserved event" characterized by the absence of a consequence. Rolider and Van Houten (1990), however, cogently described conditions under which differential reinforcement may function as punishment, and Cowdery, Iwata, and Pace (1990) recently provided data showing that differential reinforcement can be associated with the side effects (e.g., crying, withdrawal) typically attributed to punishment.

Treatment hierarchies derived solely from social acceptability ratings of procedures do not account for behavioral function, treatment effectiveness, and a variety of other characteristics that determine the outcome of therapy, and the selection of treatments according to this model will result in success only if therapists are fortunate enough to guess right. Such an approach is not likely to produce either initial behavior change or any lasting benefit for the majority of clients whose dangerous behaviors are exposed to those procedures.

Selection Based on Differential Effectiveness

In contrast to treatment selection based on whether or not a defined sample of raters "likes" or "dislikes" a given procedure, the effectiveness model takes into account data from research on the clinical outcomes associated with different treatments. These data are used as a basis for selecting procedures that also meet other minimum criteria (for risk, cost, etc.). The advantages of having information on the relative effectiveness of treatments are obvious, and two recent reviews of the literature on destructive behaviors in the developmentally disabled have addressed this issue. Carr, Taylor, Carlson, and Robinson (1989) reviewed reinforcement approaches to behavior reduction, whereas Cataldo (1989) reviewed the punishment literature. There was general agreement that reinforcement-based interventions were less effective than those based on punishment.

Although the conclusion that punishment is more effective than reinforcement in reducing behavior is an accurate summary of research findings, two factors limit its generality. First, an unknown proportion of the literature consists of studies in which initial poor results were obtained with reinforcement-based interventions whose failure might have been predicted from the outset. For example, the "ignoring" variant of extinction could be expected to have little therapeutic effect on behavior not maintained by social consequences. Similarly, DRO procedures in which stimulus delivery does not involve the presentation of a reinforcer (i.e., a consequence was provided, but it had no reinforcing value to the client) will not change behavior. And ironically, procedural extinction and DRO are particularly prone to such failures because of their status as least restrictive interventions. The second limiting factor is that the effects of punishment are not dependent on reinforcement. A punishing stimulus can suppress behavior that continues to be reinforced (as was elegantly demonstrated by Azrin & Holz, 1966); therefore, the development of effective punishment programs does not require knowledge of a behavior's maintaining variables. When these factors interact, it is easy to see how arbitrarily selected reinforcement procedures will usually be less effective than punishment procedures selected in a like manner, although it is impossible to determine the extent to which this problem has affected research outcomes.

Selection Based on Structural (Topographical) Analysis of the Target Behavior

As treatment data continue to accumulate on the effects of a range of procedures on an equally wide range of behavior problems, it becomes possible to develop a more sophisticated version of the effectiveness model by constructing a procedure-topography matrix with outcome as the variable of interest. The resulting data might answer two questions related to treatment selection—whether treatment A is more effective than treatment B when applied to behavior 1 and whether treatment A is more effective with behavior 1 than with behavior 2. If the answer to either question is yes, behavioral topography might be a useful predictor of procedural effectiveness.

Several attempts have been made to match treatment procedures with behavioral topography based on outcome. Schroeder, Schroeder, Rojahn, and Mulick (1981), for example, reviewed the treatment literature on success rate for seven treatments applied to eight topographies of SIB. They found that punishment was the most effective treatment for hitting, scratching/ gouging, and hair pulling; time out was most effective for biting; overcorrection was most effective for pica/mouthing and feces ingestion; and satiation was most effective for vomiting/rumination. These conclusions sometimes were based on small subject samples for a given topography (e.g., only two cases of gouging/scratching), and it is not clear that the same results would be obtained from a meta-analysis of the current literature. It is interesting to note, however, that punishment (aversive stimulation, overcorrection, and contingent restraint) was the most generally effective intervention both within and across response topography, a finding consistent with the more recent review conducted by Carr et al. (1989).

The major limitation in selecting treatment based on response topography is that topography reveals little about function. Multiple behavioral topographies can be maintained by the same reinforcement contingency; aggression, destruction, and SIB uniformly produce social consequences, such that one behavior may be substituted for another. It is also possible that the same topography is subject to control by different maintaining contingencies: SIB, for example, can produce both attention and escape.

The Communication Model

One approach to treatment selection containing elements of the functional analysis model is based on the assumption that behavior disorders represent attempts by individuals to communicate either general or specific needs (Donnellan, Mirenda, Mesaros, & Fassbender, 1984). Thus, using the functions previously described, behavior problems can be translated into verbal response classes: "I want attention" (social-positive reinforcement), "I'm bored" (automatic-positive reinforcement), "Please stop this activity" (social-negative reinforcement), and "I'm hurt" (automatic-negative reinforcement). Using the communication model as a basis for treatment, the focus of intervention becomes the differential reinforcement of alternative behavior (DRA) with the consequence that currently maintains the behavior problem. Carr and Durand (1985) provided an interesting example of this approach. They found that the inappropriate behavior of some students was maintained by teacher attention, whereas that of others was maintained by escape from difficult tasks. Treatment involved teaching the former children a response ("Am I doing good work?") that produced teacher attention and the latter children a response ("I need help") that produced escape from the difficult task in the form of assistance.

The communication model is a significant improvement over other approaches to treatment selection because interventions derived from it are consistent with the functional properties of a behavior disorder—they take into account the source of reinforcement. Moreover, because the reinforcer for alternative behavior is not arbitrarily selected, one would expect training to generalize to similar types of situations. Nevertheless, as a description of behavioral function and as a prescriptive approach to treatment, the model has several limitations.

First, the analysis of behavior disorders as communication places emphasis on the illusive concept of "intention," which attributes the cause of behavior to mental process (desires and motives) within the individual instead of to the action of consequences (environmental contingencies). A more parsimonious model of communicative function can be found in Skinner's extensive interpretation (1957) of verbal behavior, according to which problems such as SIB and aggression might sometimes function as *mands*—

behaviors maintained by specific, socially mediated reinforcers. The "I want attention" and "Please stop this activity" functions of behavior disorders could be considered mand equivalents, because reinforcement is socially mediated and directly related to the form of the response. Yet even this class of verbal behavior does not include or account for automatically reinforced behavior. Although from a lay standpoint it may be convenient to view SIB maintained by its own consequences as analogous to "I'm bored," this interpretation does not describe a maintaining contingency. Likewise, "I'm hurt" and the consequences provided by others when an individual actually is hurt do not maintain head banging that directly attenuates pain from an ear infection. Thus, the communication model provides both an inaccurate and an incomplete account of behavioral function.

A second limitation of the model is directly related to one of its strengths. By emphasizing the establishment of mands through communication training, the model is superior to approaches in which arbitrarily selected behaviors are strengthened with arbitrary reinforcers (e.g., as in DRO using food reinforcement). Yet it would be a mistake to assume that reinforcement contingent merely on the absence of inappropriate behavior would be ineffective, an assumption that might be derived by exclusively focusing on communication training. For example, if SIB is maintained by contingent attention, procedures such as DRO (using attention or even food as the reinforcer) might be particularly effective as initial forms of treatment with high-rate behavior in individuals with severe language deficits, until such time that an alternative behavior can be strengthened.

Third, elimination of the current reinforcement for behavior problems (extinction) is not an explicit component of communication training. For example, if an individual's aggressive behavior has a significant history with escape as negative reinforcement, it is unlikely that all instances of aggression will be eliminated as a function of reinforcing the alternative behavior of "Please stop" with escape, unless aggression is concurrently extinguished by no longer allowing it to produce escape. This example is particularly relevant because it is difficult to tolerate aggressive acts by adults, and communication training without extinction can produce a situation in which such individuals now have two escape behaviors (the newly taught mand for escape, and aggression).

Finally, as important as communication training is to the development of an individual's social control over the environment, there is no inherent provision for teaching individuals how to control their environment directly (i.e., automatically). A logical extension of teaching "I'm hurt" as a means of soliciting relief from discomfort would be to teach the individual how to eliminate discomfort directly through another behavior (e.g., self-medication). Although the latter response is not incompatible with the former, it is not explicitly derived from the communication model.

THE FUNCTIONAL ANALYSIS MODEL OF ASSESSMENT AND TREATMENT

A comprehensive approach to treating behavior disorders based on the functional analysis model is comprised of two elements: (a) behavioral assessment, which consists of identifying the source of reinforcement for a behavior disorder; and (b) treatment selection and implementation, which are accomplished by altering the behavior's maintaining contingencies. Each of these elements, in turn, can be composed of several different procedures, all of which are directly tied to behavioral function.

Behavioral Assessment: The Functional Analysis of Behavior Disorders

Iwata, Vollmer, and Zarcone (1990) recently provided a detailed review of three general approaches used to identify the function(s) of a behavior disorder: indirect (anecdotal) methods, descriptive analyses, and functional analyses. Although complementary, these methods differ with respect to the type of data collected and the degree of control exerted over situational events. Indirect methods rely on self-report, whereas descriptive and functional analyses are derived from direct observation of behavior. Indirect and descriptive approaches require little environmental control, whereas functional analyses are defined by specific manipulations of social or other environmental contingencies. A brief description of each method is provided here.

Indirect Methods

A number of interview, questionnaire, and rating-scale techniques have been developed to assist therapists in gathering verbal reports about the target behavior, the circumstances under which it does and does not occur, and the consequences that usually follow it. Although questionnaires are easy to administer, the task presented to the responder is actually quite complex. Accurate reporting requires clear description of the relative frequency and distribution of past events (when and where episodes of the behavior occurred), the temporal sequencing of events (what came before and after the behavior) and apparent functional relationships among events (which consequences were reinforcers). Because questionnaires rely on highly subjective, abbreviated, and delayed verbal reports that are so far removed from the events of interest, their reliability and validity are often questionable. In an attempt to increase the objectivity of verbal report measures, Durand and Crimmins (1988) developed a 16-item, Likert-type rating scale (the Motivation Assessment Scale, or MAS) to identify which of four contingencies maintained SIB: social-positive reinforcement (two sources—social versus materials), social-negative reinforcement (escape from demands) and automatic-positive reinforcement ("sensory" reinforcement). Although Durand and Crimmins reported adequate interobserver reliability correlations for the MAS, results of a more detailed reliability analysis (Zarcone, Rodgers, Iwata, Rourke, & Dorsey, 1991) yielded agreement scores averaging only 20%. The MAS and similar instruments may be useful as screening devices (i.e., for structuring subsequent observations), but are inadequate for diagnostic or prescriptive purposes. Because informal methods are unlikely to yield reliable information about behavioral function (diagnosis), they cannot be used as a basis for treatment selection (prescription).

Descriptive Analysis

Direct observation of ongoing behavior eliminates many problems associated with informal methods. Objective behavioral definitions serve as guides for systematic observation that can be repeated across time and setting, resulting in quantitative data on behavior across a number of situations. The most common methods used for actual data collection are based on interval or time-sampling procedures (e.g., Bijou, Peterson, & Ault, 1968; Touchette, MacDonald, & Langer, 1985). Although much more reliable and accurate than informal methods, descriptive analyses are time-consuming and do not allow very good control over the environmental contexts in which behavior occurs. Thus, detection of important but intermittent events may require extensive observation, and correlated events may not reveal behavioral function (e.g., as in escape from tasks accompanied by teacher attention contingent on inappropriate behavior).

Functional Analysis

The most direct way to identify a functional relationship between behavior and another event is to expose an individual to the event and a suitable control condition. Response differentiation indicates functional control over behavior by the event in question. This basic approach has been used for many years to establish new environment-behavior relationships; it also can be used to reveal current relationships. Two general models have evolved. The first involves testing for the effects of a single variable; for example, Lovaas and Simmons (1969) isolated adult attention as a positive reinforcer for SIB, and Carr, Newsom, and Binkoff (1980) used a similar approach to identify escape from tasks as a negative reinforcer for aggression. The second model provides a test for multiple functions using either reversal (Carr, & Durand, 1985) or multielement (Iwata, Dorsey, Slifer, Bauman, & Richman, 1982) designs. The specific model or design used is probably less important than the type of test that is run for a given contingency. Table 1 shows, for a

TABLE 1.   Basic Test and Control Conditions Used in a Functional Analysis of
Behavior Disorders

Behavioral Function	Behavior Increases (Test)	Behavior Decreases (Control)
Positive reinforcement (Sr+):		
Social	Deprivation from specific Sr+ Contingent Sr+	Noncontingent Sr+
Automatic	General deprivation	Noncontingent stimulation
Negative reinforcement (Sr−):		
Social	Aversive stimulation Contingent Sr− (escape)	No aversive stimulation
Automatic	Biological condition	No biological condition

given behavioral function, the basic test and control conditions that should produce high and low levels of behavior, respectively. Additional conditions can be designed based on the manipulation of discriminative stimuli, reinforcement schedules, and so forth. The "automatic" functions are most difficult to identify because, by definition, the reinforcing event is produced by the behavior and might not be amenable to direct observation. In fact, a functional analysis of behavior maintained by automatic-negative reinforcement will rarely be possible because of our general lack of control over events that occasion such behavior (e.g., headaches).

Treatment Selection and Behavioral Function

Behavior reduction procedures that do not entail the use of punishment achieve their effects in one of three ways. First, some interventions temporarily alter the susceptibility of behavior to reinforcement by eliminating an establishing operation. Second, other interventions eliminate reinforcement for the behavior through extinction. Finally, still other interventions are based on differential reinforcement for the absence of the target behavior (DRO) or for the occurrence of an alternative behavior (DRA). These general classes of intervention do not specify any particular therapeutic operation, and herein lies the relevance of a functional analysis approach to behavioral assessment. When the reinforcing function of a behavior is known, it becomes possible to construct procedures based on establishing operations, extinction, and differential reinforcement so that there is a "functional match" between behavior and treatment.

Treatments Based on the Alteration of Establishing Operations (EOs)

Michael (1982) described a class of antecedent events that alters the effectiveness of reinforcement and changes the frequency of behaviors that produce reinforcement. Events having these effects are called *establishing operations* (EOs) because they set up, or establish, a stimulus as a reinforcer. In the case of behavior maintained by positive reinforcement, the EO often is some form of deprivation (e.g., from food or water); for escape and avoidance behavior, the EO usually is aversive stimulation (e.g., intense light, noise). The effects of EOs are diminished through responding, as in food-seeking behavior that terminates when food is eaten or as in covering the eyes to block out light, but EOs also can be attenuated prior to responding merely by providing access to the reinforcer (e.g., food or shade). For example, Vollmer and Iwata (1991) recently demonstrated how operant performance maintained by commonly used reinforcers—food, social interaction, and music—could be increased or decreased by limiting or providing access to these events prior to experimental sessions.

The EOs for a behavior disorder are directly related to the behavior's maintaining contingency and can be altered to reduce the frequency of the behavior temporarily. Examples of treatment based on EO manipulations for the four primary functions of behavior disorders are outlined in Table 2.

EOs and Behavior Maintained by Social-Positive Reinforcement. Noncontingent access to positive reinforcers such as attention, materials, or food (noncontingent reinforcement, or NCR) reduces the frequency of behavior problems maintained by these events and at the same time decreases behavioral susceptibility to reinforcement even though it is available. The minimum schedules of NCR necessary to produce behavioral decrement have not been identified formally, but a reasonable starting point might be to match reinforcement delivery to the interresponse time of the behavior. NCR delivered to the point of satiation may produce rapid and large reductions in behavior, as demonstrated with both attention (Lovaas & Simmons, 1969) and material items (Ayllon & Michael, 1959).

Table 2.   Treatment Approaches Based on the Alteration of Establishing Operations

Behavioral Function	Treatment Procedure
Positive reinforcement	
Social	Noncontingent reinforcement (Lovaas & Simmons, 1969)
	Satiation (Ayllon & Michael, 1959)
Automatic	Noncontingent stimulation (Bailey & Meyerson, 1970)
	General enriched environment (Horner, 1980)
	Satiation (Rast et al., 1981)
Negative reinforcement	
Social	Reduced demand complexity (Weeks & Gaylord-Ross, 1981)
	Reduced demand frequency (Pace et al., in press)
Automatic	Alleviation of medical condition or discomfort

EOs and Behavior Maintained by Automatic-Positive Reinforcement. Several studies have shown that noncontingent stimulation can produce decreases in a variety of behavior problems, such as head banging (Bailey & Meyerson, 1970) and rumination (Rast, Johnston, Drum, & Conrin, 1981). To the extent that the behaviors of interest were maintained by the stimulation provided (kinesthetic stimulation for head banging, and gustatory stimulation for rumination), the interventions described in these studies amounted to NCR. If the behaviors were not maintained by these specific events, it is possible that stimulation different than that produced by the behavior may nevertheless have competed with the target behavior. For example, Horner (1980) found that a general program consisting of "environmental enrichment" was effective in reducing multiple behavior disorders in an institutional setting, some of which presumedly were maintained by automatic reinforcement.

EOs and Behavior Maintained by Social-Negative Reinforcement. Situations in which a behavioral requirement is placed on a student often serve as EOs for escape behavior. These situations traditionally have been described as *discriminative* arrangements; it is assumed that events such as instructions and prompts for work are discriminative stimuli (SDs) for escape behavior. Negative reinforcement can occur only in the presence of such stimuli, however, and not in their absence (i.e., it is not possible to remove a nonexistent task contingently). Therefore, stimulus presentation is not merely correlated with reinforcement (SD), it also establishes escape as negative reinforcement (EO). Similarly, the removal of escape-provoking stimuli is not an intervention based on stimulus control or the removal of an SD (e.g., Touchette et al., 1985), but rather elimination of the EO for escape. In the absence of an aversive demand, there is no motivation to engage in the escape behavior, just as in the "absence" of food deprivation there is no motivation to seek food.

Demanding situations have been attenuated in several ways to reduce the frequency of escape behavior. Carr, Newsom, and Binkoff (1976) embedded demands within entertaining stories, which apparently reduced the aversiveness of the demands; Weeks and Gaylord-Ross (1981) reduced task complexity by substituting easy tasks in place of difficult ones; and Pace, Iwata, Cowdery, Andree, and McIntyre (in press) initially reduced task frequency by placing fewer demands on their subjects. Although additional interventions were included in each of these studies, the demand modification per se might be expected to produce a noticeable change in behavior.

EOs and Behavior Maintained by Automatic-Negative Reinforcement. Headaches, ear infections, skin irritations, and the like, all can be considered EOs for behavior (usually SIB) that attenuates stimulation associated with these conditions. Although "tolerance" to physical discomfort might be less damaging than continued occurrence of the behavior disorder, few would propose an itnervention that eliminates the behavior but leaves the physical condition unresolved (although see below under differential reinforcement). The most humane approach to reducing behavior problems that attenuate other sources of physical discomfort involves eliminating the conditions causing the discomfort. To our knowledge, there are no published studies clearly documenting the occurrence of aberrant pain-attenuating behavior that was eliminated subsequently through medical intervention.

Limitation.   Behavior reduction through modification of EOs requires knowledge about the behavior's source of reinforcement, but it is achieved without elimination of the maintaining contingency. For example, noncontingent attention produces a decrease in inappropriate attention-seeking behavior by altering the reinforcing effects of attention; thus, behavior decreases independent of whether or not its occurrence is reinforced. But deprivation from attention is a relative state and one that is likely to recur, because it is impossible to deliver noncontingent attention on a rich schedule over long periods of time. For this reason, treatments based on the modification of EOs should be viewed as temporary and only partial solutions. The behavior disorder will inevitably recur, and the extent to which this pattern is repeated is a function of the behavior's consequences. The elimination of reinforcing consequences through extinction thus becomes an important second component of treatment.

Treatments Based on Extinction

Although the basic principle of extinction—behavior reduction through termination of reinforcement—is quite simple, the procedures by which extinction is achieved cannot be arbitrarily selected; instead, they must be derived from the behavior's reinforcement contingency. A recent study in which three procedural variations of extinction were applied to three different functions of SIB showed negligible effects when there was no match between treatment and behavioral function (Iwata, Pace, Cowdery, & Miltenberger, 1993). These variations of extinction and their relevant behavioral functions are outlined in Table 3.

Extinction and Behavior Maintained by Social-Positive Reinforcement.   This type of extinction is well established in the literature and was defined succinctly by Harris and Ersner-Hershfield (1978) as the "withholding of previously given positive reinforcement following emission of the target behavior" (p. 1355). The "withholding" often takes the form of not reacting to the behavior, which has been translated roughly into "ignoring" as a specific procedural description and time out as a more general form of limited access to reinforcement. Although extinction has been reported to be a successful treatment for a wide range of behavior problems, including aggression (Mace

TABLE 3.   Treatment Approaches Based on Extinction

Behavioral Function	Treatment Procedure
Positive Reinforcement	
Social	Withholding positive reinforcement (Mace et al., 1986)
	Time out (Mason & Iwata, 1990)
Automatic	Attenuation of response-produced stimulation (Rincover & Devaney, 1982)
Negative Reinforcement	
Social	Prevention of escape (Iwata et al., 1990)
Automatic	N/A (Extinction contraindicated)

et al., 1986) and SIB (Harmatz & Rasmussen, 1969), extinction as a sole means of intervention has rarely been used and is not considered to be highly effective. This conclusion, however, is based on an unknown proportion of treatment studies in which the "ignoring" variant of extinction was applied to behavior not maintained by social-positive reinforcement.

Extinction and Behavior Maintained by Automatic-Positive Reinforcement.   It is often difficult to identify specific stimuli directly produced by behavior, because they are not under the control of a social agent. Nevertheless, when it is possible to determine a behavior's automatic reinforcers, it may also be possible to implement extinction by arranging conditions so that the consequences are attenuated. This form of extinction has been called *sensory extinction* and has been applied to stereotypic mannerisms (Rincover, Cook, Peoples, & Packard, 1979) as well as SIB (Dorsey, Iwata, Reid, & Davis, 1982; Rincover & Devany, 1982). Procedurally, sensory extinction has involved mechanical intervention that disrupts the stimulation produced by a behavior but does not interfere with the behavior per se. Examples include padding walls or furniture, or having individuals wear padded equipment. A further procedural variation specific to SIB involves the administration of opiate-blocking drugs (e.g., naltrexone) in an attempt to eliminate hypothesized reinforcement produced by endogenous opioid production. Research on the use of naltrexone has been mixed (see Szymanski, Kedesdy, Sulkes, & Cutler, 1987, for a review) and has not included any functional analysis of the SIB prior to treatment; thus, the proportion of cases with which the drug should have been effective (assuming there is merit in the underlying theory) is unknown.

Extinction and Behavior Maintained by Social-Negative Reinforcement   Completion of a functional analysis prior to treatment is particularly important when considering the use of extinction with escape behavior. The ignoring variant of extinction, when applied to escape behavior, will actually exacerbate the problem. Extinction of escape is achieved through prevention of escape. Procedurally, this requires presentation of escape-provoking stimuli (e.g., demands) and, subsequent to the behavior problem, not removing the stimuli. Examples of extinction applied to escape behavior have been reported for aggression (Carr et al., 1980), SIB (Iwata, Pace, Kalsher, Cowdery, & Cataldo, 1990; Steege, Wacker, Berg, Cigrand, & Cooper, 1989), and stereotypic behavior that was maintained by escape (Mace, Browder, & Lin, 1987).

Extinction and Behavior Maintained by Automatic-Negative Reinforcement Although in theory it is possible to arrange a situation in which behavior does not terminate ongoing stimulation (an arrangement analogous to sensory extinction for behavior maintained by automatic-positive reinforcement), there is little justification for this type of extinction, because it leaves the individual in a state of discomfort with no effective means of dealing with the problem. Furthermore, the elimination of such behavior through extinction may reduce caregivers' ability to determine that the individual is, in fact, in need of physical intervention or medical attention.

Limitation When properly designed and consistently implemented, extinction can be very effective in reducing the frequency of behavior disorders. Nevertheless, extinction does not contain any provision for strengthening alternative behaviors. As noted previously, establishing operations are recurring events; when they are in effect, behaviors that have been reinforced also will recur. Behaviors that no longer produce reinforcement (i.e., those having undergone extinction) are less likely to occur, but they will be replaced by other behaviors that may be just as intolerable as the original problem.

Treatments Based on Differential Reinforcement

Differential reinforcement complements extinction by strengthening specific appropriate behaviors as replacements for inappropriate behavior. The two most frequently used procedures based on differential reinforcement are DRO (differential reinforcement of other behavior) and DRA (differential reinforcement of alternative behavior). Several variations of both procedures have been reported in the literature, and examples of these are listed in Table 4.

DRO, like extinction, does not directly shape appropriate behavior; therefore, emphasis here is placed on DRA procedures. Although not usually described as such, a properly designed DRO procedure combines elimination of an EO (though NCR) with extinction (the rule that NCR not be delivered within a certain time following the inappropriate behavior). Thus, DRO temporarily reduces both the motivational component of the behavior disorder and reinforcement for the behavior when it does occur. If the DRO procedure does not contain extinction, or if the reinforcer delivered is not the

TABLE 4.   Treatment Approaches Based on Differential Reinforcement

Behavioral Function	Treatment Procedure
Positive Reinforcement	
Social	DRO (Steege et al., 1989)
	DRA: Establishing mands for positive reinforcement (Day et al., 1988)
Automatic	DRO (Harris & Wolchik, 1979)
	DRA: Establishing alternative (automatically reinforced) behavior (Favell et al., 1982)
Negative Reinforcement	
Social	DRO: Tolerance training
	DRA: Increased positive reinforcement for compliance (Mace & Belfiore, 1990)
	DRA: Escape as negative reinforcement for compliance (Iwata et al., 1990)
	DRA: Establishing mands for escape (Steege et al., 1990)
Automatic	DRO: Tolerance training (Cowdery et al., 1990)
	DRA: Establishing mands for physical care
	DRA: Establishing self-administration of physical care

same as or cannot compete with the reinforcer maintaining the behavior, limited results will be expected. For example, Harris and Wolchik (1979) found that food and praise were relatively ineffective when used in a DRO contingency for stereotypic behavior apparently maintained by automatic-positive reinforcement. The food and praise did not compete with reinforcement directly produced by the behavior, which also was not subjected to extinction.

DRA and Behavior Maintained by Social-Positive Reinforcement   Day, Rea, Schussler, Larsen, and Johnson (1988) described an interesting application of DRA as treatment for SIB. The investigators noticed that two subjects' SIB was apparently maintained by contingent access to toys. Treatment consisted of making these items unobtainable following SIB (extinction). Additionally, when subjects did not engage in SIB, they were required to make specific vocal and gestural responses in order to obtain toys. These responses could be considered mand equivalents because they were paired with specific, socially mediated reinforcers.

DRA and Behavior Maintained by Automatic-Positive Reinforcement   As indicated previously, extinction of automatically reinforced behavior is difficult to achieve. Still, DRA even without extinction may produce reductions in behavior. For example, Berkson and Mason (1965) and Davenport and Berkson (1963) observed reductions in several stereotypic behaviors when toys were given to subjects noncontingently. Although these effects are often attributed to noncontingent stimulation (an EO manipulation), the toys provided no stimulation unless they were handled. Thus, stimulation (reinforcement) was contingent on play behavior, qualifying the procedure as an example of DRA. Favell, McGimsey, and Schell (1982) described a more response-specific form of DRA based on the behavior's presumed reinforcer: Toys providing visual stimulation were given to an individual who engaged in eye poking, and popcorn was given to an individual who engaged in pica.

DRA and Behavior Maintained by Social-Negative Reinforcement DRA for escape behavior can take a number of forms. First, an alternative behavior (e.g., compliance) can be strengthened by providing more potent positive reinforcement. Mace and Belfiore (1990) examined this approach by identifying instructions for which there was a high probability of compliance (high-p commands). When these were presented in a 3:1 ratio with instructions for which compliance was low (low-p commands), escape behavior decreased and compliance increased. A second approach involves negative instead of positive reinforcement made contingent on compliance. Iwata, Pace, et al. (1990) observed increases in compliance while extinguishing self-injurious escape behavior during instructional sequences. Because no additional positive reinforcement was delivered during treatment, it was hypothesized that compliance increased because it provided a means of terminating an escalated prompt sequence. A third example of DRA involves reinforcement of alternative escape behaviors (mands for escape). Steege, et al. (1990) used such an approach while treating two individuals who exhibited SIB in training situations. Contingent on pressing a microswitch (activating a tape recorder that played the word "Stop"), brief (10-second) breaks from training were provided.

DRA and Behavior Maintained by Automatic-Negative Reinforcement In addition to alleviating any physical conditions that serve as EOs for pain-attenuating behavior, it would be desirable to provide individuals with other methods for coping with sources of discomfort. Initially, individuals might be taught an alternative behavior that indicates a painful state; this alternative behavior could be strengthened using either positive reinforcement (e.g., praise, materials) or negative reinforcement (alleviation of the discomfort). Individuals who are capable of learning more complex behaviors might later be taught to alleviate discomforting conditions directly through self-medication. We were unable to find any examples of this approach in the literature, although it appears consistent with general procedures used in teaching nonhandicapped individuals.

Limitation Differential reinforcement procedures can be quite effective in replacing inappropriate behavior with appropriate alternatives. To the extent that EOs recur and the inappropriate behavior is not placed on extinction, however, the inappropriate behavior may continue to compete with the newly established one. Under these conditions, differential reinforcement alone may produce limited results, because it is unlikely that a newly reinforced behavior will completely suppress another behavior that continues to be reinforced.

SUMMARY

Several models for treatment classification and selection have been proposed over the years. Each has some merit but is not based on a complete account of the functional properties of behavior disorders and how these interact with environmental changes of a therapeutic nature. Recent advances in assessment methodology make it possible to identify the maintaining contingencies for most behavior disorders by conducting a functional analysis prior to intervention. When the source of reinforcement for a behavior problem is identified, treatment procedures can be selected so as to effect behavior change maximally by (a) altering the behavior's establishing operation, (b) eliminating reinforcement for the behavior through extinction, and (c) replacing the behavior with another through differential reinforcement. An approach to treatment classification and selection based on behavioral function will result in a therapeutic technology that is analytic and firmly tied to basic principle, yet highly adaptable to individual circumstances (i.e., response and reinforcer idiosyncracies).

REFERENCES

Axelrod, S. (1990). Myths that (mis)guide our profession. In A. C. Repp & N. N. Singh (Eds.), *Perspectives on the use of nonaversive and aversive interventions for persons with developmental disabilities* (pp. 59–71). Sycamore, IL: Sycamore.

Ayllon, T., & Michael, J. (1959). The psychiatric nurse as a behavioral engineer. *Journal of the Experimental Analysis of Behavior, 2,* 323–334.

Azrin, H. N., & Holz, W. C. (1966). Punishment. In W. K. Honig (Ed.), *Operant behavior: Areas of research and application* (pp. 380–447). New York: Appleton-Century-Crofts.

Bachman, J. A. (1972). Self-injurious behavior: A behavioral analysis. *Journal of Abnormal Psychology, 80,* 211–224.

Bailey, J., & Meyerson, L. (1970). Effect of vibratory stimulation on a retardate's self-injurious behavior. *Psychological Aspects of Disability, 17,* 133–137.

Berkson, G., & Mason, W. A. (1965). Stereotyped movements of mental defectives: 4. The effects of toys and the character of the acts. *American Journal of Mental Deficiency, 70,?* 511–524.

Bijou, S. W., Peterson, R. F., & Ault, M. H. (1968). A method to integrate descriptive and experimental field studies at the level of data and empirical concepts. *Journal of Applied Behavior Analysis, 1,* 175–191.

Borthwick, S. A., Meyers, C. E., & Eyman, R. K. (1981). Comparative adaptive and maladaptive behavior of mentally retarded clients of five residential settings in three western states. In R. H. Bruininks, C. E. Meyers, B. B. Sigford, & K. C. Lakin (Eds.), *Deinstitutionalization and community adjustment of mentally retarded people* (pp. 351–359). Washington, DC: American Association on Mental Deficiency.

Carr, E. G. (1977). The motivation of self-injurious behavior: A review of some hypotheses. *Psychological Bulletin, 84,* 800–816.

Carr, E. G., & Durand, V. M. (1985). Reducing behavior problems through functional communication training. *Journal of Applied Behavior Analysis, 18,* 111–126.

Carr, E. G., Newsom, C. D., & Binkoff, J. A. (1976). Stimulus control of self-destructive behavior in a psychotic child. *Journal of Abnormal Child Psychology, 4,* 139–153.

Carr, E. G., Newsom, C., & Binkoff, J. (1980). Escape as a factor in the aggressive behavior of two retarded children. *Journal of Applied Behavior Analysis, 13,* 101–117.

Carr, E. G., Taylor, J. C., Carlson, J. I., & Robinson, S. (1989, September). *Reinforcement and stimulus-based treatments for severe behavior problems in developmental disabilities.* Background paper for the Consensus Development Conference on Destructive Behaviors in Persons With Developmental Disabilities. Bethesda, MD: National Institutes of Health.

Cataldo, M. F. (1989, September). *The effects of punishment and other behavior reducing procedures on the destructive behaviors of persons with developmental disabilities.* Background paper for the Consensus Development Conference on Destructive Behaviors in Persons With Developmental Disabilities. Bethesda, MD: National Institutes of Health.

Cataldo, M. F., & Harris, J. (1982). The biological basis for self-injury in the mentally retarded. *Analysis and Intervention in Developmental Disabilities, 2,* 21–39.

Cowdery, G. E., Iwata, B. A., & Pace, G. M. (1990). Effects and side effects of DRO as treatment for self-injurious behavior. *Journal of Applied Behavior Analysis, 23,* 497–506.

Davenport, R. K., & Berkson, G. (1963). Stereotyped movements in mental defectives: Effects of novel objects. *American Journal of Mental Deficiency, 67,* 879–882.

Day, R. M., Rea, J. A., Schussler, N. G., Larsen, S. E., & Johnson, W. L. (1988). A functionally based approach to the treatment of self-injurious behavior. *Behavior Modification, 12,* 565–589.

DeLissovoy, V. (1963). Head banging in early childhood: A suggested cause. *Journal of Genetic Psychology, 102,* 109–114.

Donnellan, A. M., Mirenda, P. L., Mesaros, R. A., & Fassbender, L. L. (1984). Analyzing the communicative functions of aberrant behavior. *Journal of the Association for Persons With Severe Handicaps, 9,* 201–212.

Dorsey, M. F., Iwata, B. A., Reid, D. H., & Davis, P. A. (1982). Protective equipment: Continuous and contingent application in the treatment of self-injurious behavior. *Journal of Applied Behavior Analysis, 15,* 217–230.

Durand, V. M., & Crimmins, D. B. (1988). Identifying the variables maintaining self-injurious behavior. *Journal of Autism and Developmental Disorders, 18,* 99–117.

Edwards, K. A. (1974). Physical restraint as time-out therapy. *Psychological Record, 24,* 393–397.

Evans, I., & Meyer, L. H. (1985). *An educative approach to behavior problems: A practical decision model for interventions with severely handicapped learners.* Baltimore: Paul H. Brookes.

Florida Department of Health and Rehabilitative Services. (1989). *Florida HRS manual 160-4.* Tallahassee: Author, Developmental Services Program Office.

Favell, J. E., McGimsey, J. F., & Schell, R. M. (1982). Treatment of self-injury by providing alternate sensory activities. *Analysis and Intervention in Developmental Disabilities, 2,* 83–104.

Foxx, R. M., & Shapiro, S. T. (1978). The timeout ribbon: A nonexclusionary timeout procedure. *Journal of Applied Behavior Analysis, 11,* 125–143.

Griffin, J. C., Williams, D. E., Stark, M. T., Altmeyer, B. K., & Mason, M. (1984). Self-injurious behavior: A state-wide prevalence survey, assessment of severe cases, and follow-up of aversive programs. In J. C. Griffin, D. E. Williams, M. T. Stark, B. K. Altmeyer, & H. K. Griffin (Eds.), *Advances in the treatment of self-injurious behavior* (pp. 1–25). Austin: Texas Planning Council for Developmental Disabilities.

Harmatz, M. G., & Rasmussen, W. A. (1969). A behavior modification approach to head banging. *Mental Hygiene, 53,* 590–593.

Harris, S. L., & Ersner-Hershfield, R. (1978). Behavioral suppression of seriously disruptive behavior in psychotic and retarded patients: A review of punishment and its alternatives. *Psychological Bulletin, 85,* 1352–1375.

Harris, S. L., Ersner-Hershfield, R., Kaffashan, L. C., & Romanczyk, R. G. (1974). The portable timeout room. *Behavior Therapy, 5,* 687–688.

Harris, S. L., & Wolchik, S. A. (1979). Suppression of self-stimulation: Three alternative strategies. *Journal of Applied Behavior Analysis, 12,* 185–189.

Horner, R. D. (1980). The effects of an environmental "enrichment" program on the behavior of institutionalized profoundly retarded children. *Journal of Applied Behavior Analysis, 13,* 473–491.

Iwata, B. A. (1987). Negative reinforcement in applied behavior analysis: An emerging technology. *Journal of Applied Behavior Analysis, 20,* 361–378.

Iwata, B. A., Dorsey, M. F., Slifer, K. J., Bauman, K. E., & Richman, G. S. (1982). Toward a functional analysis of self-injury. *Analysis and Intervention in Developmental Disabilities, 2,* 3–20.

Iwata, B. A., Pace, G. M., Cowdery, G. E., & Miltenberger, R. G. (1993). *Procedural variations of extinction with self-injury having similar topography but different function.* Manuscript submitted for publication.

Iwata, B. A., Pace, G. M., Kalsher, M. J., Cowdery, G. E., & Cataldo, M. F. (1990). Experimental analysis and extinction of self-injurious escape behavior. *Journal of Applied Behavior Analysis, 23,* 11–27.

Iwata, B. A., Vollmer, T. R., & Zarcone, J. R. (1990). The experimental (functional) analysis of behavior disorders: Methodology, applications, and limitations. In A. C. Repp & N. N. Singh, *Perspectives on the use of nonaversive and aversive interventions for persons with developmental disabilities* (pp. 301–330). Sycamore, IL: Sycamore.

LaVigna, G. W., & Donnellan, A. M. (1986). *Alternatives to punishment.* New York: Irvington.

Lovaas, I., Newsom, C., & Hickman, C. (1987). Self-stimulatory behavior and perceptual reinforcement. *Journal of Applied Behavior Analysis, 2,* 45–68.

Lovaas, O. I., & Simmons, J. Q. (1969). Manipulation of self-destruction in three retarded children. *Journal of Applied Behavior Analysis, 2,* 143–157.

Lutzker, J. R. (1978). Reducing self-injurious behavior by facial screening. *American Journal of Mental Deficiency, 82,* 510–513.

Mace, F. C., & Belfiore, P. (1990). Behavioral momentum in the treatment of escape-motivated stereotypy. *Journal of Applied Behavior Analysis, 23,* 507–514.

Mace, F. C., Browder, D. M., & Lin, Y. (1987). Analysis of demand conditions associated with stereotypy. *Journal of Behavior Therapy and Experimental Psychiatry, 18,* 25–31.

Mace, F. C., Page, T. J., Ivancic, M. T., & O'Brien, S. (1986). Analysis of environmental determinants of aggression and disruption in mentally retarded children. *Applied Research in Mental Retardation, 7,* 203–221.

Mason, S. A., & Iwata, B. A. (1990). Artifactual effects of sensory-integrative therapy on self-injurious behavior. *Journal of Applied Behavior Analysis, 23,* 361–370.

Michael, J. L. (1982). Distinguishing between discriminative and motivational functions of stimuli. *Journal of the Experimental Analysis of Behavior, 37,* 149–155.

Mulick, J. A., & Kedesdy, J. H. (1988). Self-injurious behavior, its treatment, and normalization. *Mental Retardation, 26,* 223–229.

Nelson, C. M., & Rutherford, R. B. (1983). Timeout revisited: Guidelines for its use in special education. *Exceptional Education Quarterly, 3,* 56–67.

O'Brien, S., & Karsh, K. G. (1990). Treatment acceptability: Consumer, therapist, and society. In A. C. Repp & N. N. Singh (Eds.), *Perspectives on the use of nonaversive and aversive interventions for persons with developmental disabilities* (pp. 504–516). Sycamore, IL: Sycamore.

Ontario Ministry of Community and Social Services. (1987). *Standards for the use of behavioural training and treatment procedures in settings for the developmentally handicapped.* Toronto, Ontario: Author.

Pace, G. M., Iwata, B. A., Cowdery, G. E., Andree, P. J., & McIntyre, T. (in press). Stimulus (instructional) fading during extinction of self-injurious escape behavior. *Journal of Applied Behavior Analysis.*

Porterfield, J. K., Herbert-Jackson, E., & Risley, T. R. (1976). Contingent observation: An effective and acceptable procedure for reducing disruptive behavior of young children in a group. *Journal of Applied Behavior Analysis, 9,* 55–64.

Rast, J., Johnston, J. M., Drum, C., & Conrin, J. (1981). The relation of food quantity to rumination behavior. *Journal of Applied Behavior Analysis, 14,* 121–130.

Repp, A. C., & Singh, N. N. (Eds.). (1990). *Perspectives on the use of nonaversive and aversive interventions for persons with developmental disabilities.* Sycamore, IL: Sycamore.

Rincover, A., Cook, R., Peoples, A., & Packard, D. (1979). Sensory extinction and sensory reinforcement principles for programming multiple adaptive behavior change. *Journal of Applied Behavior Analysis, 12,* 221–233.

Rincover, A., & Devany, J. (1982). The application of sensory extinction procedures to self-injury. *Analysis and Intervention in Developmental Disabilities, 2,* 67–81.

Rolider, A., & Van Houten, R. (1985). Movement suppression time-out for undesirable behavior in psychotic and severely developmentally delayed children. *Journal of Applied Behavior Analysis, 18,* 275–288.

Rolider, A., & Van Houten, R. (1990). The role of reinforcement in reducing inappropriate behavior: Some myths and misconceptions. In A. C. Repp & N. N. Singh (Eds.), *Perspectives on the use of nonaversive and aversive interventions for persons with developmental disabilities* (pp. 119–127). Sycamore, IL: Sycamore.

Schroeder, S. R., Schroeder, C. S., Rojahn, J., & Mulick, J. A. (1981). Self-injurious behavior: An analysis of behavior management techniques. In J. L. Matson & J. R. McCartney, *Handbook of behavior modification with the mentally retarded* (pp. 61–115). New York: Pelnum.

Skinner, B. F. (1957). *Verbal behavior.* New York: Macmillan.

Skinner, B. F. (1969). *Contingencies of reinforcement: A theoretical analysis.* New York: Appleton-Century-Crofts.

Steege, M. V., Wacker, D. P., Berg, W. K., Cigrand, K. K., & Cooper, L. J. (1989). The use of behavioral assessment to prescribe and evaluate treatments for severely handicapped children. *Journal of Applied Behavior Analysis, 22,* 22–33.

Steege, M. W., Wacker, D. P., Cigrand, K. C., Berg, W. K., Novak, C. G., Reimers, T. M., Sasso, G. M., & DeRaad, A. (1990). Use of negative reinforcement in the treatment of self-injurious behavior. *Journal of Applied Behavior Analysis, 23,* 459–467.

Szymanski, L., Kedesdy, J., Sulkes, S., & Cutler, A. (1987). Naltrexone in treatment of self-injurious behavior: A clinical study. *Research in Developmental Disabilities, 8,* 179–190.

Touchette, P. E., MacDonald, R. F., & Langer, S. N. (1985). A scatter plot for identifying stimulus control of problem behavior. *Journal of Applied Behavior Analysis, 18,* 343–351.

Vollmer, T. R., & Iwata, B. A. (1991). Establishing operations and reinforcement effects. *Journal of Applied Behavior Analysis, 24,* 279–291.

Weeks, M., & Gaylord-Ross, R. (1981). Task difficulty and aberrant behavior in severely handicapped students. *Journal of Applied Behavior Analysis, 14,* 449–463.

Zarcone, J. R., Rodgers, T. A., Iwata, B. A., Rourke, D., & Dorsey, M. F. (1991). Reliability analysis of the Motivational Assessment Scale: A failure to replicate. *Research in Developmental Disabilities, 12,* 349–360.

6

The Interpersonal Treatment Model

Teaching Appropriate Social Inhibitions Through the Development of Personal Stimulus Control by the Systematic Introduction of Antecedent Stimuli

AHMOS ROLIDER AND RON VAN HOUTEN

Persons with developmental handicaps and traumatic head injury often exhibit behavior problems that interfere with the acquisition of habilitative repertoires. It is sometimes noted that these individuals exhibit these problems more in the presence of some people than others; that is, the presence of some people exerts stimulus control over the occurrence of the problem behaviors. It is also noted that the behavior often occurs more in the presence of some stimuli than others. The purpose of this chapter is to illustrate how severe behavioral problems can be treated through the use of a treatment model that places primary emphasis on establishment of personal stimulus control in the presence of those stimuli previously associated with the problem behavior. This control is established through the systematic introduction of discriminative and eliciting stimuli in a highly controlled and structured treatment environment. Once interpersonal stimulus control is

AHMOS ROLIDER • Department of Psychiatry, McMaster University, Hamilton, Ontario L8N 3Z5.   RON VAN HOUTEN • Psychology Department, Mount Saint Vincent University, Halifax, Nova Scotia B3M 2J6.

Behavior Analysis and Treatment, edited by R. Van Houten & S. Axelrod. Plenum Press, New York, 1993.

established steps are taken to ensure that it is maintained in other settings whenever necessary.

The methods advocated are based on a careful analysis of the social variables influencing normal behavior in the natural setting. Although the focus of this chapter is the application of these variables to solve problems exhibited by persons with special needs, the theory applies equally well to behavioral problems with all populations. Indeed, the main premise of this approach is that people with special needs should not be treated in a qualitatively different manner than other individuals. This approach is compatible with a recent trend in behavior analysis to conduct a comprehensive analysis of social variables controlling behavior.

A complete analysis should determine not only why some individuals exhibit behavioral problems but also why most people normally do not engage in such behaviors. In other words, to teach, generalize, and maintain appropriate behavior, one must understand how such behavior is maintained by the normal social community. The problem of treating antisocial behavior is eventually a problem in the development of appropriate stimulus control relationships. One develops social contact through the actions and reactions of people rather than through the use of less natural contingencies, such as time-out rooms or a communication token. Further, one cannot develop normal social influence and inhibitions by reacting in an abnormal way to inappropriate behavior. For example, one should not expect a teacher to stand by and do nothing while students jump on his or her feet.

The interpersonal treatment model involves the following steps:

1. A comprehensive behavioral analysis is administered in order to identify the functions (functional analysis) of the problem behaviors, as well as any discriminative or eliciting stimuli that precede these behaviors (antecedent analysis).
2. A curriculum is established based on the results of the functional assessment.
3. The treatment is then initiated in a controlled and highly structured environment in order to establish a new set of interpersonal relationships with the client.
4. Procedures are introduced to promote transfer of treatment gains to natural settings.

Each of the steps is described in detail below.

PERFORMING A COMPLETE BEHAVIORAL ANALYSIS

In recent years there has been an increased interest in identifying the factors responsible for maintaining problem behavior (Axelrod, 1987; Iwata, Dorsey, Slifer, Bauman, & Richman, 1982). This work has primarily focused on the identification of possible sources of positive and negative reinforcement (Carr & Newsom, 1985; Iwata et al., 1982; Mace, Page, Ivancic, & O'Brien, 1986) that might serve to maintain these behaviors. This analysis has tended to neglect two important factors influencing the occurrence of problem behavior. First, little attention has focused on the role of possible elicited or adjunctive factors in maintaining these behaviors. An adjunctive reinforcer is one that acquires its reinforcing characteristics as a result of some other ongoing reinforcer system (Falk, 1966). It has been long known that extinction-correlated stimuli can serve to establish the opportunity to engage in aggression as an adjunctive reinforcer (Azrin, Hutchinson, & Hake, 1966). Second, the role of important antecedents such as discriminative stimuli and eliciting stimuli in maintaining these behaviors has been virtually ignored. This oversight seriously undermines the development of effective treatment programs, because one cannot regulate the behavior in manageable units unless one understands how it is controlled.

The Role of Operant and Respondent Processes

Much antisocial behavior is maintained by positive and negative reinforcement. A *positive reinforcer* is any form of stimulation and/or activity that increases the frequency of a behavior that it follows. Typically, positive reinforcers involve the delivery of more than one type of stimulation; for example, playing ball with a child may involve providing social forms of attention, activity, and a tangible item (the ball). Studies have demonstrated that antisocial behavior can be maintained by access to social stimulation (Thomas, Becker, & Armstrong, 1968), sensory stimulation (Rincover & Devany, 1982), and tangible reinforcers (Durand & Kishi, 1987).

A *negative reinforcer* is any form of stimulation and/or activity that increases the frequency of a behavior that terminates it. Typically, negative reinforcers also involve a complex combination of factors. Studies have demonstrated that antisocial behavior can be maintained by the termination of teaching (Carr & Durand, 1985; Iwata, Pace, Kalsher, Cowdery, & Cataldo, 1990; Sailor, Guess, Rutherford, & Baer, 1968) and the termination of responsibilities associated with daily living (Iwata et al., 1990).

Although the roles of positive and negative reinforcement have received considerable attention, the roles of respondent- and schedule-induced phenomena have received significantly less. Many problems in these populations have been referred to as being associated with anger, frustration, and other emotional phenomena (Zarkowski & Clements, 1988). Typically, these behaviors are associated with the delivery of negative reinforcers, waiting for the delivery of positive reinforcers, the termination of positive reinforcers, or stimuli associated with extinction (e.g., the presentation of extinction-correlated stimuli or the denial of requested positive reinforcers). These events have been shown in the animal learning literature to elicit aggression and other antisocial behavior (Azrin et al., 1966; Azrin, Hutchinson, & Sallery, 1964; Gentry, 1968; Hutchinson, Azrin, & Hunt, 1968; Ulrich & Azrin, 1962). It is important to note that these behaviors have been shown to persist even though they do not receive any form of positive or negative reinforcement. Flory, Smith, and Ellis (1977) have shown that extinction plus a DRO schedule was effective in reducing operant aggression, but was relatively ineffective in reducing schedule-induced aggression. These data suggest that functional analysis programs that ignore possible elicited causes of severe behavior may be destined to failure in some cases.

Even individuals engaging in attention-seeking behavior may have problems with waiting for attention, accepting the termination of attention, and the denial of attention. Therefore, these individuals may engage in aggression or tantrum behaviors that are more elicited than operant in nature (i.e., associated with waiting for, the termination of, or the denial of attention). Addressing the role of respondent processes in antisocial behavior requires placing greater emphasis on determining the stimuli associated with the occurrence of these behaviors. Thus, we will begin our discussion of the functional analysis phase with the identification of unconditioned stimuli, conditioned stimuli, and discriminative stimuli associated with the occurrence of antisocial behavior.

Identifying Precursor Stimuli

One way to identify precursor stimuli is to ask individuals who are familiar with the person questions that will help to identify the specific situations associated with the target behavior. Although laypersons may not be reliable in determining the function of a behavior, one would expect them to be much more reliable in describing the situations in which the behavior occurs. It is relatively easy to discriminate whether someone throws a tantrum when attempting to brush his or her teeth, but more difficult to discriminate whether he or she is doing so in order to escape tooth brushing, to obtain attention, or simply in response to some painful aspect of the activity (meaning that the behavior would continue even if no escape were possible).

For this reason, the checklist presented in Figure 1 places primary emphasis on determining the specific stimuli associated with a behavior. For example, if one suspects the behavior is being maintained by attention, one would want to determine the discriminative stimuli, setting, and motivational events associated with the behavior of concern. One would therefore wish to identify specific situations, staff, and activities associated with the behavior. If one suspects the behavior is maintained as an escape response, one would want to identify the specific negative reinforcers associated with it; these could include the type of task, its difficulty, or the pace with which it is being taught. If one suspects the behavior to be elicited, one would want to identify the specific stimuli eliciting the behavior. Therefore, if a problem

STIMULUS CONTROL CHECKLIST

Client: _____   Date: __/__/__
                                             d / m / y
Respondent: _____

Relationship to Client: _____

Please describe the nature of your involvement with the client. For example: Mother and client lives at home, Nurse working on the unit with the client three times per week.

_____

_____

Behavioral Difficulties: _____

_____

_____

NOTE: Please fill out this assessment scale in regards to client.

1. If the person lacks full range of voluntary movement, does the behavior   [ ] YES
   occur more when the individual is in the same position for an extended   [ ] NO
   period of time?

   If YES, briefly describe the specific position.

   _____

   _____

   _____

2. Was the onset of the behavior associated with a change in medication?   [ ] YES
                                                                             [ ] NO

   If YES, what was the change in medication?

   _____

   _____

   _____

FIGURE 1. A stimulus control checklist for administration to parents and other mediators. (1991).

3. Does the behavior occur more often just before the menstrual period or is it associated with the onset of menopause?

[ ] YES
[ ] NO

4. Does the behavior occur more often toward the end of a long, busy day, or, following a prolonged activity, or does the individual show signs of being tired before the occurrence of the behavior?

[ ] YES
[ ] NO

If YES, describe briefly.

_____

_____

_____

5. Does the behavior occur more often after consumption of alcoholic beverages?

[ ] YES
[ ] NO

If YES, please describe the client drinking pattern.

_____

_____

_____

6. Does the behavior occur more often just prior to, during or after seizure activity?

[ ] YES
[ ] NO

a) If YES, please describe the behavior of the individual during the seizure.

Facial expression _____

Typical body movements _____

Verbal behavior _____

Other _____

_____

7. Does the behavior occur in relation to inability to remember recent events?

[ ] YES
[ ] NO

If YES, please provide some examples.

_____

_____

_____

8. Does the behavior occur more when the environment is noisy?   [ ] YES
                                                                    [ ] NO

    If **YES**, what kind of noise?

_____

_____

_____

9. Does the behavior occur more in a crowded room?   [ ] YES
                                                        [ ] NO

    If **YES**, please describe crowded setting in detail.

_____

_____

_____

10. Does the behavior occur more when the individual has to wait for an item   [ ] YES
    or activity such as waiting for a meal, waiting in line,   [ ] NO
    waiting for scheduled activity?

    If **YES**, please list these items in descending order of importance.

    1. (most) _____

    2. _____

    3. _____

    4. (least) _____

11. Is the behavior often associated with the termination of specific   [ ] YES
    activities for example: the end of a show; the end of a scheduled   [ ] NO
    activity; at the end of a conversation.

    If **YES**, please list these activities in descending order of importance.

    1. (most) _____

    2. _____

    3. _____

    4. (least) _____

(continued)

12. Does the behavior occur when the person is denied something they asked for or want?　　[ ] YES　[ ] NO

If **YES**, please list the items denied in descending order of importance.

1. (most) _____

2. _____

3. _____

4. (least) _____

13. Does the behavior reliably occur during specific self-care activity, such as, brushing teeth, taking a bath, getting dressed, etc?　　[ ] YES　[ ] NO

If **YES**, please list in descending order of importance.

People

1. (most) _____　　5. _____

2. _____　　6. _____

3. _____　　7. _____

4. _____　　8. (least) _____

14. Does the behavior appear to be related to the individuals inability to communicate their needs because of impaired speech?　　[ ] YES　[ ] NO

If **YES**, please list those needs.

_____

_____

_____

_____

15. Does the behavior occur more often when you begin to teach a new skill?　　[ ] YES　[ ] NO

If **YES**, please list these skills, starting with skill most associated with the behavior.

1. (most) _____

2. _____

3. _____

4. (least) _____

16. Does the behavior occur more often when the difficulty of a task is increased?

[ ] YES
[ ] NO

    If **YES**, please briefly describe a task.

_____

_____

_____

17. Does the behavior occur more often when you increase the amount of work to be done?

[ ] YES
[ ] NO

18. Does the behavior occur less often when the individual is receiving a lot of attention from volunteers, professional, or others?

[ ] YES
[ ] NO

19. Does the behavior occur more often when you are short staffed?

[ ] YES
[ ] NO

20. Does the individual engage in the behavior in order to obtain, something he/she wants such as cigarettes, snacks, loud music, etc.

[ ] YES
[ ] NO

    If **YES**, please give example.

    1. (most) _____

    2. _____

    3. _____

    4. (least) _____

21. Often times a behavior is more likely in the presence of some persons than others. List all of the people who interact with the client and circle the item that best describe, how often the behavior occurs in their presence.

Name	Relationship to Client	Not at All	Just a Little	Pretty Much	Very Much
_____	_____	0	1	2	3
_____	_____	0	1	2	3
_____	_____	0	1	2	3
_____	_____	0	1	2	3
_____	_____	0	1	2	3
_____	_____	0	1	2	3
_____	_____	0	1	2	3

behavior was associated with waiting for a reinforcer (i.e., is schedule induced), questions would focus on the types of items a person has difficulty waiting for, as well as how long he or she could typically wait. Similar questions would be asked in regard to termination of events as well as denial of events.

It is particularly important here, as well as with escape, that respondents to these questions provide a wide range of examples that vary from reliably producing a strong reaction to producing little reaction so that a hierarchy can be established as part of the treatment plan. A checklist designed to collect more detailed information on the precursor stimuli associated with the presence of antisocial behavior is presented in Figure 1. These items also allow one to identify a hierarchy of mediators associated with the presence and absence of the behaviors of concern. It should be noted that the information obtained on the *antecedent* stimuli related to the behavior should be of value to the behavior analyst even when his or her guess about the probable *function* of the behavior proves incorrect.

Identifying the Function of the Behavior

One way to identify the function of a behavior is to ask people familiar with the client questions designed to distinguish the various functions of antisocial behavior. For example, Durand and Crimmins (1988) devised a brief reinforcer assessment instrument, the Motivational Assessment Scale (MAS), designed to determine whether behavior was maintained by sensory, escape, attention, and tangible reinforcers. This scale was supposed to allow one to determine the relative ranking of each of the four reinforcer categories by having respondents rate 16 questions on a 6-point scale. The results of recent research found interrespondent agreement to be unacceptable, however, and that the results of the questionnaire did not correlate well with the results of an experimentally determined functional analysis (Rodgers, Zarcone, & Iwata, 1990; Zarcone, Rodgers, & Iwata, 1990).

One reason why the MAS may have been unreliable is that family and staff may not have sufficient background in behavior analysis to make the required discriminations accurately based on their memory of events. It is also possible, though, that the questions in the MAS were not specific enough. More carefully selected questions might help provide a more useful questionnaire. At the moment, however, no questionnaire has been demonstrated to be sufficiently reliable to substitute for an experimental analysis of the function of the behavior.

Whereas the MAS was devised to determine the function of a behavior, the checklist presented in Figure 1 was designed to determine possible antecedents to behavior. Although unvalidated, this scale may prove useful in generating hypotheses concerning the function of antisocial behavior (these hypotheses, however, must be confirmed by some form of experimental analysis). Examples of questions designed to determine whether a behavior is being emitted in order to produce attention are as follows: Does the individual typically approach you immediately preceding the behavior? Does he or she smile or show signs of being relaxed while engaging in antisocial behavior? Examples of questions designed to determine whether a behavior is functioning as an escape response are as follows: Does the behavior occur more often following attempts to teach a new skill? Does the behavior occur more often when a task is associated with a higher ratio of incorrect/correct responses?

A similar approach is employed in determining elicited and adjunctive causes. Examples of questions designed to identify elicited, and adjunctive causes of behavior are as follows: Does the behavior occur more when the individual has to wait for an activity or is told he or she has to wait for an activity that he or she likes? Is the behavior often associated with the termination of specific activities? Does the behavior occur when the person is denied something he or she wants? Does the individual show signs of being upset, angry, or otherwise agitated immediately prior to, as well as while engaging in, antisocial behavior?

Note that communication does not receive its own category in this checklist. This is because we do not view communication factors as a function or cause of a behavior, although teaching behaviors that facilitate communication can be a useful strategy in remediating a problem. Of course, one could consider all operant and elicited behavior as communicative in function; in our view, however, such a use trivializes the term. Perhaps more importantly, it can lead to an adoption of the more cognitive term of *purpose* over the more behavioral term of *function*.

We suspect that accurately identifying the function of a behavior may be less important to treatment outcome than identifying the antecedent stimuli associated with the occurrence of the behavior. Once the antecedents are correctly identified, one can usually employ gradual change techniques along with effective consequences to teach alternative means of responding.

Conducting a Structured Validation

Having people familiar with the person respond to a structured questionnaire can help to formulate some hypotheses about the stimuli associated with antisocial behaviors as well as their functions. The next step in the assessment process is to conduct a structured validation of these hypotheses. This validation is carried out in three phases. First, staff are instructed to record incidents of antisocial behavior using an incident reporting form. An example of an incident reporting form is shown in Figure 2. This form has space to record the time of the incident, the form of the behavior, the precursors to the behavior, the location, the people present, and the staff's reactions following the behavior. This procedure is followed for several days

INCIDENT REPORT

Client's Name: _____ Observer/Recorder: _____ Date: _____.

Time	Behavior	Antecedent	Location	Persons Present	Person's Reaction

FIGURE 2. An incident report form filled out by parents and other mediators.

in order to determine whether the hypotheses derived from the functional interview appear valid, as well as to detect any functions that may have been missed during the interview. These data can also provide information about which persons are most associated with the occurrence of the behavior.

The second step in the validation process is to conduct a structured clinical assessment. Prior to beginning the clinical assessment, a script is prepared from the information acquired from the functional interview and by validation observations. This script consists of a precise sequence of events that includes the presentation and removal of each precursor a predetermined number of times in a highly controlled and structured situation. In the final phase, the behavior analyst revises the script if necessary based on results obtained in the previous step, and the procedure is replicated with each of the significant mediators interacting with the client in the natural setting.

Such an assessment was performed on the behavior of five children with developmental handicaps who participated in a group treatment program. Each of five possible functions was assessed in the following manner: In the ignore condition, each trial lasted 5 minutes. During this condition the mediator was alone in the room with the child. Toys were present in the room, and the mediator sat in a chair reading a book or engaging in any other insular behavior that was reported to be associated with the child's inappropriate behavior on either the functional analysis checklist or the incident reports. Anytime the child approached the mediator, the latter attempted to redirect the child; if the child became aggressive or engaged in self-injury, the mediator restrained the child. Four trials of the ignore condition were conducted each session.

In the demand condition, the mediator conducted 10 trials per session. During each trial the mediator sat opposite the child in a knee-to-knee seating arrangement (Van Houten & Rolider, 1989), with a table at the mediator's side. At the start of each trial, the mediator initiated one of several behaviors that was reported to be associated with the inappropriate behavior on the functional analysis checklist and/or the incident reports. Each trial was scored for the presence or absence of inappropriate behavior.

In the termination condition, the mediator conducted 5 trials per session. The mediator engaged the child in an activity whose termination was reported to be associated with the occurrence of the behavior on the functional analysis checklist or incident reports. After several minutes, the mediator attempted to redirect the child to a neutral activity. Each trial was scored for the presence or absence of inappropriate behavior.

In the wait condition, the mediator again sat in the knee-to-knee seating arrangement, presented (out of reach) an item that was reported to be associated with the occurrence of the behavior, and told the child to wait. At the end of 5 seconds, the mediator gave the item to the child. The child was only given the item on trials during which inappropriate behavior did not occur. Each child was scored for the presence or absence of the inappropriate behavior.

The denial condition was only conducted if the child was able to request the items. As in the wait condition, an item was placed in the child's sight. If the child requested the item or otherwise attempted to obtain the item, the mediator told the child, "No, you can't have that" and prevented him or her from obtaining it by moving the item. Each trial was scored for the presence or absence of inappropriate behavior. If no behavior occurred within 5 minutes, the trial was terminated. Five trials of this condition were conducted each session. (Sensory reinforcement was not assessed in this study, because the results of the functional analysis checklist and the incident reports did not suggest that it was a factor with any of these five cases.)

Data collected in the structured clinical assessment are presented in Figure 3. These data show the percentage of trials that the target behavior occurred for each precursor of the problem behavior in the presence of the therapist and one or more natural mediators in the clinic and home situation over five assessment sessions. Problem behaviors treated included aggression, self-injury, and severe tantrums. All assessment sessions were video-taped, and data were scored from the videotapes.

The results for subject 1 showed that inappropriate behavior occurred in the presence of the boy's mother but not in the presence of his father or the therapist. In the home situation, however, inappropriate behavior occurred in the presence of both his mother and father, but not in the presence of the therapist. For both parents the behavior tended to occur in situations where their son had to wait for a reinforcer, had reinforcers terminated, was denied reinforcers, or was presented with various demands. The behavior did not occur at all in the ignore condition; therefore, ignoring the child's approach behavior was not a reliable antecedent for his behavior. It is interesting to note that in the clinic environment, the behavior was most probable when the mother denied her son something, whereas in the home setting the behavior was most probable when the mother terminated reinforcers. In this case, most of the behavior seemed to be related to frustrating situations associated with extinction or periods without reinforcement. This trend is repeated in the data of several of the other subjects.

For subject 2, the behaviors occurred in the presence of waiting, denial, termination, and demand, but not in the ignore condition. The data also reveal that the behavior occurred in the presence of all conditions with the father (who was a single parent) and the therapist, although the behavior occurred somewhat less often in the therapist's presence. For subject 3, the behavior also occurred only in the waiting, denial, termination, and demand conditions. The behavior also occurred somewhat less in the clinic in the presence of the mother (who was also a single parent). It is interesting to note that this subject was better able to accept denial from the therapist in the home than in the clinic, whereas the reverse was true in the parent's presence.

For subject 4, the behavior was more probable in the clinic setting than in the home setting for most of the factors for the mother, whereas the behavior was more probable in the home setting than in the clinic setting for all factors for the therapist. For subject 5, the behavior did not occur in the presence of his mother or the therapist in any of the conditions in the clinic or home, but did occur in all conditions in the presence of his father. In this case the ignore condition was associated with the behavior 100% of the time in both settings for the father.

An examination of these data reveals several important points. First, for all of the children, the behavior problem had more than one eliciting or operant function. Second, the functions of much of the antisocial behavior of each of the children were predominantly elicited or adjunctive in nature (waiting, termination of reinforcers, and denial). Third, the function of the behaviors often varied across persons. *These data support the assertion that treatment may not need to be based on the function of the behavior in many cases.* It may be more important to identify the antecedent stimuli (whether condi-

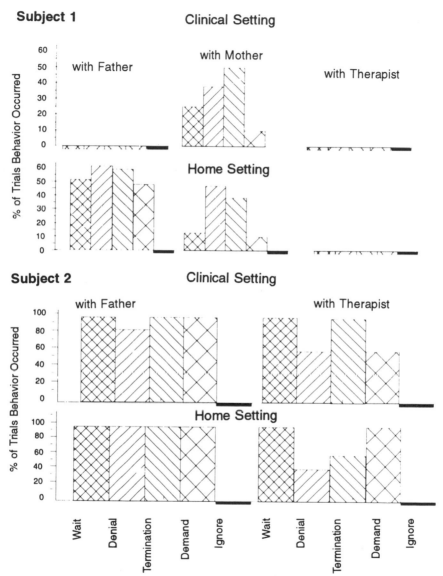

FIGURE 3. Data collected on five children during structured clinical assessment sessions under a variety of analogue conditions.

(continued)

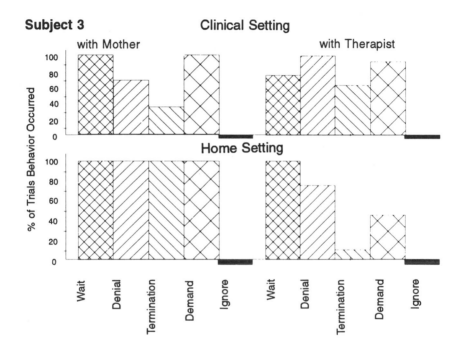

Subject 3 — Clinical Setting / Home Setting

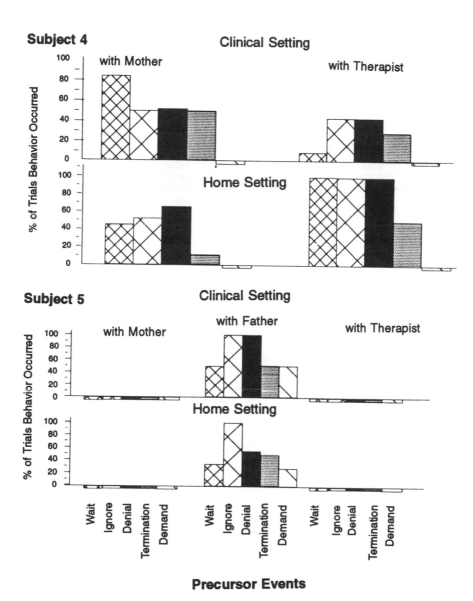

tioned stimuli, unconditioned stimuli or discriminative stimuli) than to identify the function of these stimuli.

SELECTING A CURRICULUM

The selection of the treatment curriculum is perhaps one of the more important decisions in developing the treatment plan. The curriculum must be closely related to the precursors of the problem behavior and usually will take one of two forms. First, the curriculum can involve providing graded exposure to a variety of stimuli that elicit inappropriate social reactions (Schloss, Smith, Santora, & Bryant, 1989). These curriculum materials are used to help teach normal social inhibitions that everyone needs in order to handle the everyday frustrations of life. Second, the curriculum can involve teaching behavior that is appropriate and yet functionally equivalent to the problem behavior (Bird, Dores, Moniz, & Robinson, 1989; Carr & Durand, 1985; Day, Rea, Schussler, Larsen, & Johnson, 1988). These strategies of teaching social inhibitions and functionally equivalent behavior are not mutually exclusive and are usually employed together.

Establishing Treatment Priorities

It is important to weigh three factors when setting treatment priorities. First, one must evaluate the seriousness of the behavior related to the precursors. Second, one must evaluate the seriousness of the behavior related to the mediators. Third, one must evaluate the seriousness of the behavior in relation to the environment. The general rule to follow here is to begin with the precursor, mediator, and environment that produce the least severe reaction from the individual.

The purpose of this approach is to allow many treatment trials while minimizing the likelihood of serious problem behaviors. One can increase the magnitude of the precursor gradually so as to shape the desired social responses in progressively more difficult or complex situations. For example, one might begin by having someone wait for something that is mildly important for a short period of time. Gradually the amount of time can be increased, and then the reinforcing value of the thing the client is waiting for can also be increased. Similarly, one can be taught to handle the occasional denial of relatively unimportant reinforcers before moving on to more significant reinforcers.

A similar approach can be taken to mediator involvement in the program. The first mediator to work with the person on a particular problem should be the one who initially encounters the least difficulty in the initial clinical assessment. Next, other significant mediators can be introduced in the presence of the first mediator, who will be gradually faded out. The same approach is taken in regard to the treatment environment; however, here the environment associated with the least severe behavior will almost always be the relatively novel and highly structured treatment environment. Only after favorable results are obtained in this environment does treatment progress to one of the natural settings.

A major advantage of this approach is that it allows one to obtain favorable results with the use of relatively unobtrusive social consequences. Thus, social learning takes place in a relatively natural social setting.

Establishing a Precursor Hierarchy

There are essentially three ways to arrange a precursor hierarchy. First, one can vary the level of motivation for the behavior or the intensity of the eliciting stimulus. One can vary the level of motivation for attention-seeking behavior by varying the amount of social deprivation. In the case of escape-motivated behavior, one can vary motivation by increasing or decreasing the aversiveness of a task along a relevant dimension (e.g., task difficulty or pacing). If the precursor is the termination, denial, or waiting for a reinforcer (e.g., food), one could vary the level of motivation by introducing trials after a fixed amount of satiation in regard to the reinforcers.

In the second case, one can vary the stimulus properties of the discriminative or eliciting stimulus. If the behavior is escape motivated, one can vary the type of task. If the precursor is termination, denial, or waiting for a reinforcer, one can vary the item waited for, terminated, or denied. For example, someone may be able to wait reasonably well for a raisin but not for a chocolate chip cookie.

In the third case, one can vary the schedule thought to induce the problem behavior. An example of this would be to increase gradually the amount of work required when the function of the behavior is to escape demands. Another example would be to increase the time that someone has to wait for attention or other reinforcers, the length of time that attention or the preferred item has to be given up, or the percentage of trials that someone is denied something he or she requested.

Selecting Functional Alternatives

The next step in selecting a curriculum is to identify functionally equivalent alternative behaviors, or socially appropriate ways to engage in functionally nonequivalent alternatives, while waiting or following the termination of an important reinforcer. When selecting functionally equivalent alternative behaviors, it is important that the behaviors taught will produce the desired consequence in a relatively reliable manner. An example would be to teach a nonverbal individual who attacks other residents to obtain staff attention to tap staff members on the shoulder instead. This would represent an effective strategy because the person's behavior would be difficult to miss or to ignore. An individual who becomes aggressive when reinforcers are terminated could be taught to ask for more time with the reinforcer. A person with a developmental handicap can be taught to say "Stop it" to terminate an aversive event rather than to behave aggressively or throw a tantrum, or to say "No, I don't want to" in an assertive tone of voice if he or she does not want to engage in a task.

Teaching Appropriate Social Inhibitions

No matter how successfully one teaches functionally appropriate alternative behaviors, these behaviors will not always be reinforced in the natural setting. Like everyone else, the client with developmental handicaps must also learn that good things must sometimes come to an end, that you cannot always get what you want, that you sometimes have to wait, and that you sometimes have to perform tasks that you do not enjoy. For example, one could teach a handicapped person who engages in severe tantrums and self-injury to sign that she wants to go to a fast-food restaurant. If she is in a special education classroom and she emits this sign at 10:30 a.m., the teacher might sign back, "Later, when it is lunchtime." Alternatively, the teacher might offer her an early recess snack.

This strategy will not be effective if the client cannot inhibit the emotional reactions associated with the immediate denial of going to the restaurant or with waiting until lunch. If a person cannot react appropriately to these normally occurring "frustrating" events the prognosis for long-term community integration will remain poor. Although everyone experiences these same frustrations to some degree, those who remain out of prisons or institutions have learned to inhibit aggression or tantrum behavior, at least in public places. For this reason, teaching social inhibitions should be a primary focus of successful treatment. *The curriculum for teaching waiting involves teaching the client to wait for progressively longer periods of time, or for progressively more reinforcing items or activities. The curriculum for teaching someone to accept the termination of a reinforcer involves teaching someone to give up a reinforcer for progressively longer periods of time, or to give up progressively more reinforcing items or activities. The curriculum for teaching someone to accept denial of a reinforcer would be to deny increasingly more reinforcing activities.*

Teaching Cooperation

Although it is important to teach behaviors that can be immediately useful to the client, many behaviors are important because they open up the possibility of future learning and growth. Examples are teaching motor imitation that involves object manipulation as a prerequisite to teaching toy play or other recreational activities more effectively, or motor imitation that involves body orientation as a prerequisite to teaching signing. Early attempts to teach verbal imitation can pay off nicely with many younger clients with developmental handicaps. It is difficult to initiate any program designed to teach unless the client is a relatively cooperative learner. Therefore, teaching good cooperation is an important skill for many clients. Gaining cooperation on less reinforcing educational activities that the client might be motivated to escape is important if these clients are to succeed in future learning.

THE INTERPERSONAL TREATMENT MODEL

In order to teach functional skills, appropriate social inhibitions, and cooperation in the most effective manner, it is essential that the teaching be conducted in a very systematic manner in a highly structured situation.

Establishing a Structured Environment

A structured environment is one in which the mediator is seated close to the client, has no other responsibilities, and can freely introduce at his or her discretion the antecedents controlling the behavior. One seating arrangement that can meet this requirement is the knee-to-knee arrangement reported by Van Houten and Rolider (1989). The arrangement offers many advantages over the unstructured natural setting or the more artificial laboratory setting. Only when favorable results have been produced in this seating arrangement is it possible to move to a less structured arrangement.

There are several reasons why it is important to initiate treatment in a highly structured environment. First, the highly structured treatment situation is free of distractions that can impair the ability of the mediator to react correctly and promptly. Second, it affords a high degree of proximity that allows the mediator to react with the most effective social contingencies. Third, this arrangement enables the mediator to determine better when antisocial behaviors will occur, because he or she introduces the antecedents associated with those behaviors. Fourth, the mediator can be better prepared to react to inappropriate behavior when he or she controls the presentation of relevant antecedent events. Fifth, the mediator has no other response requirements in the structured setting but to react in the most effective manner. Sixth, the structured treatment setting provides frequent opportunities to interact in an intensive manner with the client, thereby maximizing opportunities to learn. This provides the client frequent opportunities to inhibit antisocial behavior and to respond in a more socially appropriate manner. This is important because the more opportunity the person has to interact in a meaningful manner, the better the chances that the person will respond to treatment.

Structuring the Introduction of Treatment Curriculum

Before initiating treatment, one must first design the treatment curriculum. This involves preparing behavioral interaction scripts that specify how the antecedent stimuli will be presented, as well as all relevant setting events, and how the mediator should react to the client's responses. An example of an initial script used for a client who had difficulty waiting for edible reinforcers is shown in Figure 4. These scripts are prepared from the information acquired during the structured clinical assessment.

Once the client is able to wait for the reinforcer for a predetermined brief period of time, progressively more powerful reinforcers can be introduced. Once the client can wait for a short period of time for a more powerful reinforcer, the amount of time that he or she has to wait can be systematically increased. Once the client can wait for a more powerful reinforcer for a relatively long period of time, the proximity of the mediator can be progressively decreased. Next, other features can be introduced from the natural setting, such as the presence of siblings or household distractions (e.g., television). Finally, other mediators can be faded into the structured environment, and the initial mediator can be faded out.

Establishing Personal Stimulus Control

Practitioners and laypeople alike have long known that clients often behave differently in the presence of different people. For example, a child may cooperate more with one parent than another, or may engage in frequent antisocial behavior in the presence of one parent but not in the presence of the other. Similarly, a resident in a treatment center may engage in a high level of self-injury in the presence of one staff member and a low level of self-injury in the presence of a second staff member (Touchette, MacDonald, & Langer, 1985). If a change in behavior occurs the moment a person is introduced or removed, it is likely that the person exerts stimulus control over the client's behavior. The presence of such *personal stimulus control* can be exploited by beginning treatment with the mediator who initially obtained the best overall level of cooperation from the client. If it is not possible to identify a mediator or therapist who initially is associated with absence of antisocial behavior in the presence of its usual antecedents, one should begin treatment with a mediator whose presence is associated with the lowest frequency and intensity of antisocial behavior.

Obtaining such personal stimulus control for all important mediators is the overriding goal of the interpersonal treatment model. This goal is achieved by progressively introducing mediators who initially showed less personal stimulus control. Once one mediator acquires personal stimulus control, a second mediator carries out the program in conjunction with the first. Once acceptable results have been produced in the presence of both

SCRIPT: Wait

CLIENT: Nancy   TEACHER: Allison

TARGET BEHAVIORS: screaming, crying, whining, hitting,
                     biting, and slapping others

MATERIALS: scoring form and pencil
              reinforcers: chocolate bar, plain chips, cola
              2 chairs and a table

SETTING: A one-to-one seating arrangement in a quiet
            location, free of distractions.

INSTRUCTIONS:
1.   Sit knee-to-knee with Nancy with the table of the
therapist's dominant hand side.
2.   Arrange a few pieces of the chocolate bar, chips, and a
small glass of cola on the table out of arm's reach of
Nancy.   The scoring form should be adjacent to the teacher.
3.   Begin a trial by instructing Nancy to place her hands on
your knees and saying: "Look at me".   Reinforce looking
with praise if necessary.
4.   While maintaining eye contact with Nancy, pick up a
piece of chocolate (or chip or the glass) and say: "Nancy,
you can have the ___, but you have to wait".   Place the
reinforcer on the table within arm's reach of Nancy.   Wait
for 5 seconds (or whatever the predetermined time is).
5.   If Nancy waits without grabbing the reinforcer, or
engaging in any of the target behaviors, give her the
reinforcer and provide copious praise.   RECORD as an
appropriate trial.
6.   If Nancy grabs for the reinforcer, physically block her
attempt and say: "NO!   You must Wait!"
    a.   If Nancy accepts the disapproval: RECORD as an
    inappropriate trial and begin the next trial immediately;
    b.   If Nancy begins to engage in any of the target
    behaviors respond as prescribed in the treatment plan;
    RECORD as an inappropriate trial.
7.   Once control has been re-established, begin the next
trial.
8.   Continue for the pre-determined number of trials.

FIGURE 4. An example of a script employed with a client who had difficulty waiting for edible
reinforcers.

mediators, the first mediator is gradually faded from the structured environment.

Social Processes Leading to Personal Stimulus Control

One way to facilitate the generalization to other settings of changes in behavior produced in the structured treatment setting is to rely as much as possible on social processes to produce the behavior change. This is because personal stimulus control develops best when the presence of a person is associated with personal reactions to behavior. Therefore, an effective way to produce durable personal stimulus control is through effective rapport-building strategy, instructions, and verbal and nonverbal approval and disapproval.

One should begin the treatment process by establishing a positive relationship with the client. This can be done by removing all of the possible antecedents for antisocial behavior and providing a large amount of interpersonal reinforcement. Examples of rapport-building strategies include sharing edibles or toys that the child likes, playing interactive games such as tickling or peek-a-boo games, helping the client to engage in reinforcing activity, engaging in a conversation on a favorite topic, playing a cooperative video game together, and providing praise. The purpose of this phase is to establish the mediator's presence as a strong conditioned reinforcer.

Once the mediator has established a reinforcing relationship with the client, the structured treatment sessions are introduced. First the mediator needs to ensure that the client will sit in the knee-to-knee seating arrangement. If the client cannot sit appropriately, the mediator needs to teach appropriate sitting behavior. First, the person is presented with a reinforcer and permitted to engage in a reinforcing activity while seated in the chair; most clients who refuse to sit probably do so because it involves the termination of some other reinforcer. Once the client is sitting and engaged in the reinforcing activity, one can begin to teach the person to accept the termination of the reinforcer for longer and longer periods of time. Because the reinforcers employed may be fairly powerful, one should begin with very brief periods of termination, perhaps as short as 1 or 2 seconds.

Structured teaching trials are always begun with a short request; it is essential that these requests be made in an assertive but pleasant tone of voice. Many factors have been shown to be related to the level of compliance with requests. First, clients are more likely to follow requests when the mediator demands eye contact before making the request (Hamlet, Axelrod, & Kuerschner, 1984). Therefore, anytime the client breaks eye contact while an instruction is being given, the mediator should demand eye contact by saying "Look at me" in a firm tone of voice. Second, one can set the occasion for following a request that is usually associated with noncompliance by providing several instructions that have a high probability of being complied with prior to making the request (Mace et al., 1988).

A third factor influencing compliance is the tone of voice used by the person making the request. In general, people are less likely to respond to a request that involves a questioning inflection (an increase in pitch on the last word) than one that employs a more assertive inflection (a decrease in pitch on the last word). Fourth, the content of a direction can influence the likelihood that the client will follow a request. In general, requests should be brief and direct and not include phrases like "Can you" or "Would you." Fifth, it is important that the mediator's gestures, body language, expression, and tone all convey to the client that they expect the direction to be carried out, in short, that the mediator means it. For example, when making a request, it is important that the mediator not raise and lower his or her eyebrows, but instead freeze their position. These are the small details that can make the difference between success and failure.

Whenever the client emits the requested response, it is important to provide immediate social reinforcement. For approval to be effective, it is important that the mediator deliver approval in a way that the person finds reinforcing. Many of the activities employed in the rapport-building phase can be paired with the approval to accomplish this goal. The best indication that the mediator has successfully delivered approval are such signs of client contentment as smiling, laughing or other pleasant sounds. It is important that the mediator view the giving of approval as an interactive process. The more the behavior of the mediator contributes to the reinforcing value of the approval, the stronger the conditioned reinforcing value of the mediator. Examples of some types of interactions that clients might find interesting are high fives, pats on the shoulder, hugs and other forms of physical contact, tickling, funny noises, telling jokes or stories, discussing activities of mutual interest, going to a mall, or sharing a snack.

When the client engages in antisocial behavior following the presentation of the antecedent stimulus, it is very important that the mediator provide correction as quickly as possible. The moment the antisocial behavior begins to occur, the mediator should immediately interrupt the behavior by establishing quick eye contact and making a brief and firm statement of disapproval, followed by immediate requests to engage in the appropriate behavior. The mediator should use a firm tone of voice when delivering disapproval. Voice pitch should drop on the last word, and it can be helpful to emphasize unvoiced consonant stops (e.g., t, k, and p sounds). The mediator should also maintain a glare and use firm gestures, such as holding up the index finger at face level. If the client does not terminate the antisocial behavior, the mediator should physically interrupt the response.

It is important that the mediator try not to provide any form of reinforcing contact while interrupting the behavior. This can be best accomplished by quick motions and abrupt release. For example, if the client attempts to strike the mediator (or himself or herself), the mediator should quickly place the client's hand on his or her lap and release the hand all in one motion. Immediately following this procedure, the mediator should reintroduce the antecedent stimulus. If the client responds in a cooperative manner, the mediator should provide enthusiastic approval.

The timing of the reaction is another factor that can influence the efficacy of disapproval. We find that it is best to deliver disapproval early in the chain, before the client can emit an effective or vigorous response. The most important skill needed to accomplish this goal is to identify the behaviors associated with the onset of the episode. For example, the mediator should deliver disapproval after the first couple of words when it is apparent that the client is saying something that is clearly inappropriate. Similarly, if a client clenches his or her fists prior to engaging in tantrum behavior, disapproval should follow clenching the fist. Even though it may be necessary to use forcefully delivered correction procedures in the initial phase, the client should not move to the next level in a hierarchy of precursor stimuli until he or she responds appropriately in the presence of pleasant requests and requires only a mild correction for occasional lapses.

Another factor that is important in the development of social control is the effective use of prompting strategies. Frequently it is helpful to remind the person how he or she should behave before presenting the precursor stimulus. For example, just prior to making a request, a person who behaves inappropriately when asked to perform a task would be told that he or she is about to be asked to do something and reminded how you expect him or her to behave. Initially the reminders would be given just prior to making the request; later, the time between the reminder and the request would be gradually increased until the reminders were no longer necessary.

Crisis Intervention

Because the stimulus antecedents are introduced in a hierarchal manner, beginning with stimuli associated with low-intensity antisocial behavior, many clients will not exhibit severe forms of antisocial behavior throughout the treatment process. On occasion, however, some clients with severe problems will engage in severe antisocial behavior that, if left unchecked, would lead to their hurting themselves or others. In these cases it is necessary to employ some type of crisis intervention procedure.

Typically, the outbursts take three forms. First, some clients might be ill, and staff may be unaware of their illness. Whenever illness is suspected, the treatment session should be suspended until either a medical examination has ruled out illness or the client is better. Second, some clients who are making very good progress will on some occasions respond out of proportion to the magnitude of the antecedent stimulus. Third, some clients exhibit such a high frequency and intensity of behavior that it is impossible to prevent severe episodes completely through the manipulation of antecedent stimuli, motivation, and mediators. In the two latter situations, the occasional application of crisis intervention may be warranted.

The first consideration in selecting a crisis intervention strategy is the safety of the client and mediators. Brief restraint procedures that safely immobilize the client and prevent him or her from injuring self or others are to be preferred to those procedures that involve struggling and risk of injury. Because some clients have been shown to find restraint reinforcing (Favell, McGimsey, & Jones, 1978), it is important that the procedure not involve prolonged holding. One can also reduce the likelihood of inadvertently reinforcing antisocial behavior by applying a restraint procedure that is mildly uncomfortable. Brief restraint has been shown to reduce the frequency of severe antisocial behavior when applied on a contingent basis (Azrin, Besalel, Jammer, & Caputo, 1988; Bitgood, Crowe, Suarez, & Peters, 1980; Griffin, Locke, & Landers, 1975; Rapoff, Altman, & Christophersen, 1980; Saloviita, 1988; Singh, Dawson, & Manning, 1981).

Factors influencing whether physical restraint functions as a positive or negative reinforcer may include how uncomfortable the restraint is and the individual's prior exposure to restraint. One effective crisis management procedure is momentary movement restraint (Rolider, Williams, Cummings, & Van Houten, 1991). This procedure involves placing the seated client's head between his or her knees, with arms held behind the back at waist level. Following a major outburst, two mediators press the client's upper back between the shoulder blades; the client is guided forward and down so that his or her chest rests against the knees. The client's arms are placed behind his or her back, with one hand on top of the other over the small of the back. In carrying out this procedure, the therapist always brings the head down toward the knees by pressing on the upper back, and never by pressing on the neck. Conditions that may preclude employing the procedure include spinal problems, Down's syndrome, high blood pressure, obesity, and asthma; therefore, a physician approval should be obtained prior to its use.

One advantage of momentary movement restraint as a crisis management procedure is that the technique readily prevents injury or escape once someone is maintained in the prescribed position. Another advantage is that the position is not as likely to prove reinforcing to an individual as other forms of restraint, because it is relatively uncomfortable and limits the degree to which the individual can see what is going on around him or her.

Because most crisis management procedures are somewhat restrictive in nature, it is important to apply them only for a brief period of time and then determine whether the client has calmed down and can resume treatment. On some occasions, it may be necessary to apply the procedure several times in succession before the person calms down. It is recommended that the procedure only be applied for 30 seconds during each application. If this procedure does not calm the client down after several consecutive applications, the mediators should discontinue the treatment session and reevaluate the appropriateness of the treatment plan. Another procedure that can be applied in a crisis situation is movement suppression (Rolider & Van Houten, 1985b).

It has been our experience that the application of an effective crisis management procedure has often been the turning point in establishing interpersonal stimulus control over antisocial behaviors. Many clients often show marked reductions in antisocial behavior following a few application of either of the above procedures, as well as marked increases in prosocial behavior (Rolider, Cummings, & Van Houten, 1991).

PROMOTING TRANSFER OF TREATMENT GAINS

Bringing the Natural Environment Into the Treatment Setting

After establishing personal stimulus control in the presence of the antecedent stimuli that previously were associated with the most severe intensity of the behavior, elements from the unstructured natural setting should be gradually introduced into the structured setting. For example, siblings, noise, and other distractions can be systematically introduced. In addition, the mediator should gradually loosen structure of the one-on-one situation by incrementally moving further away from the client.

Introducing Untrained Mediators

Once antisocial behavior has been eliminated in the presence of several mediators in both the structured setting and the natural environment, untrained mediators are directed to interact with the client in the presence of the trained mediators. If antisocial behavior occurs in the presence of the untrained mediators, the trained mediators intervene in order to establish control. This procedure is continued until the client behaves in an acceptable manner in the presence of the untrained mediators.

Using Time-Delay Procedures

One reason why behavior may fail to generalize to new situations is because the behavior is under the close control of verbal rather than nonverbal environmental stimuli. For example, a client who is taught to say "Help" rather than engage in tantrum behavior when he or she requires assistance may not transfer this behavior to situations where he or she requires help in the natural setting. The time-delay procedure is one way to transfer stimulus control to nonverbal stimuli (Charlop, Schreibman, & Thibodeau, 1985;

Ingemey & Van Houten, 1991); it is particularly useful in promoting the client's use of functionally equivalent alternatives to an inappropriate behavior.

To transfer control from verbal to nonverbal stimuli, one needs first to present the nonverbal stimulus, immediately followed by an effective verbal prompt. Next, a short delay is introduced between the presentation of the nonverbal and verbal prompt. The duration of the delay between the nonverbal and verbal prompt is then gradually increased until the behavior occurs "spontaneously" in the presence of the nonverbal stimulus.

In the example presented above, the person did not ask for help unless he or she was instructed to do so. The time-delay procedure can be employed in the one-on-one treatment situation in order to teach such an individual to ask for help in a variety of situations. For example, the therapist can give the client a clear container or jar that he or she cannot open, but that contains something he or she wants. The therapist can then immediately prompt the client to say or sign "Help" before providing assistance. Afterward, the interval between the presentation of the jar and the prompt can be increased until the client spontaneously requests help.

In addition to standard curriculum tasks, it is also important to provide practice with specific items taken from the stimulus control checklist. If the client engages in tantrum behavior when he or she requires assistance in tying shoes, or in turning on the television, he or she can receive daily practice on these tasks in the structured setting.

A similar approach can be adopted in teaching clients appropriate assertive behavior. Many clients have difficulty terminating unpleasant activities or stimulation in a socially acceptable way. Teaching these clients to say "Stop it" in an assertive manner rather than to engage in aggression or tantrum behavior is a necessary part of their functional teaching curriculum. The use of "Stop it" can be taught by first pulling lightly on the client's ear, or repeatedly nudging him or her on the shoulder; at the same time, the therapist prompts the client to say "Stop it" in an assertive tone of voice. Next, the delay between the physical stimulus and the verbal prompt is gradually increased until the behavior occurs without a prompt. A similar approach can be taken in teaching a wide range of important assertive behaviors. If the behavior occurs reliably in the one-on-one teaching situation but fails to occur in the natural environment, the use of the time-delay procedure needs to be introduced in the natural setting by a therapist who has good personal stimulus control.

Recreating the Situation

Recreating the situation is another way to promote generalization from the one-on-one situation to the natural setting (Van Houten & Rolider, 1988). This procedure involves pairing stimuli associated with a problem behavior with a decelerative consequence, such as firmly delivered reprimand or a brief restraint procedure.

There are three ways to employ the recreate-the-situation procedure: audiotape mediation (Rolider & Van Houten, 1985a); videotape mediation, and physical guidance mediation (Van Houten & Rolider, 1988). In the audiotape and videotape mediation procedures, a sample of an audiotape or videotape containing the inappropriate behavior is presented to the individual, followed by a planned consequence. The audiotape procedure can be employed when the behavior has a strong verbal component, as is typically the case with tantrum behavior; the videotape procedure is required whenever the behavior has a significant motor component. The use of both of these procedures is limited to clients who can differentially respond to audio and video feedback.

In the physical guidance mediation approach, each recreation trial is initiated by asking in a firm and disapproving tone of voice for the client to demonstrate parts of his or her inappropriate acts. If the client refuses, the behavior is manually guided. Later, a prearranged consequence follows the behavior.

The recreate-the-situation procedures are useful when the generalization from the one-on-one therapy situation to the natural setting is not complete. Typically this problem arises in situations where the mediators who have acquired personal stimulus control are not present. The use of the above procedures in these circumstances by the mediators who have personal stimulus control can greatly extend the degree of generalization.

EXAMPLES

Treatment plans based upon the interpersonal treatment model were introduced for the five children whose assessment data were reported in Figure 3. Subject 1 was provided with a program to teach him to wait, to accept termination of reinforcers, and to accept denial of reinforcers. He was taught to wait by placing edible and toy reinforcers on the table, one at a time, for progressively longer durations before he could consume or play with the reinforcer. All treatment was begun using the reinforcers that he had the least amount of difficulty waiting for, then gradually progressing to the reinforcer associated with the most difficulty. The subject did not progress to the next reinforcer until he could successfully wait for the previous reinforcer. Lavish approval was provided whenever the subject waited for the predetermined time, and the subject was able to consume or play with the reinforcer for a short period of time. Whenever the child attempted to reach for the edible or

→

FIGURE 5. The results produced using the interpersonal treatment model with subjects 1 through 5.

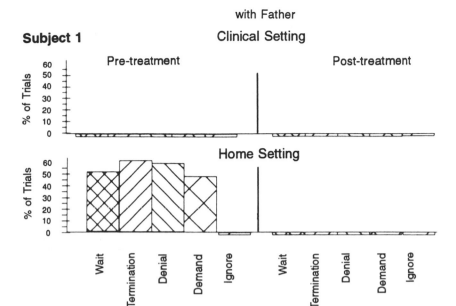

with Father

Subject 1 Clinical Setting

Pre-treatment Post-treatment

% of Trials

Home Setting

% of Trials

Wait Termination Denial Demand Ignore Wait Termination Denial Demand Ignore

Precursor Events

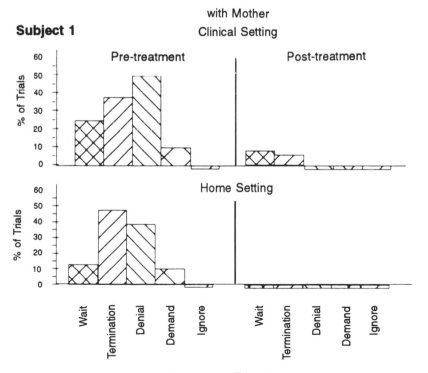

with Mother

Subject 1 Clinical Setting

Pre-treatment Post-treatment

% of Trials

Home Setting

% of Trials

Wait Termination Denial Demand Ignore Wait Termination Denial Demand Ignore

Precursor Events

157

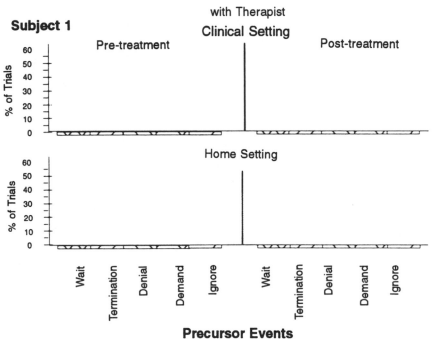

FIGURE 5. (*continued*)

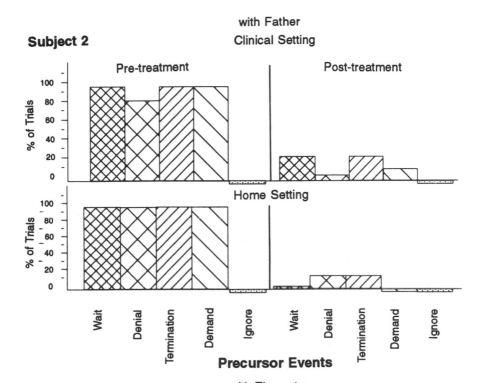

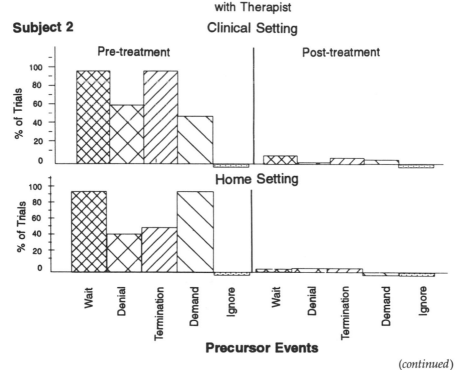

(continued)

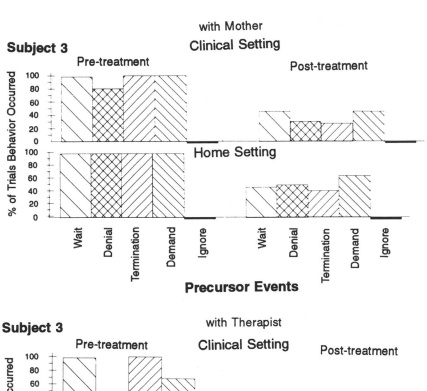

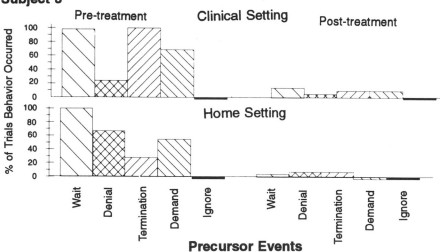

FIGURE 5. (*continued*)

160

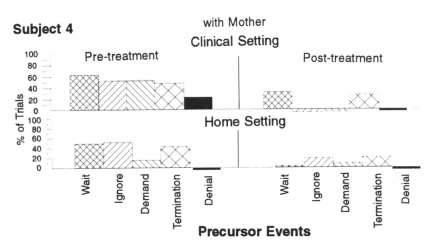

Subject 4   with Mother

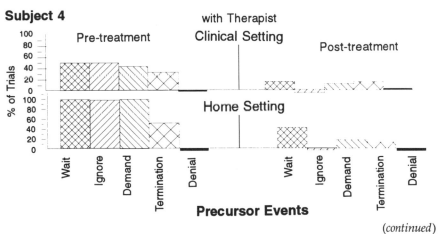

Subject 4   with Therapist

(*continued*)

161

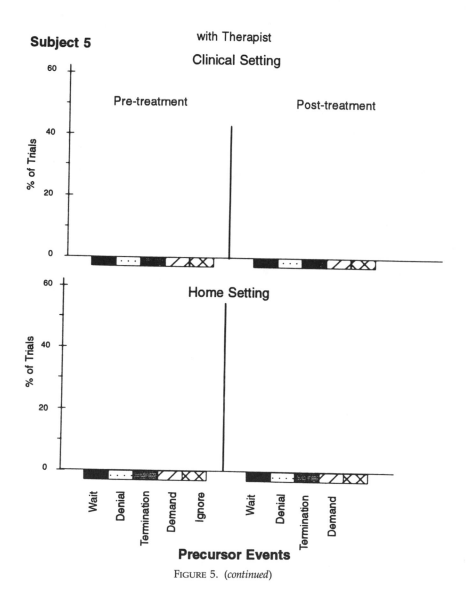

FIGURE 5. (continued)

Subject 5

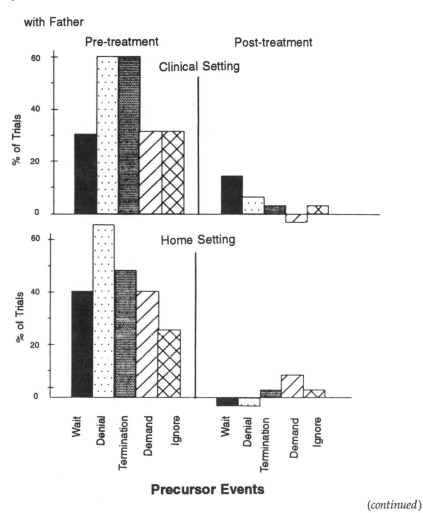

with Father

Pre-treatment   Post-treatment

Clinical Setting

Home Setting

Precursor Events

(*continued*)

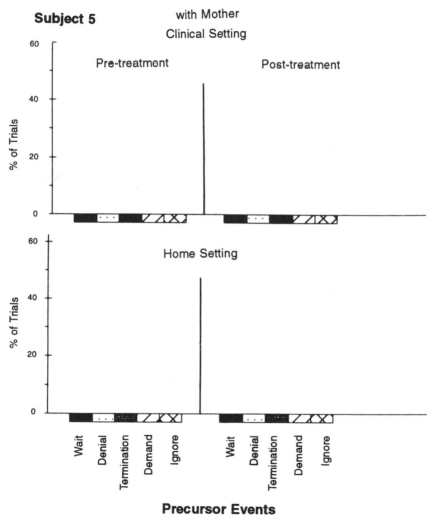

FIGURE 5. (*continued*)

the toy, the therapist mediator delivered a firm reprimand ("No, you don't touch; you have to wait") and the response was abruptly blocked. A second waiting program involved having the subject hold the reinforcer without eating or playing with it for progressively longer periods of time. Once the subject could successfully wait for the reinforcer that was previously associated with the highest frequency of the problem behaviors, the distance between the subject and the mediator was gradually increased.

The client was taught to accept the termination of reinforcers by providing him with a reinforcer such as a toy or play activity for several minutes (or, if it was an edible reinforcer, several bites). Next, the mediator firmly asked the subject to give him or her the reinforcer. The child received lavish praise when he complied with the request, and a firm reprimand if he did not give up the reinforcer. If the child did not give up the reinforcer following the first reprimand, a series of several reprimands was delivered with increasing firmness. If necessary, the mediator physically assisted the child in giving up the item on the third reprimand. The amount of time between the subject giving up the reinforcer and the reinforcer being presented again was gradually increased over time from 15 seconds to 10 minutes. As in the case of waiting, treatment was begun with a reinforcer that the child had little difficulty giving up and gradually moved to those items associated with more severe behavior. Once the subject could accept the termination of the reinforcer most frequently associated with the behavior, the distance between the mediator and the subject was gradually increased by moving the chairs further apart.

The subject was taught to accept denial in the following manner. First, various items that the child liked were placed on a table situated on the side of the mediator and subject. The mediator then waited for the child to request or reach for one of the items. If the child did not request or attempt to reach for an item, the session was terminated. If the child requested the item, he was told, "You cannot have that right now." If the child reached for the item, the mediator reprimanded the behavior while quickly grasping the child's hand and abruptly placing it back on his lap and releasing it.

This procedure was repeated each time the child attempted to grab an item. If the child sat without attempting to grab or request an item for the 2 minutes, the mediator provided lavish praise and terminated the trial and offered an alternative reinforcer. As in the case of teaching waiting and termination of reinforcers, the distance between the mediator and the subject was gradually increased once the latter could accept denial when seated in the knee-to-knee seating arrangement. The therapist was the first mediator to work with the child, followed by the father and finally the mother.

Figure 5 shows the results of this intervention with subjects 1 through 5. Subject 1's data show marked reductions in antisocial behavior in the presence of all of the precursor events in the analogue setting following the treatment condition. This change occurred in the presence of all three mediators.

Similar treatment procedures were employed for subjects 2 through 5; the results obtained for subjects 2, 4, and 5 were very similar to those produced with subject 1. Although subject 3 showed large reductions with the therapist, only moderate reductions were produced in the presence of the boy's mother. Although data were not collected by the parents throughout the day, it was the opinion of each of the parents that the behavior had improved considerably throughout the day after the treatment was introduced.

SUMMARY

This chapter presented a model for the treatment of severely inappropriate behavior in persons with acquired brain injury, developmental disabilities, and severe conduct disorders. The model is based upon the delineation and manipulation of precursor stimuli in a structured teaching environment. The first step in the treatment process is to perform a complete behavioral analysis; any behavioral analysis is incomplete unless the stimuli controlling the occurrence of the behavior are completely identified. Particular care should be taken to identify eliciting stimuli, including those associated with periods of extinction. It is also important to teach functional alternatives.

Clients often need to be taught assertive and cooperative behaviors, as well as appropriate social inhibitions. These behaviors are taught in a structured environment in the presence of the gradual introduction of the precursor stimuli controlling the inappropriate behavior. Personal stimulus control is established through the use of social contingencies to influence behavior change. Once personal stimulus control is established by several mediators in the controlled setting, the degree of control is assessed in the client's natural environment. In most cases, personal stimulus control established in one setting transfers to other settings. In some cases when it is not perfectly established by the natural mediators, procedures can be employed to assist them in achieving an adequate level of influence through the use of mediational procedures.

REFERENCES

Axelrod, S. (1987). Functional and structural analyses of behavior: Approaches leading to reduced use of punishment procedures. *Research in Developmental Disabilities, 8,* 165–178.

Azrin, N. H., Besalel, V. A., Jammer, J. P., & Caputo, J. N. (1988). Comparative study of behavioral methods of treating self-injury. *Behavioral Residential Treatment, 3,* 119–152.

Azrin, N. H., Hutchinson, R. R., & Hake, D. F. (1966). Extinction induced aggression. *Journal of the Experimental Analysis of Behavior, 9,* 191–204.

Azrin, N. H., Hutchinson, R. R., & Sallery, R. D. (1964). Pain-aggression toward inanimate objects. *Journal of the Experimental Analysis of Behavior, 7,* 223–228.

Bird, F., Dores, P. A., Moniz, D., & Robinson, J. (1989). Reducing severe aggressive and self-injurious behaviors with functional communication training. *American Journal on Mental Retardation*, *94*, 37–48.

Bitgood, S. C., Crowe, M. J., Suarez, Y., & Peters, R. D. (1980). Immobilization: Effects and side effects on stereotyped behavior in children, *Behavior Modification*, *4*, 187–208.

Carr, E. G., & Durand, V. M. (1985). Reducing behavior problems through functional communication training. *Journal of Applied Behavior Analysis*, *18*, 111–126.

Carr, E. G., & Newsom, C. D. (1985). Demand-related tantrums: Conceptualization and treatment. *Behavior Modification*, *9*, 403–426.

Charlop, M. H., Schreibman, L., & Thibodeau, M. G. (1985). Increasing spontaneous verbal responding in autistic children using a time delay procedure. *Journal of Applied Behavior Analysis*, *18*, 155–166.

Day, R. M., Rea, J. A., Schussler, N. G., Larsen, S. E., & Johnson, W. L. (1988). A functionally based approach to the treatment of self-injurious behavior. *Behavior Modification*, *12*, 565–589.

Durand, V. M., & Crimmins, D. B. (1988). Identifying the variables maintaining self-injurious behavior. *Journal of Autism and Developmental Disorders*, *18*, 99–117.

Durand, V. M., & Kishi, G. (1987). Reducing severe behavior problems among persons with dual sensory impairments: An evaluation of a technical assistance model. *Journal of the Association for Persons With Severe Handicaps*, *12*, 2–10.

Falk, J. L. (1966). The motivational properties of schedule-induced polydipsia. *Journal of the Experimental Analysis of Behavior*, *9*, 19–25.

Favell, J. E., McGimsey, J. F., & Jones, M. L. (1978). The use of physical restraint in the treatment of self-injury and as positive reinforcement. *Journal of Applied Behavior Analysis*, *11*, 225–241.

Flory, R. K., Smith, E. L. P., & Ellis, B. A. (1977). The effects of two response-elimination procedures on reinforced and induced aggression. *Journal of the Experimental Analysis of Behavior*, *25*, 5–15.

Gentry, W. D. (1968). Fixed-ratio schedule-induced aggression. *Journal of the Experimental Analysis of Behavior*, *11*, 813–817.

Griffin, J. C., Locke, B. J., & Landers, W. F. (1975). Manipulation of potential punishment parameters in the treatment of self-injury. *Journal of Applied Behavior Analysis*, *8*, 458.

Hamlet, C. C., Axelrod, S., & Kuerschner, S. (1984). Eye contact as an antecedent to compliant behavior. *Journal of Applied Behavior Analysis*, *17*, 381–387.

Hutchinson, R. R., Azrin, N. H., & Hunt, G. M. (1968). Attack produced by intermittent reinforcement of a concurrent operant response. *Journal of the Experimental Analysis of Behavior*, *11*, 489–495.

Ingemey, R., & Van Houten, R. (1991). The use of time delay to promote spontaneous speech in an autistic child during play. *Journal of Applied Behavior Analysis*, *24*, 591–596.

Iwata, B. A., Dorsey, M. F., Slifer, K. J., Bauman, K. E., & Richman, G. S. (1982). Toward a functional analysis of self-injury. *Analysis and Intervention in Developmental Disabilities*, *2*, 3–20.

Iwata, B. A., Pace, G. M., Kalsher, M. J., Cowdery, G. E., & Cataldo, M. F. (1990). Experimental analysis and extinction of self-injurious escape behavior. *Journal of Applied Behavior Analysis*, *23*, 11–27.

Mace, C., Hock, M. L., Lalli, J. S., West, B. J., Belfiore, P., Pinter, E., & Brown, D. K. (1988). Behavioral momentum in the treatment of noncompliance. *Journal of Applied Behavior Analysis*, *21*, 123–141.

Mace, F. C., Page, T. J., Ivancic M. T., & O'Brien, S. (1986). Analysis of environmental determinants of aggression and disruption in mentally retarded children. *Applied Research in Mental Retardation*, *7*, 203–221.

Rapoff, M. A., Altman, K., & Christophersen, E. R. (1980). Reducing aggressive and self-injurious behavior in institutionalized retarded blind child's self-hitting by response-contingent brief restraint. *Education and Treatment of Children*, *3*, 231–236.

Rincover, A., & Devany, J. (1982). The application of sensory extinction procedures to self-injury. *Analysis and Intervention in Developmental Disabilities, 2,* 67–81.

Rodgers, T. A., Zarcone, J. R., & Iwata, B. A. (1990). *A comparison of methods for conducting functional analysis of self-injurious behavior.* Paper presented at the 16th annual convention of the Association for Behavior Analysis, Nashville, TN.

Rolider, A., Cummings, A., & Van Houten, R. (1991). Side effects of therapeutic punishment on academic performance and eye contact of two persons with developmental handicaps. *Journal of Applied Behavior Analysis, 24,* 763–773.

Rolider A., & Van Houten, R. (1985a). Suppressing tantrum behavior in public places through the use of delayed punishment mediated by audio recordings. *Behavior Therapy, 16,* 181–191.

Rolider, A., & Van Houten, R. (1985b). Movement suppression timeout and undesirable behavior in psychotic and severely developmentally delayed children. *Journal of Applied Behavior Analysis, 18,* 275–288.

Rolider, A., Williams, L., Cummings, A., & Van Houten, R. (1991). The use of a brief movement restriction procedure to eliminate severe inappropriate behavior. *Journal of Behavior Therapy and Experimental Psychiatry, 22,* 23–30.

Sailor, W., Guess, D., Rutherford, G., & Baer, D. M. (1968). Control of tantrum behavior by operant techniques during experimental verbal training. *Journal of Applied Behavior Analysis, 1,* 237–243.

Saloviita, T. (1988). Elimination of self-injurious behaviour by brief physical restraint and DRA. *Scandinavian Journal of Behavior Therapy, 17,* 55–63.

Schloss, P. J., Smith, M., Santora, C., & Bryant, R. (1989). A respondent conditioning approach to reducing anger responses of a dually diagnosed man with mild mental retardation. *Behavior Therapy, 20,* 459–464.

Singh, N. N., Dawson, M. J., & Manning, P. J. (1981). The effects of physical restraint on self-injurious behaviour. *Journal of Mental Deficiency Research, 25,* 207–216.

Thomas, D. R., Becker, W. C., & Armstrong, M. (1968). Production and elimination of disruptive classroom behavior by systematically varying teacher's behavior. *Journal of Applied Behavior Analysis, 1,* 35–45.

Touchette, P. E., MacDonald, R. F., & Langer, S. N. (1985). A scatter plot for identifying stimulus control of problem behavior. *Journal of Applied Behavior Analysis, 18,* 343–351.

Ulrich, R. E., & Azrin, N. H. (1962). Reflexive fighting in response to aversive stimulation. *Journal of the Experimental Analysis of Behavior, 5,* 511–520.

Van Houten, R., & Rolider, A. (1988). Recreating the scene: An effective way to provide delayed punishment. *Journal of Applied Behavior Analysis, 21,* 187–192.

Van Houten, R., & Rolider, A. (1989). An analysis of several variables influencing flash card instruction. *Journal of Applied Behavior Analysis, 22,* 111–118.

Van Houten, R., & Rolider, A (1991). Applied behavior analysis. In J. L. Matson & J. A. Mulick (Eds). *Handbook of mental retardation* (pp. 574–577) New York: Pergamon.

Zarcone, J. R., Rodgers, T. A., & Iwata, B. A. (1990). *Reliability analysis of the Motivation Assessment Scale.* Paper presented at the 16th annual convention of the Association for Behavior Analysis, Nashville, TN.

Zarkowski, E., & Clements, J. (1988). *Problem behavior in people with severe learning disabilities: A practical guide to a constructional approach.* London: Croon Helm.

Providing State-of-the-Art Treatment

Ensuring the Competence of Behavior Analysts

Gerald L. Shook and Ron Van Houten

The role of an applied behavior analyst is to provide effective treatment for clients though the use of scientifically validated techniques within an ethical framework. Given the complexity of the principles governing human behavior, a competent clinical applied behavior analyst must display a large array of highly refined skills and must keep abreast of new developments in a rapidly evolving field.

Professional Training

Behavior analysts working on difficult clinical cases must be particularly well trained and perform to the highest standards. In a sense, a behavior analyst involved with a demanding case has much in common with a surgeon (R. M. Foxx, 1987, personal communication). Both of these professionals (a) conduct preintervention assessments in order to determine the variables that control the problem (or behavior) and to determine the sensitivity of the client to a variety of interventions, (b) work directly with the client, (c) do not merely prescribe procedures but rather conduct them until success is assured, and (d) are responsible for the behavior of those who are to maintain the therapeutic effect.

Gerald L. Shook • Shook & Associates/Community Environments, 310 East College Avenue, Tallahasee, Florida 32301.   Ron Van Houten • Psychology Department, Mount Saint Vincent University, Halifax, Nova Scotia B3M 2J6.

Behavior Analysis and Treatment, edited by R. Van Houten & S. Axelrod. Plenum Press, New York, 1993.

To the greatest extent possible, the behavior analyst, like the surgeon, draws upon scientific evidence to treat clients most effectively. Just as the surgeon may find during surgery that what appeared to be routine has become exploratory, however, the behavior analyst may not always find a standard program that is effective, or he or she may discover that information is not available on how best to apply a given procedure in a particular situation. In such instances, the behavior analyst must draw and extrapolate from previous training and knowledge in order to make treatment decisions. The behavior analyst working on a difficult clinical case also must often provide hands-on treatment. Just as the thoracic surgeon would not attempt to perform bypass surgery by writing out the steps in the treatment procedure (i.e., the bypass operation) and asking a parent, teacher, or aide to conduct it, neither do behavior analysts approach complex problems in this manner (R. M. Foxx, 1987, personal communication). Because behavior analysts with demanding cases are often required to employ complex hands-on skills, it would seem reasonable that training programs for behavior analysis could be modeled on the successful methods employed to train surgeons.

The training of a surgeon begins with learning anatomy and other content areas in a classroom environment. As a function of the hands-on nature of the profession, however, additional training is provided via supervised practicum. The student may begin by making a few simple incisions, suturing, assisting general surgeons with uncomplicated operations, closing at the completion of various operations, performing uncomplicated operations, assisting in complicated operations, and finally conducting complicated procedures himself or herself. After such an apprenticeship in thoracic surgery, the individual may be capable of performing coronary bypasses.

Some of the skills required of a competent behavior analyst may be acquired in the classroom through reading articles and books, by attending lectures and demonstrations, or by other similar means. Because many behavioral treatment techniques are quite complex as well as subtle, however, they may be acquired best through supervised direct experience. It is therefore essential that professionals responsible for delivering, directing, or evaluating behavioral treatment programs be given both appropriate classroom training and supervised experience. Training should result in persons having a thorough knowledge of behavioral principles, methods of assessment and treatment, research methodology, and professional ethics (Van Houten et al., 1988). Clinical competence may be developed through practicum and internship experiences with relevant client populations, with supervision being provided by qualified behavior analysts. As with the training of a surgeon, the student may begin with simple behavioral operations and systematically progress, with guidance from the supervisor, to more complex challenges.

PROFESSIONAL OVERSIGHT

One problem in the field of behavior analysis has been that untrained people often attempt to perform very difficult behavioral procedures. This is a serious problem, because small differences in how procedures are applied can make the difference between success and failure (R. M. Foxx, 1987, personal communication). To avoid this problem, it may be necessary to allow only highly qualified behavior analysts to develop, provide, and oversee behavioral treatment, especially in the initial stages of a complex intervention. When the success of the intervention has been assured, therapists who have less comprehensive behavior analysis training may be involved in the treatment.

Complex interventions should not be thought of as consisting only of those programs designed to reduce severe inappropriate behavior. Complex acquisition procedures often require equal skill and training, and even reinforcement procedures, if implemented incorrectly, can result in the development of significant behavior problems. The generalization and maintenance of appropriate behavior in the natural environment may present a greater challenge still. Thus, a well-trained, qualified behavior analyst should provide oversight of all behavioral programming to help ensure the best therapeutic effect.

The analyst responsible for overseeing a behavioral program should ensure that therapists who will conduct the program are well trained and competent in its implementation. This may be accomplished by having the therapists observe and practice the program before they are responsible for it, testing their hands-on knowledge and expertise before they are allowed to function as therapist, and collecting relevant data on therapist and client performance during the intervention.

The behavior analyst should provide supervision during all aspects of the program implementation. Supervision should include scheduled periodic direct observations of the therapist implementing the program. Components of the therapist's performance should be evaluated via a standard format, and constructive, specific feedback should be provided vocally and in writing. This process is particularly effective if it is made part of the formal staff evaluation procedure.

In difficult cases with severe problems that may be life threatening, Lovaas and Favell (1987) recommend that behavior analysts only supervise a relatively small number of cases. The right to treatment by a competent behavior analyst cannot be met unless the caregivers who deliver the treatment perform their duties in a competent manner, and this requires extensive time for training and supervision.

In addition, the supervising behavior analyst should be available to make treatment decisions when required. In some cases, possible problems can be anticipated and conditional programs can be recommended; in others, however, it will be necessary for the behavior analyst to consult about unanticipated problems in a timely fashion. Such direct consultation is particularly critical when the treatment involves dangerous behaviors or highly restrictive procedures. The right to access is part of a client's right to an effective behavior analyst.

DEVELOPING THE PROFESSION OF BEHAVIOR ANALYSIS

Members of the medical community heavily influence what constitutes ethical, effective state-of-the-art treatment in the field of medicine, and practitioners have a large degree of professional latitude. Physicians have achieved this latitude through the control exercised by the profession in training, monitoring, and regulating the practice of medicine; it ensures a minimum standard of trust and competence that allows the practitioners to discharge their duties in an efficient manner. The medical profession helps to ensure that its members are accountable, that they work from a scientific basis, and that they possess the clinical and behavioral skills required to guarantee the best treatment for their clients (R. M. Foxx, 1987, personal communication). The profession provides leadership in accrediting university medical programs and participates in the credentialing of medical professionals.

At present there is no formalized profession of behavior analysis to provide leadership in the regulation of its members. Often state governments establish systems to regulate the practice of behavior analysis (Johnston & Shook, 1987, 1993; Shook, 1988); these systems generally include manuals or guidelines that dictate what behavioral procedures may be used, under what conditions procedures may be used, and what process must be followed by a practitioner in getting approval to use a given procedure. Often, well-trained behavior analysts must obtain approval to use a procedure from a committee made up of individuals who, in many cases, have little or no training in behavior analysis. Although such a system may be helpful in protecting the client with regard to human rights issues, it is not as useful in ensuring best practice. Surely surgeons would not agree to similar constraints on their professional behavior.

Yet if behavior analysts are to enjoy the same degree of professional latitude that physicians enjoy, it is essential that they develop a profession with a comparable uniform standard and level of competence. A physician demonstrating a new surgical technique at a conference of surgeons can confidently ask anyone in the audience to suture the patient, because such a basic procedure would be familiar to everyone present. One could not be so confident at a behavior analysis conference, however, that anyone present could come forth and conduct a specific procedure. In light of this problem, behavior analysts must develop uniform standards within the profession and ensure that practitioners meet these standards. Such action will foster professional latitude and help the profession gain the general acceptance required to provide effective treatment for clients.

The profession of behavior analysis must help guarantee that practitioners possess the appropriate educational background, hands-on skills, experience with procedures and populations, behavioral diagnostic skills, and up-to-date contact with the literature and colleagues. The profession also needs to ensure that practitioners are accountable within the profession, work from a scientific basis, employ data-based decision-making techniques, and provide ethical and humane treatment.

If these goals are to be achieved, it will be necessary to establish a strong behavior analysis professional discipline. To date, behavior analysis has been a subject area spread out over a number of fields, such as psychology, education, and family studies. In order to train and develop new practitioners, behavior analysts rely upon the goodwill of the members of these discipline areas; unfortunately, goodwill has been a transient and scarce commodity. Therefore, despite the great success of applied behavior analysis, membership in the field has shown little growth in recent years.

For example, most behavioral clinicians are trained in graduate programs housed in psychology departments. The production of new behavior analysts, therefore, is directly related to the number of behavioral faculty hired by psychology departments granting graduate degrees. Because these departments are predominantly staffed by traditionally oriented psychologists, there is little inclination on the part of the department to hire behavior analysts. It is little wonder that the membership of the principal behavior analysis professional organization has not shown tremendous growth in recent years (Graf, 1991; Vargas, 1989)—even though the demand for professional behavior analysts in the marketplace has increased substantially, and positions go unfilled or are filled with less than qualified applicants.

An important question, therefore, is whether behavior analysts wish to continue being a relatively powerless subdiscipline of such other major disciplines as psychology and education, or whether they wish to move toward forming their own autonomous discipline. Some behavior analysts (Epstein, 1984; Fraley & Vargas, 1986) have made the case for establishing a separate field in the area of behavior analysis. Epstein (1984) pointed out that psychology is not likely ever to reject mentalism, and that as long as there are only a fixed number of positions in psychology departments, behavior analysis will not thrive. He further stated, however, that the promotion of a new discipline does not require the immediate withdrawal of all behavior analysts from psychology.

Fraley and Vargas (1986) pointed out that psychology departments are predominantly made up of a variety of cognitive psychologists. Because this means more cognitive psychologists are being trained in psychology departments than behavior analysts, it is impossible to shift this unfavorable ratio. Harzem (1987), on the other hand, reasons that we should not abandon the tradition of psychology, from which behavior analysis has arisen. He and others feel that behavior analysis may yet have a major impact on psychology and can benefit from its association with psychologists (Nuringer, 1991).

In time, the issue of whether behavior analysis will remain as a subdiscipline of psychology or strike out on its own will be answered by evolution within both fields. In the short run, however, it may prove useful to promote behavior analysis as a separate field at some times and as a subdiscipline of psychology at others. For example, in jurisdictions where behavior analysts cannot become licensed as psychologists and are thereby prevented by legislation from practicing their profession, a separate act to license behavior analysts would make sense. Under more favorable circumstances, it is possible that behavior analysts could collectively negotiate with psychologists so as to allow the former to become regulated under the act that licenses the latter. Even if behavior analysts decide to affirm their roots in psychology, it is not unreasonable for psychology programs to seek accreditation in applied behavior analysis (as described below).

In any event, moves to strengthen the identity of behavior analysis should work toward extending the influence and growth of the profession. In this regard, the development of departments of behavior analysis should promote its influence in society and cause more people to take favorable notice of the field's achievements. Psychology may respond to the resulting increased interest in behavior analysis by paying more attention, as well.

FORMAL MECHANISMS TO ENSURE COMPETENCE

There are several reasonable formal mechanisms that may be used by the profession to help ensure the competence of behavior analysts. First, the professional association may accredit university graduate programs that meet established training requirements. Second, professional associations may provide recognition to members who have met standards of competence established by the organization. Third, states or provinces may license practicing behavior analysts. Finally, professional organizations may provide a program of continuing education and professional development that keeps members abreast of new developments in the field. The above means are not mutually exclusive, and several might be employed together in order to achieve the goal of assuring the competence of behavior analysts.

Accreditation of Training Programs

The first way to help guarantee the competence of behavior analysts is to set standards for university training programs. This method may be thought of as ensuring the competence of behavior analysts from the front end. The assumption underlying accreditation of training programs is that appropriately trained students should be adequately qualified to practice behavior analysis.

There are several reasons why the existence of training programs meeting a quality standard is a prerequisite for establishing an autonomous profession. First, appropriate training programs could train the number of behavior analysts required both to argue persuasively for recognition as a profession and to meet society's needs. Second, the existence of specific training programs in behavior analysis within recognized institutions of higher learning would help to document its existence as a profession. Third, accreditation standards would serve a quality control function by ensuring that persons trained in behavior analysis would complete course work and other requirements in those areas that professionals in the field consider to be essential for appropriate practice. Fourth, training standards recognized by all professionals in the field would encourage consistency in licensing standards from state to state, or province to province.

The Association for Behavioral Analysis (ABA), in response to reports from two of its task forces (Hopkins et al., 1991; Shook et al., 1988) established a six-person board to accredit programs of study in behavior analysis at the master's and doctoral level. At the master's level, the course of study must provide instruction in behavior analytic approaches to research and/or conceptual issues and behavioral interventions. The program also must include a thesis, review paper, or general examination based on a behavior analytic approach to problems or issues. At the doctoral level, the course of study must provide instruction in behavior analytic approaches to research and/or conceptual issues and include advanced curriculum topics in a specialized area of nonhuman and/or human basic research literature, research methods, and in one or more applied areas. In addition, a dissertation is required in which questions and methods are based on a behavior analytic approach to problems and issues.

The accreditation board evaluates applications for accreditation by studying detailed information on the content of all courses, the methods and standards of evaluation, and the credentials of the faculty members. In addition, board members visit sites to meet with faculty and students and to inspect facilities. Subsequent to a site visit, an accreditation hearing is conducted at the annual meeting of the ABA, and the board recommends to the ABA executive council that the program be either accredited or denied accreditation. All accreditation is to be reviewed every 5 years. Accreditation standards, however, are to be reviewed annually; such a mechanism is essential if an accreditation program is to keep pace with new developments in the field. Without such a review process, there would be a danger that the discipline would stagnate, becoming more like a guild and less scientifically oriented.

Although this accreditation process makes a significant contribution toward standardizing training in the field of behavior analysis, it does not address adequately the specific coursework or hands-on performance required by behavior analysts working directly with clients in such areas as developmental disabilities and behavioral medicine. It is hoped that the standards will be expanded to address these important issues in the future in order to reflect current behavior analysis research on teaching clinical and other behavior analytic skills most effectively.

Diplomate in Behavior Therapy

A second way to help ensure the competence of behavior analysts is to recognize individuals demonstrating a senior level of competence in a specialty area by establishing diplomate status within the broader profession of psychology. The American Board of Behavioral Psychology was established by the Association for the Advancement of Behavior Therapy to award diplomate status to licensed psychologists who have attained excellence in the behavioral field. The diploma in behavior therapy is intended to cover subspecialization in behavior analysis as well as behavior therapy, cognitive therapy, or cognitive-behavior therapy (American Board of Behavioral Psychology, 1989).

Applicants must be licensed psychologists and submit an application for candidacy with documentation that they meet a number of criteria. prior to taking an exam, the candidate must pay a fee and submit one or more work samples reflecting his or her typical practice. The candidate may also send in a videotape of treatment sessions to accompany the description of a case and the data obtained. The work sample is then examined by a three-person examining committee that generally consists of diplomate-level psychologists from the same subspecialty field. The work sample review is followed by an oral examination that comprises an observation of skills in realistic problem assessment, effectiveness research, and sensitivity to ethical implications of professional practice. It is also possible to expand upon this procedure by requiring the candidate to generate a work sample in the presence of the evaluation panel as a form of clinical simulation. The tone of the examination is intended to be one of professional interaction among peers and colleagues, as opposed to an interrogation of the candidate by the examination committee.

Behavior analysts who are licensed psychologists and who meet the qualifications for diplomate status should apply for it. If a number of behavior analysts attain diplomate status, it will certainly add support to the behavioral movement within psychology.

Licensure of Professionals

As mentioned above, another way to assure the competence of behavior analysts is by licensing individuals who practice behavior analysis (Shook,

1993). Licensure programs are established at the state or provincial level through legislation and are administered by the state or province in the form of either a title act or a practice act. A *title act* protects and limits the use of professional title. Under such an act, individuals could not call themselves behavior analysts unless they were so licensed, although they could practice behavior analysis without limitation. A *practice act*, in contrast, includes title protection but extends limitations into the practice of behavior analysis, as well. Under a behavior analysis practice act, unlicensed individuals could neither call themselves behavior analysts nor do any of the things the act defined as the practice of behavior analysis. Both title and practice acts usually apply only when individuals charge for their services, so parents, for instance could apply behavior analysis principles without a license. Both title and practice acts generally have a number of exemptions as to who is required to have a license; certified teachers, social workers, and any number of other professionals could be exempted.

Licensure acts regulating a profession typically specify educational and experience requirements, and they require individuals to pass a written examination. The educational requirement in most acts usually specifies the degree required, the course work required in the specialty area, and the amount of practical or field training required. For example, a bill introduced before the Florida legislature to license behavior analysts requires 27 semester hours of graduate course work. Among the courses required are those in behavior analysis research designs and behavioral research methods, as well as behavioral courses in 3 out of 10 areas of study. The proposed act also requires a course on ethics, and a minimum of one supervised practicum, internship, or field experience in the area of behavior analysis.

Licensing acts typically also require an amount of experience supervised by a qualified individual. The supervisor generally must possess the credential of the profession involved and may need to meet additional requirements, such as a specified number of years of active practice within the profession.

Some form of written examination is a part of all licensing programs, and it is occasionally supplemented with a performance component. The written examination is developed by professional test construction firms with considerable input from professionals working in the content area. The content of the examination is taken both from a job analysis (essentially a task analysis) of what practitioners do and from survey work and consultation from professionals in the field to be tested. A written examination without a performance component generally is the preferred format of test construction professionals (Johnston & Shook, 1987); however, the notion of performance testing holds obvious appeal for behavior analysts and is most certainly in an area in which the field can make significant contributions. For example, such basic skills as reinforcement of a behavior or providing instructions might be evaluated through the direct observation of treatment sessions or through videotapes or simulations of clinical sessions.

Licensure programs generally have provisions for disciplining persons licensed under the act who engage in unethical or illegal behavior. Licenses must be renewed periodically, usually by documenting the completion of continuing education requirements and paying a renewal fee. Most licensure programs are primarily or wholly funded through fees paid by those being licensed.

Behavior analysts will need to work with their state association for behavior analysis and various branches of their state government to obtain a licensing program. This process will have political and fiscal requirements beyond those usually encountered by behavior analysts and will demand a multiyear commitment for those who wish to establish such a program.

Continuing Education

A continuing education program within the professional organization is a fourth way to help ensure the competence of behavior analysts. The intent of continuing education requirements is to ensure that professionals remain current in the content of their profession after their primary education has been completed, thereby maintaining a high level of professional competence. Professional organizations such as the Association for Behavior Analysis can help to ensure that members stay abreast of developments by providing a balanced program at their annual meetings and by offering continuing education courses or workshops just prior to the start of such conferences. Of course, they should also take the measures necessary to make sure that attendance at these courses will be accepted by state licensing boards.

The ABA might consider providing a membership category that would require that a specific amount of continuing education be completed in order for the member to continue in that category. This membership category approach might evolve into a more formal diplomate status through the addition of education, experience, professional reference, and perhaps even performance requirements as the program developed toward a professional registration program.

SUMMARY

The protection of the right of persons to treatment by a competent behavior analyst is intertwined with the development and regulation of behavior analysis as a profession. Surgeons do not have to contend with state-generated manuals, procedure review committees, or untrained bureaucrats who dictate how they will practice their profession. They can avoid these indignities because their profession has taken it upon itself to ensure the competence of its own membership by taking the initiative to regulate the profession. Several methods have been discussed in this chapter that together perhaps represent what needs to be accomplished if behavior analysts wish to ensure true competence within their own profession. Certainly the client would be the ultimate benefactor.

REFERENCES

American Board of Behavioral Psychology. (1989). *Procedures and regulations for the creation of the diplomate in behavior therapy.* New York: Author.

Epstein, R. (1984). The case for praxis. *Behavior Analyst, 7,* 101–119.

Fraley, L. E., & Vargas, E. A. (1986). Separate disciplines: The study of behavior and the study of psyche. *Behavior Analyst, 9,* 47–59.

Graf, S. (1991). ABA membership reaches record level. *ABA Newsletter, 14,* 1.

Harzem, P. (1987). On the virtues of being a psychologist. *Behavior Analyst, 10,* 175–181.

Hopkins, B., Bailey, J. S., Blase, K., Bushnell, D., Cuvo, T., Fuqua, W., Heward, W. Johnston, J. M., Lattal, K., Salzburg, C. & Schreibman, L. (1991). *Second report of the task force on accreditation.* Kalamazoo, MI: Association for Behavior Analysis.

Johnston, J. M., & Shook, G. L. (1987). Developing behavior analysis at the state level. *Behavior Analyst, 10,* 199–233.

Johnston, J. M., & Shook, G. L. (1993). A model for the state-wide delivery of programming services. *Mental Retardation, 31,* 127–139.

Lovaas, I. O. & Favell, J. E. (1987). Protection for clients undergoing aversive restrictive interventions. *Education and Treatment of Children, 10,* 311–325.

Nuringer, A. (1991). Behaviorism: Methodological, radical, assertive, skeptical, ethological, modest, humble, and evolving. *Behavior Analyst, 14,* 43–47.

Shook, G. L. (1988). Managing behavior management: The Florida system. *Advocate, 1,* 8–9.

Shook, G. L. (1993). The professional credential in behavior analysis. *Behavior Analyst, 16,* 87–101.

Shook, G. L., Johnston, J. M., Cone, J., Thomas, D., Greer, D., Beard, J., & Herring, R. (1988). *Credentialing, quality assurance, and right to practice.* Kalamazoo, MI: Association for Behavior Analysis.

Van Houten, R., Axelrod, S., Bailey, J. S., Favell, J. E., Foxx, R. M., Iwata, B. A., & Lovaas, O. I. (1988). The right to effective treatment. *Journal of Applied Behavior Analysis, 21,* 381–384.

Vargas, J. S. (1989). The road less traveled. *Behavior Analyst, 12,* 121–130.

A Decision-Making Model for Selecting the Optimal Treatment Procedure

Saul Axelrod, Scott Spreat, Brian Berry, and Lynn Moyer

In delineating the rights due to all persons receiving treatment, Van Houten et al. (1988) indicated that each individual has a right to the least restrictive effective procedures that are available. In further delineating this right, the authors specified that a practitioner should not employ restrictive procedures unless it could be shown that such tactics were necessary to produce safe and meaningful behavior change. On the other hand, the report stated that it was unacceptable to expose people to nonrestrictive procedures that were unlikely to work. Thus, it becomes a delicate balancing act to choose a procedure that is as nonrestrictive as possible, yet is effective enough to solve a person's problem.

This chapter will present a decision-making model to guide practitioners in choosing procedures that will achieve these dual aims when dealing with excess behaviors. A decision-making model formalizes the judgment process and increases the likelihood that treatment procedures are derived in a logical manner (Evans & Meyer, 1985, p. 110). The present model has the following characteristics:

1. It was made as simple as possible. The model described in Figure 1 has only seven major steps. Models with an abundance of steps (e.g.,

Saul Axelrod, Brian Berry, and Lynn Moyer • Special Education Program, Temple University, Philadelphia, Pennsylvania 19122.   Scott Spreat • The Woods School, Langhorne, Pennsylvania 19047.

Behavior Analysis and Treatment, edited by R. Van Houten & S. Axelrod. Plenum Press, New York, 1993.

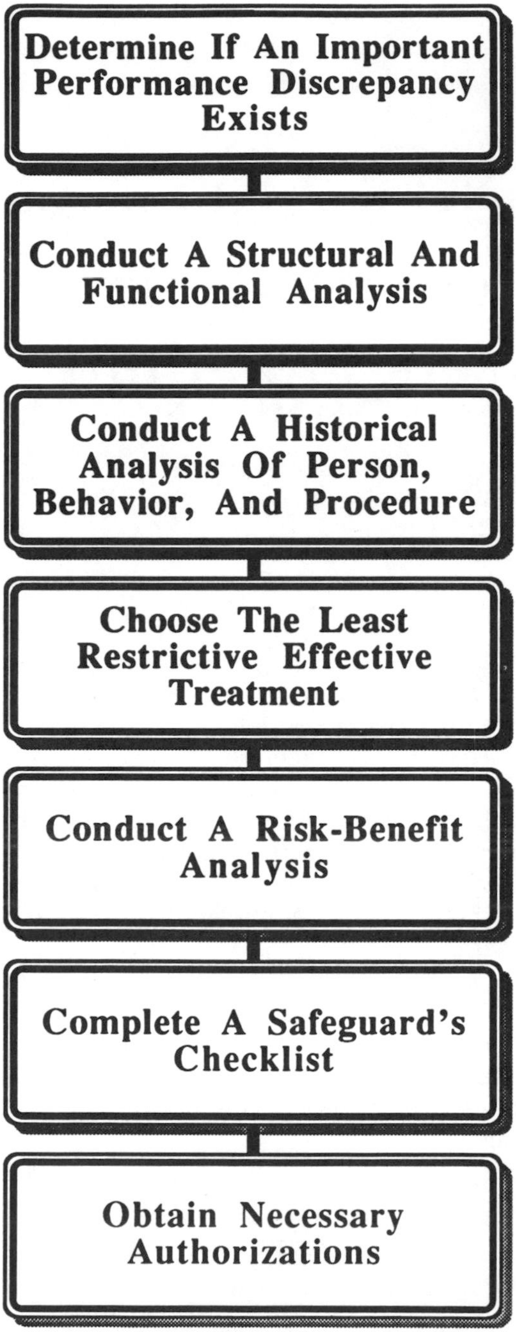

FIGURE 1. Flowchart of a recommended model for selecting the optimal procedures to reduce excess behavior.

Evans & Meyer, 1985) may have some merit in an abstract sense, but are of limited practical value.

2. It is based on science wherever possible. As a result, practitioners should refer to existing research literature whenever deciding on the parameters of treatment.

3. The model recognizes the importance of professional judgment, particularly in cases in which there is no research to guide a practitioner's efforts. Such judgments, however, should be behavior analytic rather than based on personal preference or intuition.

4. No distinction is made in the need for the approval process for restrictive and nonrestrictive procedures. This position is based on the following: (a) any procedure can be applied properly or improperly, and thus people's rights must be safeguarded in all cases; (b) both restrictive and nonrestrictive procedures can result in undesirable side effects (Balsam & Bondy, 1983); (c) any treatment can be regarded as restrictive (e.g., positive reinforcement procedures can be considered restrictive because they limit a person's access to favored events); and (d) the distinction between restrictive and nonrestrictive procedures is nontechnical and is often blurry.

5. The model does not rule out procedures (e.g., lavish amounts of positive reinforcers, time-out procedures on an a priori basis.) Rather, judgments are made on a case-by-case basis to determine which procedures are in the best interests of a person receiving treatment.

Figure 1 depicts the components of the decision-making model we are recommending. The proposal is not meant to be the final word on the topic, but rather as a possible model for guiding the practices of behavior analysts and for generating discussion on the issue. As with any model, the present one should be further refined as new treatments evolve and as intervention philosophies change. In the pages that follow we describe the components of each step.

Components of Decision-Making Model

Determine If an Important Performance Discrepancy Exists

The initial step in the decision-making process is to determine whether intervention is needed. This is decided by first identifying a discrepancy between actual and expected performance. If a self-injury rate of 1.5/min exists, for example, and a zero rate of self-injury is expected, a performance discrepancy exists. The existence of a performance discrepancy, however, does not necessarily mean that intervention should take place (Mager & Pipe,

1970). In order for a performance discrepancy to warrant intervention, a decision on the importance of the discrepancy for the individual needs to be made. Simply being different in performance is not a cause for intervention unless the deviation detracts from the person's quality of life or, in some cases, detracts from someone else's quality of life.

In evaluating the social significance of a performance discrepancy, it is important to distinguish differences that are based on the personal preference of the individual from those that are attributable to a lack of skill development. *Deviance*, with regard to behavior, implies a choice in being different (Robinson & Robinson, 1983). Often, however, performance discrepancies do not exist out of choice, but rather because the person has not learned the desired skill. Thus, people who greet others in an unusual manner but are capable of greeting them more traditionally are in a different educational situation from people who are only capable of greeting others in an unusual manner.

In order to isolate performance discrepancies of people with handicaps, Brown, Shiagra, York, Zanella, and Rogen (1984) recommend the process of comparing the performance of students with handicaps with the performance of people without handicaps. Such a comparison yields precise information about the components of any discrepancy.

Once performance discrepancies have been identified and deemed to be of social relevance, the final step is to prioritize various performance discrepancies according to the learning needs of the individual. Intervention should begin with the behavior that, if left unattended, would have the greatest negative impact on the individual's (or, in some cases, other people's) quality of life. Thus, if a person both swallowed dangerous substances and called out frequently in class, the behavior analyst would first intervene regarding the inappropriate swallowing behavior. The discrepancy analysis does not identify an instructional strategy, but it does encourage a behavior analyst to consider whether a behavior interferes with an individual's access to a better quality of life sufficiently to warrant some intervention.

Conduct a Structural and Functional Analysis

After a performance discrepancy has been identified and determined to be of sufficient significance for the individual to warrant intervention, a structural and functional analysis of the behavior needs to be done. An extensive examination of structural and functional analyses can be found in several chapters in this text. Axelrod (1987b) defined this approach as a means of determining the factors that occasion or reinforce a particular behavior so that one may intervene on those factors to eliminate or reduce the performance discrepancy. Simple identification of a learning need does not scientifically direct one toward remediation (Evans & Meyer, 1985); behavior is identified as being part of a system for the individual, with intervention on one behavior inevitably affecting other behaviors. Therefore, comprehensive knowledge of people's behaviors and their ecology is vital for making appropriate decisions.

Structural and functional analyses assist in identifying the reason(s) for performing a certain behavior. Structural analysis involves the examination of antecedent variables within the internal (i.e., biological) or external environment of the individual that may be occasioning a behavior. Functional analysis, on the other hand, is the means by which the consequences for a behavior can be determined. Structural and functional analyses are important in determining intervention because they allow identification of the cause of a performance discrepancy. Groden (1989) states that to perform some type of consequence manipulation without first carefully scrutinizing the variables that might be responsible for the behavior is both potentially inefficient and unethical. Attempts to identify the functional and structural bases for serious behavior problems demonstrate a commitment to the notion that performance is not isolated and that causation is of vital importance for making sound decisions.

Despite the demonstrated importance of completing a structural and functional analysis for selecting interventions (Iwata, Dorsey, Slifer, Bauman, & Richman, 1982; Steege, Wacker, Berg, Cigrand, & Cooper, 1989), such analyses are not always carried out. Matson and Taras (1989), in conducting a review of decelerative intervention strategies, concluded that insufficient research has been done on functional analysis when dealing with problem behaviors. Lennox, Miltenberger, Spengler, and Efranian (1988) echo this position in their review of the literature. The authors found that only about one-third of studies reported any pretreatment functional analysis, and only 6% conducted analyses more stringent than staff reports or cursory type analyses. Rather than attempting systematically to identify biological or environmental controls for performance, decisions may have been based on intuition or past experience with certain interventions.

An examination of several tools used for functional assessment yields a wide variety of methods for conducting structural and functional analyses (Durand & Crimmins, 1983; Evans & Meyer, 1985; see chapter 6). The common element is to use a multidimensional approach investigating more than a single aspect of an individual's performance. Evans and Meyer (1985) liken the process to detective work, combining the technical knowledge of the behavior with the intimate knowledge of the individual. This provides the basis on which to develop a hypothesis about conditions affecting individual performance. Steadfast rules about the reasons for performance can be deceptive at best, and overreliance on assumptions about performance without careful examination of individual conditions can be inefficient and ineffective. The use of structural and functional analyses within a decision-making model helps to determine the least restrictive effective intervention by identifying the controlling factors for a behavior.

Conduct a Historical Analysis of the Person, Behavior, and Procedure

A person whose behavior is to be modified has a behavioral and programmatic history that precedes present intervention efforts. Thus, prior to initiating new treatment, it is necessary to review the behavioral and medical records of the individual and to interview people such as parents, teachers, and others who are close to the case. To obtain a more complete picture, the practitioner should also interact with the person receiving treatment. The historical analysis of the person should reveal one or more procedures that have been useful with other behaviors and are likely to be beneficial in the present situation. The analysis should also specify the probable side effects of each procedure. Thus, if it is found that the delivery of tokens embarrasses a person, or that a time-out procedure is likely to result in injury, this information should be taken into account in making treatment decisions.

Although past information on a person is helpful, it can also be useful to determine which procedures have been effective in altering similar behaviors of other individuals. This information can be obtained from a relevant literature search. The rationale for this component of programming is that although no two people have identical behavioral histories, procedures that have been effective in modifying the behavior of one person have a reasonable probability of altering similar behaviors exhibited by another person.

In some cases, it may be necessary to expose people to procedures they have not previously experienced. In those cases it is essential to peruse the literature to determine the outcome of such procedures when applied to the behavior of other individuals. Thus, a practitioner will be able to make reasonable predictions on the likelihood and speed with which the procedure will work, the requirements for implementing it properly, and its level of social acceptability. The treatment that will emerge from the historical analysis of the person, behavior, and procedure will therefore be a combined function of specific information regarding the individual and general knowledge of the behavior and procedure under consideration.

On the basis of a historical analysis of the individual, the behavior, and the treatment under consideration, reasonable predictions can be made. The predictions should concern not only treatment effects but side effects; the risks of the procedure to the individual and the program implementer; the time away from social, educational, and vocational activities; the likelihood of implementing the procedure properly; the degree to which the treatment will generalize across settings; and the probability that the procedure can be successfully eliminated, if necessary.

Choose the Least Restrictive Effective Treatment

As mentioned earlier, Van Houten et al. (1988) asserted that people have a right to receive the least restrictive effective treatment that is available. Typically, this means that other factors being equal, a behavior analyst should use a positive reinforcement procedure rather than a punishment procedure in reducing aberrant behavior. If praise is effective in reducing inappropriate behavior, for example, it should be selected over a more intrusive procedure (e.g., a reprimand).

Choosing the least restrictive procedure is not always a simple matter. When evaluating the restrictiveness of an intervention, it should be realized that a "procedure's overall level of restrictiveness is a combined function of its absolute level of restrictiveness, the amount of time required to produce a clinically acceptable outcome, and the consequences associated with delayed intervention" (Van Houten et al., 1988, p. 114). Thus, it may superficially appear that counseling is a less restrictive procedure than a 30-minute detention for disruptive classroom behavior. One might reevaluate the position, however, if it takes 2 years for counseling to be effective, whereas a detention is effective after one episode. Likewise, positive reinforcement procedures might appear to be universally less restrictive than punishment procedures. A young adult with mild mental retardation might be more embarrassed, though, by publicly receiving a token for appropriate actions than by encountering a raised eyebrow for inappropriate behavior. Also, the general category of a procedure does not determine its level of restrictiveness. Thus, a reprimand can vary from a mild correction to a strong statement of disapproval (Favell, 1990).

In attempting to isolate the least restrictive treatment for destructive behavior, a number of recommendations have been made (e.g., Axelrod, 1983, p. 29; Evans & Meyer, 1985, p. 57; May et al., 1975). Some have advised that punishers only be used in cases where positive reinforcement of alternative behaviors has failed. LaVigna and Donnellan (1986, p. 187) were more exact in suggesting that punishment procedures only be used when three attempts at positive reinforcement had failed. Matson and Taras (1989) recommended that punishment procedures be used as a last resort.

All of the above recommendations miss the basic point: *In the case of dangerous behaviors, people are entitled to the least restrictive effective treatment from the outset.* People should not be exposed to a hierarchy of treatments that are likely to be ineffective when there are treatments available that are likely to be effective. A hierarchical decision-making model stating that a number of "nonrestrictive" procedures be used first fails to hit the target, because it implies that there is nothing wrong with several failures before an effective procedure is identified. This does not make sense in cases of serious self-abuse and aggression. There is an urgency to eliminating some problems; therefore, finding an effective procedure from the outset is crucial. Gast and Wolery (1987) properly summarize this position by stating, "If the choice of treatments is between procedures that are equally effective, then the least aversive (intrusive) should be selected. If the choice is between a less intrusive, but *in*effective procedure, and a more aversive but effective procedure, then the effective procedure should be selected" (p. 422).

Some (e.g., LaVigna & Donnellan, 1986, p. xiii) would prohibit all restrictive procedures, whereas others (see *AuClair Behavior Management Guidelines*, 1988, pp. 27–28) have banned specific procedures. Procedures, however, should not be banned on a priori basis; rather, procedures should be banned in specific cases where effective, less restrictive procedures are available. Banning procedures in an a priori manner can potentially hinder applied behavior analysts in cases where extraordinary behaviors emerge. Such a ban implies a less than total commitment to solving the most dangerous behaviors that the field encounters.

In deciding on the restrictiveness of a procedure, a number of factors should be considered. These include the following

- The urgency with which the behavior must be changed
- The speed with which the procedure works
- The likely side effects of the procedure, a prediction of which should be made according to the individual's past history and the history of the procedure and behavior with other people
- The amount of embarrassment, deprivation, or discomfort the procedure causes
- The likelihood that the procedure can be applied correctly in normalized environments
- The social acceptability of the procedure
- The potential for harm to the individual and program implementers when applying the procedure
- The degree to which the procedure removes the individual from educational, social, and vocational opportunities

Conduct a Risk-Benefit Analysis

After deciding on a procedure that meets the condition of being the least restrictive procedure that is likely to be effective, a behavior analyst must decide whether the potential cost of treatment is worth the benefit the person is likely to experience. In other words, a risk-benefit analysis must be done.

Judicial rulings, accreditation standards, and common sense dictate that in weighing treatment alternatives, practitioners must consider the likely benefits and possible risks that are associated with a proposed treatment plan. Roos (1974) stated that professionals must realize that their goal is to select a strategy that has a reasonable probability of success, while minimizing the disadvantages of the intervention.

This process has typically been operationalized in terms of a relatively fixed hierarchy of treatment alternatives, accompanied by peer review of all proposed procedures that exceed a specified limit (Spreat & Lipinski, 1986). Griffith (1980) described such a system in his article on legally safe treatment environments. Although a hierarchical approach of treatment restrictiveness may satisfy legal regulations and standards, it is possible that it leads to an oversimplification of the decision-making process. It also minimizes the role of professional judgment in making treatment decisions.

In order to balance the risks and benefits of a proposed treatment, the practitioner must consider a large number of factors that go beyond the simple notion of a restrictiveness-intrusiveness continuum. Reese (1982) noted that the task of balancing these factors was typically assigned to a human rights committee (HRC). More recent judicial rulings (e.g., *Youngberg v. Romeo*, 1982), however, suggest that the responsibility is more appropriately placed with the professionals who are designing the program. In choosing among behavior treatment options, it is the role of the behavior analyst to select the treatment that achieves the most reasonable balance between likely benefits and potential risks.

Spreat (1982) proposed a mathematical model for treatment selection that weighted various relevant factors. These factors included (a) probability of treatment success, (b) the length of time until the behavior was eliminated, (c) the distress of the procedure to the individual, and (d) the distress to the individual caused by the emission of the target behavior. Various authors (e.g., Mulick, 1989; Reese, 1982) have proposed more elaborate or inclusive systems, but most elements can be subsumed within this simpler model. Each of the four elements will be discussed below.

Probability of Treatment Success

Estimates of treatment effectiveness are essentially probability statements about the likelihood of achieving a certain goal. These probabilities are admittedly unknown, but can be estimated from the literature and from professional experience. The limitations of the literature knowledge base are discussed elsewhere in this chapter. These limitations force the general acknowledgement that the assessment of likely treatment effectiveness is, in large part, professional judgment (i.e., the behavior analyst's best estimate). Reese (1982) suggested that in considering treatment effectiveness, one should also consider the durability and generalizability of the anticipated positive changes.

The Period of Time It Takes to Eliminate a Behavior

A simple probability statement may be insufficient, because it generally fails to consider the amount of time it takes for treatment to be effective. It is conceivable that two effective treatments will vary widely with respect to celerity. For example, the experimental literature indicates that although both procedures may be effective, a punishment program will reduce a specified behavior more quickly than will extinction. It should be clear that the longer people require treatment, the longer they are exposed to the potential risks of the treatment and to the risks of the target behavior. This factor must be taken into account in selecting among treatment alternatives. Of course, with a behavior that is not dangerous and an intervention that is not intrusive, longer treatment procedures become acceptable.

The Distress Caused by the Procedure

Employing any treatment procedure is introducing an element of risk to the person. There are obvious physical and emotional risks associated with the use of restrictive procedures (e.g., physical restraint; see Spreat & Baker-Potts, 1983). There are also many more subtle risks associated with various treatment forms. These include embarrassment, discomfort, and the extent to which the program promotes segregation of the person receiving treatment. It should also be noted that even such "positive" approaches as DRO-based programs are capable of inducing considerable distress, as seen in the typically negative reaction of people who have been informed they have not earned their reinforcers for a given time period. In fact, a number of authors (see Axelrod, 1987a; Champlin, 1989) consider programs such as DRO to be punishment procedures. The point is that any treatment procedure has the potential to cause both physical and emotional distress to an individual. One must also be aware that this distress is idiosyncratic to the particular individual. Practitioners must be cognizant of the common physical risks associated with a treatment and must consider the likely emotional response of each individual receiving treatment.

The Distress Caused by the Behavior

A final factor that is often ignored is the level of discomfort caused by a behavior. There can be little doubt that a person who causes tissue damage through head banging, or blindness through eye gouging, is in serious distress. Procedures that allow the target behaviors to continue for long periods of time require the individual to continue to experience this distress repeatedly. In addition, the persistence of a socially aberrant behavior serves to segregate the persons receiving treatment further from the mainstream of society. There is clearly a value to treatment that has a relatively quick impact. In the case of behaviors that are not dangerous, speed becomes a less crucial consideration.

The four-step process outlined above relies on a number of subjective factors. Both the probability of treatment success and the amount of time it takes a procedure to work are unknown, even when these estimates are formulated by the most experienced practitioners. The other two factors, the distress caused by the procedure and the distress caused by the behavior, can only be quantified in terms of some subjective measure. Spreat (1982) suggested that subjective units of distress (SUDs), much like those used to quantify phobic response for desensitization hierarchies, be used to quantify the two dimensions. They would have to be individualized for each person. Reliance on subjective factors in the decision-making process in no way minimizes a commitment to a scientific approach to the practice of behavior analysis; it merely recognizes that our science is incomplete.

It is unlikely that practitioners will actually employ a mathematical model in the near future, although such a model does exist (Spreat, Lipinski, Dickerson, Nass, & Dorsey, 1989a). It reflects the manner in which practitioners make professional judgments about various treatment options. Although individual behavior analysts may be unable to verbalize the actual process through which they assign weights to various factors associated with different treatments, it is clear that the process occurs. According to the literature on treatment acceptability (Spreat et al., 1989a; Spreat, Lipinski, Dickerson, Nass, & Dorsey, 1989b), clinicians do consider a variety of factors in reaching decisions about the acceptability of any proposed treatment. It is evident that the task of balancing risks and benefits is an essential and complex part of providing appropriate treatment for persons with behavioral disorders. The model that we have outlined above serves to prompt the practitioner to consider each of the four constituent areas.

Complete a Safeguards Checklist

When serving people who exhibit severely disruptive behaviors, it is important to maintain safeguards protecting their rights. The process of decision making concerning the treatment choice, the manner of implementation, and the evaluation of results is critical to ensure these safeguards. Informed consent is often a recommended means of providing protection (Singer & Irvin, 1987; Spreat & Lanzi, 1989). A checklist for meeting objective criteria of appropriate treatment is one way to increase the likelihood that all areas are addressed and met prior to implementing any intervention procedure. A checklist devised for this purpose appears in Figure 2.

Treatment Checklist

Name _____   Date _____

A.   Determination of the target behavior, treatment environments   <u>Yes</u>   <u>N/A</u>
**   and procedures.**

1.   Does an important performance discrepancy exist?   ____   ____
2.   Has the target behavior been identified?   ____   ____
3.   Has the target behavior been operationally defined?   ____   ____
4.   Has the baseline level of behavior been determined?   ____   ____
5.   Has the intensity/severity of the behavior been considered?   ____   ____
6.   Have structural and functional analyses been conducted?   ____   ____
7.   Have the treatment environments been identified?   ____   ____
8.   Have alternative functional skills that can be taught been identified?   ____   ____
9.   Has generalization of appropriate behaviors across time and settings   ____   ____
      been planned?
10.   Have all materials and apparatus necessary for implementation   ____   ____
      been determined and provided?
11.   Have all other ancillary resources (speech, physical therapy,   ____   ____
      cooperative employment settings) necessary for implementation
      been determined and provided?
12.   Has a historical analysis of the person been conducted?   ____   ____
13.   Has a historical analysis of the behavior been conducted?   ____   ____
14.   Has a historical analysis of the procedure been conducted?   ____   ____
15.   Has the individual's least restrictive effective treatment been   ____   ____
      identified?
16.   Has a risk-benefit analysis been conducted?   ____   ____

B. Review of Proposed Procedures

1.   Has the intervention plan been approved by an Interdisciplinary   ____   ____
      Committee?
2.   Has the intervention plan been approved by a Peer Review Committee   ____   ____
      (when requested by Interdisciplinary Committee)?
3.   Has the intervention plan been approved by a Human Rights Committee   ____   ____
      (when requested by Interdisciplinary Committee)?

C. Informed Consent

1.   Has the individual, parent, or guardian been notified?   ____   ____
2.   Have signatures from the appropriate parties been obtained?   ____   ____
3.   Have the beginning and end dates of treatment been determined?   ____   ____
4.   Has a description of the program been developed?   ____   ____
5.   Has the individual, parent, or guardian been informed of   ____   ____
      procedures for the due process, grievances, amendments, and
      withdrawal from treatment?

FIGURE 2. Checklist of conditions that must be met before modifying excess behaviors.

<u>Yes</u>   <u>N/A</u>

D. Implementation

1. Is there an adequate number of staff for safe and effective treatment? ____ ____
2. Have all involved staff been trained for proper implementation? ____ ____
3. Has a supervisor of program implementation been identified? ____ ____
4. Has a supervision schedule been identified? ____ ____

E. Review of Proposed Procedures

1. Is there an adequate number of staff for safe and effective treatment? ____ ____
2. Have schedules for data collection and display been determined? ____ ____

F. Evaluation of the Procedure

1. Has a date for evaluation of effectiveness been determined? ____ ____
2. Has criterion for determining effective treatment been determined? ____ ____
3. Has a list of alternative treatment plans been compiled? ____ ____

* An explanation is always required for selections N/A (Not Applicable).

Explanation of all Sections Rated as N/A.

_____

_____

_____

_____

_____

_____

_____

_____

_____

Components of the checklist are divided into the following categories: (a) determination of the target behavior, treatment environment(s), and procedure; (b) review of the proposed procedures; (c) informed consent; (d) implementation; (e) documentation and reporting; and (f) evaluation of the procedure. These components, however, are not an all-encompassing list. Some sections may need to be combined or expanded, depending upon the people served, the site of implementation, the program, resources, and other mitigating factors. These suggested components, however, will be looked at in greater detail to generate discussion of a proposed list of considerations.

The first area involves determining target behaviors, the treatment environment, and the intervention. A severely disruptive behavior must be described in rate and severity (*AuClair Behavior Management Guidelines*, (1988) and undergo a functional analysis (Lovaas & Favell, 1987; Van Houten et al., 1988). The chosen environment needs to be specified and determined as therapeutic (i.e., one that promotes personal welfare and provides positive reinforcement, generalization, and the learning of appropriate functional skills; Van Houten et al., 1988). Materials, apparatuses, and other necessary resources need to be specified and available in all places where treatment will be carried out (*Behavioral Programming and Management Manual*, 1982). Perhaps most importantly, the environment should be identified as being the least restrictive setting for the individual (Lovaas & Favell, 1987; Singer & Irvin, 1987).

In addition, an intervention must be determined. Research support should be found, if possible, for the method's prior effective use with the behaviors serving similar functions (Lovaas & Favell, 1987; Singer & Irvin, 1987; Van Houten et al., 1988). This provides a justification for treatment selection. Also, any prior treatment techniques that have been used with the individual for the targeted behavior should be identified and analyzed (Lovaas & Favell, 1987).

Once the behavior, environment, and procedure are selected, they should be submitted to review committees. Such committees are commonly used for behavioral programs, yet their role with respect to selection, evaluation, and monitoring of procedures remains controversial (Spreat & Lanzi, 1989). Regardless of how committees are formed and titled, review of proposed programs by peers, parents, and members of the community helps to promote the rights of the people served (Griffith & Henning, 1981; Lovaas & Favell, 1987; Matson & Taras, 1989; Spreat & Lanzi, 1989; Van Houten et al., 1988). Recommendations have also been made to form a separate committee responsible for reviewing any emergency procedures that have been used or that need to be implemented before a scheduled review by the standard review committees (Brakman, 1985).

In all cases, informed consent must be obtained from parents, guardians, and the individuals being served, if possible. Consent to treatment, however, involves more than simple notification and signatures. A beginning and ending date for treatment, as well as positive and negative procedural consequences, should be listed (*Behavioral Programming and Management Manual*, 1982). Procedures for due process, grievances, amendments, and withdrawal from treatment should also be specified (Griffith & Henning, 1981; Singer & Irvin, 1987; Spreat & Lanzi, 1989). The issue of obtaining approval for treatment will be more thoroughly discussed in the following section of this chapter.

The next component of program safeguards involves procedural implementation. An adequate number of trained, qualified staff is necessary for safe and effective intervention. Staff must be trained not only in implementation of the particular procedure, but in behavior analysis principles in general (Lovaas & Favell, 1987; Van Houten et al., 1988); at times, direct involvement may be required by a high-level, certified professional (Matson & Taras, 1989; Van Houten et al., 1988). Treatment should be continually monitored and supervised to ensure correct and exact delivery (Lovaas & Favell, 1987; Spreat & Lanzi, 1989; Van Houten et al., 1988). Data recording needs to be continuous, objective, accurate, clearly reported, and visually displayed (Lovaas & Favell, 1987).

The final component for providing program safeguards is regular evaluation of (*Behavioral Programming and Management Manual*, 1982), and responsiveness to collected data. This increases the likelihood of correct implementation of and a rationale for continuing or discontinuing treatment. If program effectiveness is not evident, one of the previously identified alternative treatment plans should be implemented.

The component areas of determining the target behavior, treatment environment, procedure, review committees, informed consent, program implementation, documentation and reporting, and evaluation provide the basis for creating a safeguards checklist. One can be drafted to suit individual organizations, providing a systematic treatment plan that offers safe and effective treatment for the individual needs of each person served.

Obtain Necessary Authorizations

In their review of state policies regulating the practice of applied behavior analysis with persons who exhibit mental retardation, Spreat and Lipinski (1986) identified several common trends with respect to review processes. It was noted, however, that there was considerable state-to-state variation in the implementation of review procedures. In a later study, Spreat and Lanzi (1989) found considerable overlap in the role of the various review committees. Because there are differences in the review processes affecting applied behavior analysis, we are proposing a model that will more clearly delineate the responsibilities of each review component. This proposed model has three key elements, each of which will be described below.

Interdisciplinary Development

Behavior analysis procedures should be developed with significant input from an interdisciplinary team. This, however, does not imply a democratic approach to program development. The development of a specific behavior analysis program is not a simple group decision any more than the selection of the amount and type of medication a person will receive is a team decision. The team has input, but there must be one thoroughly qualified behavior analyst who is responsible for the actual development of the program. Barring the development of a professional certification program for behavior analysts, we suggest that this person be a licensed psychologist who has significant training and expertise in applied behavior analysis.

Under the direction of this competent behavior analyst (see Chapter 7), the team should thoroughly evaluate the possible risks and likely benefits of the proposed treatment plan. If the risks are judged to be more than minimal, the program should be submitted for additional review by a peer review committee (PRC). If the program restricts the individual's basic rights, human rights committee (HRC) approval should be attained.

Peer Review Committee

Behavior analysis programs that expose a person to more than minimal risk should be submitted to a body of peers for review. The PRC should be composed of persons with expertise in applied behavior analysis; it is the function of the PRC to determine the clinical appropriateness of the proposed program.

An obvious question is what constitutes appropriate treatment. A number of policies (e.g., State of New Jersey, 1988) make reference to support from the existing body of literature. A treatment has been considered clinically appropriate if it appeared in the literature several times. This guideline, however, is overly stringent. Most behavioral literature is derived from the idiographic research paradigm: Individual subjects are studied, and the uniqueness of the individual is considered to be an integral component of the study. Sidman (1960) suggested that this approach to science requires some form of meta-analysis to aggregate the findings of numerous replications of related studies employing several different single subjects. Yet a review of the literature rarely finds such meta-analyses, and one seldom sees numerous studies on related phenomena. To base a determination of clinical appropriateness on available literature seems overly restricting, because the available literature is too limited.

It is perhaps more reasonable to rely upon the expertise and professional judgment of the members of the PRC. A program derived from basic principles of behavior analysis need not have appeared elsewhere in the literature in order to be judged clinically appropriate. The task of the PRC is to determine if a program is derived from the basic principles of behavior—not whether the specific procedure has appeared elsewhere in the literature. Although reference to the professional body of knowledge is essential, the practitioner should be able to extract principles, rather than rigidly follow past research. To do otherwise would cause stagnation of the field. Of course, when the practitioner proposes to employ a novel but reasonably derived program, there is a professional responsibility to implement that treatment in a manner that affords subsequent scientific analysis.

Human Rights Committee

Although the PRC is charged with evaluating the clinical appropriateness of a proposed behavior analysis program, there are at least three areas that fall outside the domain of clinical appropriateness. All of these are human rights issues. We suggest that these be evaluated by an independent HRC that is constituted in the manner outlined by Griffith (1980) and Griffith and Henning (1981).

The first issue is consent. Consent is crucial when the procedure is nonroutine, involves significant personal risk, or restricts a person's basic rights. Consent is clearly the most appropriate mechanism with which to protect the rights of persons receiving treatment. It is the responsibility of the treatment team to develop a meaningful consent form that can be presented to an appropriate person for purposes of giving or denying permission to employ the treatment. A minimally adequate consent form should provide a thorough delineation of the risks and benefits associated with proposed and alternative treatments in a manner that is easily understood. It should describe the planned treatment program, and it should indicate that consent can be withdrawn at any time without prejudice. The Code of Federal Regulations standards (United States of America, 1983) for research consent forms could be adopted with respect to behavior analysis programs, and HRCs could serve to ensure that these standards are followed. In addition, the HRCs would have to deal with the more troublesome issue of who may appropriately give consent for the treatment of an adult who displays developmental disabilities and who lacks the capacity to make an informed decision about treatment.

The second issue pertains to treatment acceptability (Spreat et al., 1989a). The HRC functions as society's representative in the treatment process, and it gives society's sanction for various proposed treatments. It is possible that some treatments are clinically effective but not socially acceptable; an extreme example of this situation might be the use of physical punishment for off-task behavior. The HRC could review the social acceptability of each proposed procedure, considering not only the procedure itself but how the procedure might affect the person's life. Individualization is the key to this process, and the individualization must be done in a manner that ensures equality and fairness across different persons receiving treatment.

The third HRC responsibility would be to ensure that each program that involves significant risk or restricts basic rights is the product of professional judgment. This can be done by guaranteeing that no procedure receives HRC sanction without prior approval from the interdisciplinary team, the PRC, and the person's physician (where appropriate). In this manner, the HRC would ensure that the facility did exercise clinical judgment in developing the treatment program. *The HRC would not, however, be responsible for evaluating the quality of that clinical judgment or for attempting to exercise that judgment itself.* Spreat and Lanzi (1989) have reported that most HRCs lack the expertise to actually exercise professional judgment, and that it is not their role to exercise such judgement.

Summary

As indicated earlier, we are proposing a decision-making model that has relatively few steps, is based on science wherever possible, and recognizes the importance of professional judgment in accordance with the present state of behavioral technology. The model emphasizes the necessity of structural and functional analyses of behavior and historical analyses of the person receiving treatment, the behaviors of concern, and the procedure under consideration. The model underscores the importance of choosing procedures that are likely to work *at the start* when dealing with dangerous behaviors. It also requires the use of risk-benefit analyses to be certain that the advantages of treatment outweigh the disadvantages. In order to increase the likelihood that people are receiving state-of-the-art treatment, we recommend that the conditions of a safeguards checklist be satisfied.

The model we are proposing differs from existing models in several respects. First, the model rejects the use of hierarchies of treatment intrusiveness. Such hierarchies are seen as nonscientific and arbitrary. Also, procedures are not rejected in advance of the behavioral analyses, but only when a superior one is available. In addition, the model does not require one type of review for procedures seen as nonrestrictive and another for those seen as restrictive. Rather, all programs are viewed by an interdisciplinary committee and are referred to a PRC when the interdisciplinary committee regards the risks to the individual to be more than minimal, or to an HRC if significant rights of the individual are restricted. In order for the model to work, no factor is more crucial than the presence of a competent behavior analyst on the interdisciplinary committee.

As indicated earlier, we are not suggesting that either the proposed model or the safeguards checklist be the final words on these topics. Rather, we see each as a product that will be further developed as improved behavioral technology emerges and new treatment philosophies evolve.

ACKNOWLEDGMENTS.   The authors gratefully acknowledge Dr. John Parrish, University of Pennsylvania and Dr. Ron Van Houten for their helpful comments on the preparation of this manuscript.

REFERENCES

AuClaire Behavior Management Guidelines. (1988). Bear, Delaware: AuClair, Inc.

Axelrod, S. (1983). *Behavior modification for the classroom teacher* (2nd ed.). New York: McGraw-Hill.

Axelrod, S. (1987a). Doing it without arrows: A review of LaVigna and Donnellan's alternatives to punishment: Solving behavior problems with non-aversive strategies. *Behavior Analyst, 10*, 243–251.

Axelrod, S. (1987b). Functional and structural analyses of behavior: Approaches leading to reduced use of punishment procedures? *Research in Developmental Disabilities, 8*, 165–178.

Balsam, P. D., & Bondy, A. S. (1982). *Behavioral Programming and Management Manual*. Tallahassee, FL: Department of Health and Rehabilitative Services.

Balsam, P. D., & Bondy, A. S. (1983). The negative side effects of reward. *Journal of Applied Behavior Analysis, 16*, 283–296.

Brakman, C. (1985). A human rights committee in a public school for severely and profoundly retarded students. *Education and Training of the Mentally Retarded, 20*, 139–147.

Brown, L. J., Shiagra, B., York, J., Zanella, & Rogen, P. (1984). *The discrepancy analysis technique in programs for students with severe handicaps*. Madison: University of Wisconsin and Madison Metropolitan School District.

Champlin, G. (1989). On the aversive techniques/punishment controversy. *Psychology in Mental Retardation and Developmental Disabilities, 14*, 5–6.

Durand, V. M., & Crimmins, D. B. (1988). Identifying variables maintaining self-injurious behavior. *Journal of Autism and Developmental Disorders, 18*, 99–117.

Evans, J., & Meyer, L. (1985). *An educative approach to behavior problems*. Baltimore: Paul H. Brookes.

Favell, J. E. (1990). Issues in the use of non-aversive and aversive interventions. In S. L. Harris & J. S. Handleman (Eds.), *Aversive and nonaversive intervention: Controlling life-threatening behavior by the developmentally disabled* (pp. 36–56). New York: Springer.

Gast, D. L., & Wolery, M. (1987). Severe maladaptive behaviors. In M. E. Snell (Ed.), *Systematic instruction of people with severe handicaps* (3rd ed.). Columbus, OH: Charles E. Merrill.

Griffith, R. G. (1980). An administrative perspective on guidelines for behavior modification: The creation of a legally safe environment. *Behavior Therapist, 1*, 5–7.

Griffith, R. G., & Henning, D. B. (1981). What is a human rights committee? *Mental Retardation, 19*, 61–63.

Groden, G. (1989). A guide for conducting a comprehensive behavioral analysis of a target behavior. *Journal of Behavior Therapy and Experimental Psychiatry, 20*, 163–169.

Iwata, B. A., Dorsey, M. F., Slifer, K. L., Bauman, K. G., & Richman, G. S. (1982). Toward a functional analysis of self-injury. *Analysis and Intervention in Developmental Disabilities, 2*, 3–20.

LaVigna, G. W., & Donnellan, A. M. (1986). *Alternative to punishment: Solving behavior problems with non-aversive strategies*. New York: Irvington.

Lennox, D. B., Miltenberger, R. G., Spengler, P., & Efranian, N. (1988). Decelerative treatment practices with persons who have mental retardation: A review of five years of the literature. *American Journal on Mental Retardation, 92*, 492–501.

Lovaas, O. I., & Favell, J. E. (1987). Protection for clients undergoing aversive/restrictive interventions. *Education and Treatment of Children, 10*, 311–325.

Mager, R. F., & Pipe, P. (1970). *Analyzing performance problems: or "You really oughta wanna."* Belmont, CA: Fearon.

Matson, J. L., & Taras, M. E. (1989). A 20 year review of punishment procedures and alternative methods to treat problem behaviors in the developmentally disabled. *Research in Developmental Disabilities, 10.*

May, J. G., Risley, T. R., Twardosz, S., Friedman, P., Bijou, S. W., Wexler, D., et al. (1975). Guidelines for the use of behavioral procedures in state programs for retarded persons. *Mental Retardation Research, 1,* 1–73.

Mulick, J. (1989). *Restrictive behavioral interventions and their alternatives.* Presented at symposium, "Ensuring Quality of Life From Infancy Through Adulthood," Young Adult Institute, New York City.

Reese, M. (1982). Helping human rights committees and clients balance intrusiveness and effectiveness: A challenge for research and therapy. *Behavior Therapist, 5,* 95–99.

Robinson, C. C., & Robinson, J. H. (1983). Sensory-motor functions and cognitive development. In M. E. Snell (Ed.), *Systematic instruction of the moderately and severely handicapped* (3rd ed.). Columbus, OH: Charles E. Merrill.

Roos, P. (1974). Human rights and behavior modification. *Mental Retardation, 12,* 3–6.

Sidman, M. (1960). *Tactics of scientific research.* New York: Basic Books.

Singer, G. S., & Irvin, L. K. (1987). Human rights review of intrusive behavioral treatments for students with severe handicaps. *Exceptional Children, 54,* 46–52.

Spreat, S. (1982). *Weighing treatment alternatives: Which is less restrictive?* Woodhaven Center E & R Technical Report 82-11-(1). Philadelphia: Temple University.

Spreat, S., Baker-Potts, J. (1983). Patterns of injury in institutionalized residents. *Mental Retardation, 21,* 23–29.

Spreat, S., & Lanzi, F. L. (1989). The role of human rights committees in the review of restrictive/aversive behavior modification procedures: Results of a national survey. *Mental Retardation, 27,* 375–382.

Spreat, S., & Lipinski, D. P. (1986). Survey of state policies regarding the use of restrictive/aversive behavior modification procedures. *Behavioral Residential Treatment, 1,* 57–71.

Spreat, S., Lipinski, D., Dickerson, R., Nass, R., & Dorsey, M. (1989a). A paramorphic representation of the acceptability of behavioral programming. *Behavioral Residential Treatment, 4,* 1–13.

Spreat, S., Lipinski, D., Dickerson, R., Nass, R., & Dorsey, M. (1989b). The acceptability of electric shock programs. *Behavior Modification, 13,* 245–256.

State of New Jersey. (1988). *Behavior modification programming for the treatment of maladaptive behavior.* Division Circular No. 34. Trenton: New Jersey Department of Human Services, Division of Developmental Disabilities.

Steege, M., Wacker, D., Berg, W., Cigrand, K., & Cooper, L. (1989). The use of behavioral assessment to prescribe and evaluate treatments for severely handicapped children. *Journal of Applied Behavior Analysis, 22,* 23–33.

United States of America. (1983). *Code of Federal Regulations* (Title 45, Part 46, March 8, 1983). Washington, DC: Government Printing Office.

Van Houten, R., Axelrod, S., Bailey, J. S., Favell, J. E., Foxx, R. M., Iwata, R. A., & Lovaas, O. I. (1988). The right to effective behavioral treatment. *Behavior Analyst, 11,* 111–114.

Youngberg v. Romeo, 102 S. Ct. (1982).

9

Coordinating the Treatment Process among Various Disciplines

Naomi B. Swiezy and Johnny L. Matson

Considerable debate has occurred in recent years over what constitutes effective treatment. Furthermore, many have argued about what psychologically based procedures should be allowed as treatments for problem behaviors. A number of authors have laid out the various techniques, policy procedures, and potential for interventions. But after one has determined techniques one considers appropriate, if and how these methods should be put into practice is still in question. The purpose of this chapter is to discuss some of these pragmatic issues. Specifically, we discuss how to coordinate various disciplines in the treatment process and the implication of these administrative issues on selecting treatments.

CHANGES IN PROFESSIONAL ROLES

Until the late 1970s, professional decisions were rarely challenged. Whatever method the psychologist, psychiatrist, teacher, or other professional felt should be tried was routinely employed with little dissent. Informed consent, handicapped-person advocates (to represent those who could not make their own decisions), treatment team reviews, human rights committees, and all the other characteristics of the present checks-and-balance system of treat-

Naomi B. Swiezy and Johnny L. Matson • Department of Psychology, Louisiana State University, Baton Rouge, Louisiana 70803.

Behavior Analysis and Treatment, edited by R. Van Houten & S. Axelrod. Plenum Press, New York, 1993.

ment were nonexistent. This situation changed dramatically in 1970 with the *Wyatt V. Stickney* case in Alabama (Marchetti, 1987). This ruling was the first large-scale effort involving the cooperation of the federal government, professionals, parents, and politicians to develop a comprehensive system of checks and balances in the mental retardation delivery system. With human rights committees and the other checks and balances noted above, cooperation became an extremely important factor for professionals. Without good working relationships and a division of responsibility, the process of treatment development and monitoring would not work.

Coordination of treatment has also been related to research and training developments in recent years. Given the tremendous increases in knowledge, more specialty areas in assessment and treatment have emerged, as well as specialty areas within disciplines. These changes, and the recognition that groups of individuals have more expertise than any one individual, have led to the need for a more multidisciplinary approach. Further, with more legal challenges to treatment and the stress on accountability, efforts of this sort have become a necessity.

Finally, to address the issue of accountability, professionals in the area of medicine and mental health should not be considered to have opinions that are irrefutable merely by virtue of their having a specific professional degree (e.g., M.D., Ph.D.). Rather, data must be collected on individual cases, and assumptions of probable treatment effects determined. In other words, an observable rationale for treatment decisions should be outlined prior to intervention.

Along with the changing roles of professionals have been changes with regards to goals and targets of interventions. These changes will be discussed, especially with regard to the use of aversive procedures.

Changes in Treatment Goals

In program development, treatment goals are an important variable to consider. It is reasonable to assume that the objective of every intervention is to provide the most effective treatment possible. But over the last decade or so it has become apparent, especially in the treatment of severely disturbed individuals, that this objective is often not being met. Specifically, since the introduction of behavior modification to the treatment of autistic individuals, a worldwide controversy regarding the use of punishment as a behavioral treatment has ensued (Rimland, 1978).

Those against aversive procedures have maintained that all aversives except possibly saying "No" to a client should be restricted (e.g., LaVigna & Donnelan, 1986). The advocates of aversives (e.g., Rimland, 1978) agree that the use of positive procedures is preferable when they are likely to be effective and should be attempted before employing aversives. In addition, however, those favoring the selective use of punishment procedures propose that aversives should be utilized in cases where less intrusive procedures have been found ineffective and for cases in which extreme and immediate physical harm is likely (Matson & DiLorenzo, 1983). In fact, supporters of the aversive position suggest that it is our professional obligation to utilize whatever treatment is effective, given that only a select number of studies have demonstrated the effectiveness of positive procedures in the area of severe behavioral problems of the developmentally disabled (despite claims by some professionals to the contrary; Matson & Gorman-Smith, 1986). If we wish to suggest that the goal of intervention is to provide the most effective treatment, aversives are an important option.

A recent position statement of the Association for Behavior Analysis (Van Houten et al., 1988) does note that exposure of an individual to restrictive procedures is unacceptable unless it can be shown that such procedures are necessary to produce safe and clinically significant behavior change. They further note, however, that it is unacceptable to employ a less restrictive intervention if the assessment results or available research indicate that other procedures would be more effective.

This way of thinking follows the philosophy of the least restrictive alternative. According to this philosophy, the selection of the treatment that is both most appropriate to the individual's needs and least restrictive and/or intrusive is mandated. Therefore, the decision to use aversive strategies must occur after it has been documented that all alternative and nonintrusive techniques have been fully explored (Herr, 1990). Furthermore, any decision to use a nonrestrictive approach should follow the consideration of whether the use of such a strategy will actually be more restrictive by prolonging treatment, which would then increase the risk, inhibit or prevent participation in needed training programs, delay entry into a more optimal social or living environment, lead to the adaptation and eventual use of a more restrictive procedure, or expose the client to undue injury (as in the case of self-injury; Matson & Swiezy, 1990). That is, nonaversives may not be considered completely devoid of aversive components, because deprivation and other restrictions are often embedded in these strategies (Mulick & Linscheid, 1988). Thus far, there have been only speculations as to the harm caused by aversive procedures, whereas harm from *not* using these procedures has been demonstrated (Rimland, 1978).

Therefore, it is important for clinicians to keep in mind that the goal of intervention is to provide the most effective *and* least restrictive alternative. In some cases, using aversives as an alternative may be justified (B. F. Skinner, 1988), either alone or in combination with other less restrictive techniques (e.g., Foxx, Bittle, & Faw, 1989).

Although treatment efficacy is a significant goal of any proposed intervention, researchers have recently identified other goals for their treatment approaches that involve issues of prevention, treatment acceptability, side effects, maintenance and generalization. A major advance of modern treatment of problem behavior has been the focus on early detection and intervention. Treatment packages including such a focus are preventative in nature in that not only are the clients exhibiting improvement in certain skill areas, but the development of more serious problem behaviors is also being circumvented. Furthermore, early identification not only helps prevent the further development of problem behaviors, but also allows the already existing problems to be ameliorated with less invasive means than might be necessary should those behaviors be allowed to escalate (Favell, 1990). Such early intervention has proven effective in research by Lovaas (1987).

Treatment acceptability has also become an important goal in the development of intervention programs. In order that a treatment program be maximally effective, the individuals who are to give consent for the use of the procedures (e.g., parents, courts) and those who are to implement the program on a daily basis (e.g., teachers, psychiatrists, attendants) must agree that the treatment is acceptable. This topic has been one of considerable dismay for those favoring aversives. Those who wish to prohibit the use of aversives contend that aversive procedures are inhumane, unethical, and immoral. As a result, these individuals have made many perhaps false allegations and precipitated numerous court battles and rulings that have not supported their views (Matson & Swiezy,1990). With this type of resistance, no treatment program will be efficacious, and clients' rights to effective treatment may be neglected. Therefore, it is necessary that those in favor of aversives educate the public and let the data speak for themselves.

Researchers have also learned that an important goal of treatment programs should be the minimization of treatment side effects. All interventions designed to treat one aspect of an individual's behavior may be expected to produce concomitant behavior changes as well (Lichstein & Shreibman, 1976). Aversive procedures have often been cited for causing negative side effects, though beneficial collateral changes have been cited as well (Matson & Taras, 1989; Newsom, Favell & Rincover, 1983). Positive and negative side effects have also occurred with positive treatment. It is important to monitor and report on these side effects to assess more accurately whether treatment goals are being adequately satisfied.

Finally, maintenance and generalization of treatment effects have become important goals in treatment. *Maintenance* refers to treatment effects or improvements that remain stable even after intervention is removed. *Generalization* refers to the treatment effects being evident even in the settings and behaviors not involved in treatment (Favell, 1990). Aversive approaches have been assumed to produce improvements only in the specific situation where they are employed and for only as long as the intervention is in effect, thus exhibiting low generalization and maintenance (Favell, 1990). Problems with maintenance and generalization are associated with all interventions (Favell, 1990; Matson & Taras, 1989), however, and these effects will continue unless some form of maintenance is systematically programmed (Kazdin & Esveldt-Dawson, 1981). Monitoring of behavioral improvement over all situations and for long time periods is necessary for better research regarding ways to program pervasive and durable treatment effects (Favell, 1990). Ultimately, the efficacy of treatment depends on whether the behavioral improvements result in an enhanced quality of life for the individual (Lovaas & Favell, 1987).

Presently, methods receiving a great deal of clinical emphasis focus on utilizing functional analysis to assess the environmental conditions that differentially control problem behaviors and the contingencies that maintain these behaviors (Favell, 1990). For example, methods have been derived to explore behavior changes in the face of various activities, people, and times of the day to identify specific situations controlling the intensity and frequency of the problem (e.g., Touchette, MacDonald, & Langer, 1985). In addition, certain methods help researchers and clinicians identify whether the maintaining factors include positive reinforcement (e.g., attention from others, sensory stimulation) and/or negative reinforcement (e.g., escape from task demands; Iwata, Dorsey, Slifer, Bauman, & Richman, 1982).

The importance of an adequate assessment cannot be minimized. Many serious behavior problems may be prevented or diminished nonaversively if the performance of the attending caregivers is appropriately managed (Favell, 1990). For instance, if clients are frequently prompted and reinforced for exhibiting acceptable and functional behaviors in both structured (e.g., Dyer, Schwartz, & Luce, 1984; Martin, Pallotta-Cornick, Johnstone, & Goyos, 1980) and leisure (Parsons, Reid, & Cash, cited in Reid, Parsons, & Schepis, 1990) situations, then the clients are less likely to engage in incompatible maladaptive behaviors. If staff or the caregivers do not interact with clients in this fashion, then the clinician should intervene by managing caregiver performance as well as client behavior. To address only the latter when there is a nontherapeutic environment, especially when using aversive treatments, is bound to be ineffective and is clearly abusive (Favell, 1990).

Following the full assessment of the situation, the qualified mental retardation professional (QMRP) is responsible for devising a suitable treatment program (taking into consideration the constraints of the situation), educating relevant caregivers in behavioral principles and the specifics of the treatment program, supervising and giving feedback regarding the implementation of the intervention, and monitoring treatment effects. In that much of their responsibility involves the direct training, observation, and feedback of nonprofessionals regarding treatment implementation, behavior analysts can easily tend to lose their identity as clinicians and become professional supervisors of caregiver performance (Favell, 1990).

Changing Targets of Interventions

As mentioned previously, the behavior analyst's role in treatment intervention has changed. The progression has been from intervening directly with the client exhibiting problem behavior to intervening more indirectly by using the behaviors of parents, teachers, inpatient staff, and/or peers, as well as the individual client, as targets for intervention.

Training Parents

The lack of competency of parents regarding child management may be a major factor in the development of behavior problems (Blechman, 1984). Therefore, it seems to follow that these problems would be best rectified through the education and training of parents (O'Dell, 1985). In fact, the excessive number of parents requiring such services has led to the development of group training (Dangel & Polster, 1984). These groups typically focus on educating the parents (Dangel & Polster, 1984) and tend to take one of three forms: (a) didactic methods relying on oral or written materials prepared by trainers, (b) didactic methods using visual input (e.g., modeling), or (c) interactive methods involving the direct shaping of parent behavior. The latter methodology has proven most effective (O'Dell, 1985), with the didactic approaches often failing to result in skill acquisition (Rickert et al., 1988; Ziarnik & Bernstein, 1982).

More recently, competency-based procedures have been utilized as alternatives to didactic strategies (e.g., Budd & Fabry, 1984; Budd, Riner, & Brockman, 1983). With this approach, parents are required to demonstrate that they have mastered the targeted skills in order to complete training. Changes in parents' perceptions of the child's home adjustments and the parents' general attitudes are observed to follow such training (e.g., Rickert et al., 1988). Parents, however, indicated equally high levels of satisfaction whether didactic or competency-based training was utilized, though only the latter led to skill mastery (Rickert et al., 1988).

Parent training techniques have been effective in modifying a wide variety of problem behaviors (e.g., Hughes, 1985; Matson & Ollendick, 1977; Patterson, Chamberlain, & Reid, 1982; Schmitt, 1985), and a variety of techniques have been trained to accomplish this modification. The effectiveness of child management techniques utilized in controlling behaviors, however, most probably is influenced by the parents' acceptance of those techniques. For instance, Heffer and Kelley (1987) determined that lower-income parents considered time out as far less acceptable than positive reinforcement and response-cost procedures, and as equal in acceptability to spanking and medication. Conversely, these authors determined that middle- and upper-income parents viewed time out, response cost, and positive reinforcement equal in acceptability, whereas spanking and medication were viewed as less so. Such findings have important implications particularly in the training of aversive procedures. Many advocates for the prohibition of aversives include some parents who view these procedures as barbaric and immoral (these tend not to be parents of children with severe behavior problems). It is not likely that such parents will commit themselves to carrying out such procedures.

Despite the effectiveness of parent training procedures in modifying child behavior problems (Nay, 1979), the maintenance and generalization of these interventions have been less adequately investigated (Sanders & James, 1983). Rather, researchers have focused on the maintenance and generalization of child behaviors, even though parents have been the targets for intervention.

Though the psychologist will often be responsible for treatment implementation (i.e., parent training), social workers and nonprofessional volunteers, as well as the parent himself or herself, could be important in programming maintenance. The maintenance of parenting skills may be programmed by scheduling periodic therapist contact (e.g., Patterson, 1974); however, trained nonprofessional volunteers could also be utilized to meet regularly with families and provide support and reinforcement for their efforts (Nay, 1979). Further, self-control training with parents could provide for their own support and reinforcement (e.g., Wells, Greist, & Forehand, 1980).

Various factors have been cited as predictive of poor maintenance of parent and child behavior change. Not all families benefit from the proposed parent training programs, and attention to predictors of outcome should help identify families for whom alternative interventions should be developed (Clark & Baker, 1983). Predictors of poor outcome in parent training that have been cited in the literature include lower socioeconomic status (Clark & Baker, 1983), less previous experience with behavior modification (Clark & Baker, 1983), more reactive life stresses (Webster-Stratton, 1985), marital discord (Dadds, Schwartz, & Sanders, 1987), more coercive interchanges with others (Dumas & Wahler, 1983), and greater insularity of the mother (Dumas & Wahler, 1983). These predictors are especially important when considering the implementation of aversive procedures. When utilizing such a procedure, the importance of consistency and treatment integrity is tantamount. There exists a high potential for abuse should the procedure be carried out inappropriately. Therefore, parents with negative outcome predictors such as those cited above would be inappropriate candidates for a program utilizing such procedures.

The generalization of parenting skills is another important consideration in treatment planning and intervention. Few studies, however, have been conducted in this area. One such study includes investigating response generalization (Koegel, Glahn, & Nieminen, 1978), where training in one skill does not generalize to improvement in other skills; therefore, parents should be trained on all skills relevant to treatment implementation (Sanders & James, 1983). Regarding setting generalization, however, clinic training can generalize to the home (Sanders & James, 1983), and homework assignments have been shown to facilitate this effort (e.g., Forehand & King, 1977). In addition, generalization to other nontraining settings may be facilitated by teaching self-management skills (Sanders & James, 1983).

Further, parents rarely apply their parenting skills spontaneously to nontargeted behaviors. Training across various behaviors and/or settings or reinforcing generalized responding to nontargeted behaviors and/or settings are other means of programming generalization (Stokes & Baer, 1977). Regardless of the specific method used for promoting generalization, this concept is important for coordinating a treatment team in that various individuals (e.g., parents, teachers) may potentially be involved in promoting the generalization.

Training School Personnel

Behavioral procedures should be taught to and implemented by the teacher and other school personnel who have control of the environmental contingencies in the school setting. Few studies have investigated the effects of various means of training teachers in the use of behavioral techniques; however, a review of the literature contained the following conclusions (Allen & Forman, 1984). First, didactic training alone does not appear to be an effective means of training, though it may be important when combined with other procedures. Furthermore, cueing, role playing, role playing plus modeling, feedback, and reinforcement all seem to be effective in training teachers in behavioral skills. Feedback has been noted as the most effective procedure, and its success is influenced by the frequency with which the feedback is provided (i.e., the more frequently feedback is given, the more potent it becomes as a training procedure; Allen & Forman, 1984).

Again, regardless of the specific training methods utilized, treatment team coordination is essential in that not only must someone (e.g., the teacher) implement the devised behavioral programs, someone (e.g., the school principal) must also supervise the intervention, and another individual (e.g., the behavior analyst) must evaluate the integrity with which the program is being implemented. Various behavioral programs have been implemented in the classroom with great success. Such programs have included instructions in study skills (e.g., Alexander, 1985; C. H. Skinner, Turco, Beatty, & Rasavage, 1989), response-cost procedures (e.g., Forman, 1980; Witt & Elliott, 1982), differential reinforcement procedures, time out, overcorrection (Lentz, 1988), group contingencies (e.g., Harris & Sherman, 1973; Saigh & Umar, 1983), and home-school contingencies (e.g., Lahey et al., 1977; Witt, Hannafin, & Martens, 1983).

Commitment to the program is essential in the effectiveness of any of these treatments. Therefore, before the QMRP may initiate teacher training, he or she is first responsible to "sell" the techniques by addressing the limited staff time necessary to implement such plans (and the possibility of hiring an aide, if necessary) and the potential usefulness of these techniques with other problem children.

Though researchers typically recognize the necessity for maintenance and generalization of trained behavioral skills, few have programmed for these variables (Allen & Forman, 1984). General means for enhancing maintenance and generalization, however, may be adapted for use in teacher/staff training. For example, training should incorporate examples of various behavioral skills and situations to program for generalization across behaviors and settings (Stokes & Baer, 1977). Also, training materials should be utilized that will also be present and be able to serve as discriminative stimuli in the posttraining environment (Marholin & Steinman, 1977). Principals and other school personnel may also be taught the procedures, and they can serve to reinforce intermittently the teacher's utilization of the techniques (Allen & Forman, 1984; Karoly, 1980). Moreover, the clinician or trained nonprofessionals may provide occasional follow-up training sessions as a means of fading reinforcement and support (Kazdin & Polster, 1973). Finally, training teachers in self-management procedures might improve maintenance and generalization (Kanfer, 1975).

The "selling" responsibilities of the QMRP are often particularly necessary to convince the teacher and school personnel that aversive procedures are warranted in a specific situation. Though positive procedures for reducing the problem behaviors have been well investigated and are typically accepted better than aversive procedures, there are some inherent problems with these procedures. For instance, these procedures may be time-consuming, requiring short monitoring periods and frequent resetting of timers. In addition, teachers often find it difficult to be consistently positive and ignore misbehavior while providing differential attention for other behaviors (Lentz, 1988). Rather, punishment techniques are more often employed in the natural setting to reduce maladaptive behaviors (e.g., time out, loss of privileges). Also, teacher attention may not be a potent enough contingency for severe behaviors and for some individuals (e.g., Baer, Rowbury, & Baer, 1973).

Finally, and most importantly, if the positive procedures have proven ineffective with a behavior and/or the behavior is sufficiently severe to warrant an immediate and effective solution, then aversives should be the treatment of choice. Lentz (1988) provides a list of recommendations to ensure that the time-out procedure is not used abusively. These guidelines could also be applied to all aversive procedures: (a) Progress in an hierarchical fashion from positive to the more aversive techniques; (b) conduct a thorough analysis of variables and potential effectiveness of the aversive procedure; (c) use aversive procedures along with positive procedures; (d) carefully define target behaviors and adequately train staff to carry out the process for these behaviors; (e) carefully monitor the progression of treatment; and (f) ensure the safety of the patient and evaluate treatment integrity.

Because of the limited number of QMRPs relative to the demand for these individuals, it has often been suggested that volunteer nonprofessionals be trained in data collection so that the treatment program may be monitored on a regular basis. Another option, though, is to train the teacher not only in the requisite skill for implementing the plan, but also in observational skills. R. V. Hall et al. (1971) conducted a series of experiments in which they investigated this option. Teachers were effective both in implementing a program to modify problem behaviors and in monitoring the rates of these behaviors while also attending to academic responsibilities. Similarly, an innovative training approach was utilized by Bornstein, Hamilton, and Quevillon (1977). Because the teacher and student both resided in an isolated rural environment, professional involvement was restricted to a long-distance consultative approach (i.e., phone contacts and letters). The results of the investigation clearly demonstrated the effectiveness of the positive practice program, which was applied through a long-distance consultation format.

Training Institutional Staff

Treatment to be implemented in inpatient or residential settings has the most potential for success, because the QMRP has a captive audience in terms of both the clients and staff. Unfortunately, however, the potential for success is not maximized, in that the resources are not utilized effectively. For instance, staff training programs have often been unsuccessful.

Several methods for staff training in large institutional settings have been devised (e.g., Grabowski & Thompson, 1972; Panyan & Patterson, 1974; Pizzat, 1974), whereas smaller residential facilities and group homes still need methods for staff training that have been empirically validated (O'Connor, cited in Schinke & Wong, 1977). Many of the previous staff training programs have been based on operant principles (e.g., Panyan & Patterson, 1974). Conventional teaching methods including verbal and written directions often fail to modify staff behavior (Carpenter & Baer, cited in Schinke & Wong, 1978; Quilitch, 1975).

Training procedures used in teaching staff in institutional settings have typically be unsatisfactorily described and empirically validated in behavior modification articles (e.g., R. V. Hall, 1971; Kazdin, 1974). Further, studies involving multiple training methods often fail to provide information on the efficacy of the methods separately or as a package (e.g., Cheek, Laucius, Mahncke, & Beck, 1971). It is important that the procedures be consistently reported and validated so that we are sure to make optimal use of the clinician's consultative efforts and the staff's potential effectiveness with behavior modification.

Training procedures typically rely on establishing discriminative stimuli or using reinforcing consequences to maximize trainer performance (Loeber & Weisman, 1975). A number of materials may be utilized as discriminative stimuli and assist the trainer in maintaining control over his or her behavior. Such stimuli include instructions, lectures, prompts, protocols, manuals, and equipment used in treatment programs (e.g., hand counters and timers). In addition, the appearance and past performance history of the client may serve as discriminative stimuli for trainer responding. Client behaviors may also precipitate responses from staff that are not always therapeutic; both desirable and undesirable client behaviors may be either reinforced or ignored by staff (Loeber & Weisman, 1975). Finally, a widely used and complex form of discriminative stimulus is modeling, either live or filmed (Schinke & Wong, 1978). It is as yet unclear, however, whether psychologists or fellow staff are the best models (Loeber & Weisman, 1975).

The use of reinforcing consequences for staff responding has been another method utilized in staff training. Among the most potent reinforcers for staff responding are desirable changes in patients' problematic behaviors (Benberich, 1971) and nontarget responses such as smiling and positive verbalizations (Loeber & Weisman, 1975). Staff supervisors also provide various forms of consequences for training appropriate staff responding. For example, feedback has been noted as an effective means of staff training. Supervisors may monitor staff on a variable interval schedule (Loeber & Weisman, 1975) and provide feedback in descriptive or graphic form (Schinke & Wong, 1978). Alternatively, verbal feedback may be provided during behavior rehearsal sessions (e.g., Carpenter & Baer, cited in Schinke & Wong, 1978).

Supervisors have also made use of delayed contingencies such as providing social reinforcement during conferences (Loeber & Weisman, 1975), providing time off (Watson, Gardner, & Sanders, 1971), giving a promotion (Martin, cited in Loeber & Weisman, 1975) or monetary reward (Pomerlau, Bobrove, & Smith, 1973), or designating an "aide of the week" (Pomerleau et al., 1973). Use of these reinforcing contingencies, however, may often be hampered by the fact that some staff (e.g., nurses, ward supervisors) who are to be trained do not report directly to the supervisor or QMRP but to other administrators (Hall & Baker, 1973). Therefore, the training supervisor must either convince other administrators of the necessity of staff contingencies or rely on natural reinforcers to achieve success (Loeber & Weisman, 1975). The latter is more likely to be successful, in that administrators typically ignore staff concerns and fail to provide adequate training or evaluations of procedures to alleviate staff frustrations (Repp & Deitz, 1978).

Perhaps the most effective staff training method involves multiple procedures combined in a treatment package. Designing packages of training techniques allows training to be tailored to unique staff needs for specific programs. Such packaging allows one to account for variations in staff size, professional level, time limitations, and organizational constraints of specific programs (Schinke & Wong, 1978).

Regardless of the training method, staff should receive information on such basic behavioral principles and methods as antecedent control, behavioral consequences, differential reinforcement, and data collection. Research by Repp, Barton, and Brulle (1982) demonstrates that simple changes in antecedent events can greatly affect client responding. In this case, instructions to mentally retarded persons served as the antecedents. The authors found low natural rates of interaction between staff and residents. They also determined that nonverbal instructions typically generated higher rates of appropriate responding than verbal instructions. Therefore, it is important for staff to recognize that change in behavior may be produced by manipulating simple antecedent events as well as by manipulating behavioral consequences (Repp et al., 1982).

The other method for invoking behavior change is through behavioral consequences. In order for behavioral contingencies to be effective, it is important that staff be advised to apply them immediately contingent on the targeted behavior and consistently following each instance of the behavior. Though reinforcement as a consequence may seem more straightforward than punishment and to have less potential for misuse, several errors may be committed. For example, staff may delay reinforcer presentation, deeming it less effective (Loeber & Weisman, 1975). Alternatively, staff may present a reinforcer with very limited potency (Kazdin, 1974) or one that actually has undesired effects (Abidin, 1971). Other problems involved with this procedure might involve the tendency to give reinforcers to make an undesirable behavior (e.g., crying) cease, to satiate individuals by giving reinforcers too often (Loeber & Weisman, 1975), or to give a reinforcer a negative connotation by presenting it in the form of "If you do this, then you can get that" (O'Leary, Poulos, & Devine, 1972).

Finally, staff should be trained in data collection to evaluate the effectiveness of the methods they are using to modify patient behaviors. As noted previously, the study by R. V. Hall et al. (1971) indicates that individuals cannot only carry out prescribed behavior plans, but also collect observational data while still functioning adequately in their primary professional role.

It has been hypothesized that if a staff training program is effective, one should expect several positive changes in the treatment environment. As a result of successful staff training, it is hoped that increased knowledge of behavioral principles and improved attitudes toward the job and residents will occur (Schinke & Wong, 1977). How, then, do we evaluate the effectiveness of these training programs? Loeber and Weisman (1975) suggest that a desirable change in patient behaviors reflects effective training. Also, they suggest that staff who have been trained effectively will be able to teach their learned skills successfully to others.

Maintenance of trained skills is also an important factor in considering the effectiveness of training. Maintenance is often difficult to achieve, given that discriminative stimuli and reinforcements that were present during regular training are often not operative afterward. Perhaps the answer to this problem is the implementation of self-control procedures for staff following regular training (Loeber & Weisman, 1975). Finally, the authors maintain that the generalization of trainer responses to situations, behaviors, and patients other than those involved in training is important in the evaluation of staff training programs. At the time of Loeber and Weisman's review (1975), no attempts at programming for generalization had been conducted.

Training Peers

Another viable means of treatment intervention involves the utilization of peers as trainers and providers of contingencies. There are several potential benefits to involving peers in treatment intervention. First, therapist cannot be available to monitor and instruct appropriate behaviors most of the time. In addition, once the treatment is under way, peer involvement allows teachers and aides to attend to other obligations. Also, the social prompting and consequences of peer interactions are naturally occurring contingencies in the environment and serve to improve the maintenance of appropriate behaviors after the termination of training (Matson & Zeiss, 1979). Further, it has been shown repeatedly (e.g., Klingman, Melamed, Cuthbert, & Hermecz, 1984) that individuals tend to imitate and, hence, to learn the behaviors of others who are most similar to the individual.

Benefits to the peer helper include an added sense of responsibility. Potential risks, however, are also involved. For instance, the peers may become involved in various disputes (Greenwood, Carta, & Hall, 1988). Also, peer pressure might result, including verbal harassment (Harris & Sherman, 1973), threats (Pigott & Heggie, 1986), gestures, and grimaces (Schmidt & Ulrich, 1969). Given the likelihood of such negative encounters and the potential for abuse with aversive procedures (Newsom & Rincover, 1989), it seems reasonable to preclude peers form being in the position of using such contingencies.

Peer strategies are typically utilized in the modification of mild problem behaviors. For example, peers have been trained to (a) teach target individuals academic skills (e.g., Dinwiddie, cited in Greenwood et al., 1988), (b) help target individuals develop appropriate social skills and disciplined behaviors (e.g., Greenwood et al., 1984; Maheady & Sainato, 1985), and (c) enhance the interpersonal relations of target individuals (e.g., Greenwood et al., 1988; Johnson & Johnson, 1983; Johnson, Johnson, Warring, & Maruyama, 1986).

Training of peers often involves the use of instructions, modeling, rehearsal and feedback. The peers are taught not only methods for monitoring and recording the target person's behavior, but also how to provide adequate feedback, modeling, and reinforcement. The teacher's aides are usually called upon to monitor behaviors of the target individual and peer, as well as to provide feedback and social reinforcement (Matson & Zeiss, 1979).

Likely candidates for peer trainers have mastered the skill to be taught, can carry out training independently, can provide reliable and accurate feedback to the patient, and have adequate social skills to form a long-term training relationship (Greenwood et al., 1988). Therefore, peer-mediated procedures are potentially useful in the application of behavioral techniques. Treatment integrity, however, has not been sufficiently assessed. In addition, the peer-mediated procedures have not been adequately validated empirically, have not been carefully scrutinized in relation to alternative procedures (Greenwood, et al., 1988), and would not appear to be suitable candidates in cases where positive procedures have not been effective and/or the severity of the problem necessitates the use of aversive procedures.

Training Individual Clients

Self-control strategies where the client himself or herself is trained to implement the intervention have become popular. The technique originated with a study of Meichenbaum and Goodman (1971) in which hyperactive children were trained to think before they acted. This feat was accomplished successfully by means of a treatment package including modeling, overt and covert rehearsal, prompts, feedback, and social reinforcement procedures typically involved in such training programs.

Individuals involved in self-control training programs are taught to monitor and record their own problem behaviors as well as to reinforce appropriate responding. Ollendick (1981) found that sometimes problem behaviors are severe enough to warrant self-administered punishment, in this case the use of overcorrection. Therefore, individuals may become actively involved in their own treatment, even so far as to self-administer negative consequences (Ollendick, 1981). Self-instructional training has been effective in establishing self-control over problem behaviors with a number of populations, including hyperactive (Bornstein & Quevillon, 1976), disruptive and socially unskilled (Gottman, Gonso, & Schuler, 1976), mentally retarded (Burgio, Whitman, & Johnson, 1980), emotionally disturbed (Kendall & Finch, 1978), and learning disabled (Kapadia & Fantuzzo, 1988) individuals. Other studies, however, have offered less than compelling results (e.g., Friedling & O'Leary, 1979; Ollendick, 1981).

These strategies are appealing to consider, though they are limited in efficacy. In addition, research has not sufficiently advanced for us to determine which individuals will respond favorably to such training and which will not (Bornstein, 1985). Bornstein (1985), however, proposed patient variables that would be expected to influence treatment success when utilizing this technique. First, Borstein (1985) suggested that age considerations are important in effectively implementing self-control strategies, given that older children are capable of independently generating effective verbalization strategies, whereas younger children are less capable of doing so (Bornstein, 1985; Denney, 1975). In addition, Bornstein (1985) suggested that individuals may need more structured guidance and direction to utilize self-instructional strategies effectively.

Pretraining experiences are also important predictors of treatment success; that is, those individuals with a history of failure and of attempts to control the problem behaviors by external means (e.g., medication) tend to be less successful in utilizing self-control strategies (Bornstein, 1985). Finally, individuals with an internal locus of control typically respond more favorably to self-control programs, whereas those with an external locus fare better with programs conducted by others (Bugental, Whalen, & Henker, 1977). Maintenance and generalization of this technique is decidedly good in that the individual is naturally reinforcing to himself or herself, the contingencies are easily administered in an immediate rather than a delayed fashion, and as suggested by Bornstein and Quevillon (1976), covert rehearsal may facilitate the development and maintenance of appropriate behaviors.

In sum, self-control strategies have proven effective with many individuals and not so effective with others. Researchers in this area must concentrate on developing, refining, evaluating, and explicitly reporting their methodology and results of studies involving self-control training. This will allow us to identify the necessary components for the successful application of these training procedures.

COORDINATING AMONG DISCIPLINES TO ESTABLISH A TEAM APPROACH

As noted previously, a variety of individuals from various disciplines may potentially be involved in every intervention program. As such, it is important that efforts of these individuals be coordinated to result in the most efficient and effective intervention possible. Individuals who may potentially be involved in multidisciplinary efforts will be discussed, as well as the duties that might be assigned to each individual on the treatment team based on his or her particular work setting and area of expertise. Recommendations for how best to approach and establish rapport with other professionals are offered. In addition, the sequence of steps involved in the coordination of efforts is mentioned briefly.

Disciplines Typically Involved in Multidisciplinary Efforts

Many psychological problems (e.g., severe self-injurious behaviors requiring treatment with aversives) warrant treatment from highly trained professionals (e.g., clinical psychologists). Some considerations, however, prohibit the sole involvement of professionals (Kazdin, 1984). One consideration is the relative deficit of adequately trained professionals compared to the number of clients in rehabilitation (Sobey, 1970). This shortage of professionals necessitates the involvement of other individuals in the intervention process so that persons who desire and need treatment may receive it on an individual basis (Kazdin, 1984). A second consideration is that professionals often intervene by seeing the client in an office, thus removing the client from the naturalistic, problematic situation. Though this approach is more time efficient for the therapist, problematic behavior is unlikely to manifest itself in the office in the same way as it exists in the natural environment. Therefore, we again must recruit other individuals to be involved in the treatment process so that the professional may still work efficiently and yet have treatment carried out in the natural environment (Kazdin, 1984).

One answer to the shortage of professionals and the preference for providing treatment in the natural environment is the utilization of paraprofessionals, including parents, teachers and other school personnel, peers, institutional staff, and staff supervisors (Kazdin, 1984). These individuals are normally in contact with the client daily. Those in frequent contact with the client have the greatest opportunity to regulate the environmental contingencies controlling the behavior; also, these individuals are best able to observe behavior in the naturally occurring situations in which they are performed (Kazdin, 1984). Further, the individuals the client interacts with in the natural environment often contribute to or reinforce the problem behaviors (Patterson, 1982; Wahler, 1976). Therefore, the first step in intervention often involves training the behaviors of these individuals (Kazdin, 1984).

As mentioned previously, by training and consulting with various individuals, the QMRP may indirectly and effectively modify the client's problem behaviors. Depending on the setting, different individuals will have a greater or lesser impact on the client. It is important, however, that all individuals with significant client contact be trained in behavioral principles to program better for maintenance and generalization. Training may include lectures, modeling, feedback, role playing, and incentives (Kazdin, 1984).

In the home setting, the primary change agent is the parent. In school, however, many more disciplines are involved in treatment. For example, the consultant may work directly with the teacher in devising a suitable treatment plan for an individual student. Alternatively, several administrators who are interested in the effects of an in-service program for teachers might benefit from consultation. The consultation often works with both teachers and administrators in formulating objectives, plans, and evaluations. Furthermore, the school psychologist may be instrumental in evaluating the effectiveness of psychological services (Kratochwill & Bergan, 1978).

In traditional settings, the QMRP must coordinate services with not only psychiatric aides who are in frequent contact with the patients, but also the staff supervisors, social workers, and psychiatrist who play an integral part in patient treatment. It is important that the psychologist or other trained professional coordinate services with staff supervisors to whom the psychiatric aides are directly responsible by describing the proposed intervention to them. It is important that these individuals favor the treatment, because they may be instrumental in providing incentives and encouraging aides to carry out the plan with integrity. Further, in the traditional settings, the QMRP must coordinate with the unit social workers. Because they are typically responsible for management of individual cases, it is important that social workers be aware of the treatment so that they may provide social reinforcement to staff for using treatment integrity and may implement the procedures themselves when necessary. Also, psychiatrists are often the treatment team leaders in traditional settings and should be abreast of behavioral principles in general, as well as specific treatments to be implemented with particular clients. In addition, the primary form of treatment in such settings often involves medical or drug treatment. Therefore, it is important that the psychiatrist and QMRP discuss the coordination of the behavioral and medical technologies. In so doing, the QMRP should empirically determine the behavioral tendencies with and without the prescribed drug treatment. The notion is to identify whether the medication in any way may affect the problem behaviors. If so, the QMRP and psychiatrist should then confer and either decide to alter the treatment by changing medication in kind or dosage or adapt the behavioral procedures to be implemented.

In a coordinated approach to treatment, it is also important to have a legal representative on the team who will be available to consult with and inform the other team members as to the potential legal concerns and ramifications of utilizing various treatment programs. Many separate legal decisions have been implemented regarding the treatment of particularly institutionalized patients. Examples of these decisions include the *Morales v. Turman* and *Wyatt v. Stickney* cases, where the court decided that institutionalized patients, mentally retarded individuals, and juvenile delinquents are entitled to rights that include receiving nutritious meals, receiving visitors, having a comfortable bed, and having a closet for personal belongings. They also have the right to exercise, watch television, and interact with the opposite sex (Kazdin, 1984). Such rulings are part of a more general concept of the least restrictive alternative (Ennis & Freidman, cited in Kazdin, 1984). This doctrine requires that institutions justify their actions and contingencies implemented with patients. If there is any question as to the lawfulness of a treatment procedure, legal counsel should be contacted.

Cases where implementation of legal counsel may be particularly important are in those cases involving aversives. These procedures have a great potential for abuse, and often physical restraint, corporal punishment, and inhumane conditions are passed off as treatment (Kazdin, 1984). Specific court rulings have included *Hancock v. Avery, Morales v. Turman,* and *Wyatt vs. Stickney,* which specify the admissible conditions for the use of time out and isolation (Kazdin, 1984). Rulings (e.g., *Wyatt v. Stickney*) have also been offered regarding use of electric shock. Several forms of punishment (e.g., overcorrection, positive practice, response cost), however, have not been addressed by the courts; perhaps these procedures are considered relatively mild (Kazdin, 1984).

Finally, informed consent is another area that has legal ramifications. Consent involves competence (the ability to make a well-informed decision based on an understanding of the choices available), knowledge (the understanding of the treatment, its alternatives, and the risks and benefits involved) and volition (the uncoerced agreement to undergo treatment). The client may withdraw consent at any time (*Knect v. Gillman;* Kazdin, 1984). This issue may have even more bearing in cases involving the use of aversives. For example, should the patient not be competent enough to give consent, one may question whether it is lawful to allow others (i.e., parents or guardians) to give consent for such procedures.

In sum, several disciplines are involved in the implementation of treatment services. Once team members have been chosen it is important to continually evaluate whether there are gaps in the services and whether other disciplines (e.g., occupational therapy, speech therapy) are missing and are essential in order to provide comprehensive treatment. Should deficiencies be present, new team members should be added as appropriate and necessary.

Recommendations for Establishing Coordinated Efforts Between Team Members

When acting as a consultant to a multidisciplinary team, it is important to derive input and support from all team members during the various stages of intervention. This will help to ensure the coordination, cooperation, and efficiency of the services provided. No data have been provided regarding the most effective methods for achieving this necessary support from team members. A number of informal recommendations, however, have been offered.

First, in achieving support for proposed plans of action, it is important that the consultant secure support from the professional in charge (e.g., staff psychiatrist, school principal), given that this individual ultimately decides whether a plan will be implemented. Eventually, however, it is important that all team members support the proposed ideas. Support may be best achieved by presenting the similarities in interests and goals of all team members. It is also important to present clearly the rationale behind the proposals and the way in which the proposed plan of action will be beneficial to all involved. Finally, the consultant should encourage involvement from all team members throughout treatment planning and intervention to maximize opportunities for the members to express comments and concerns regarding the plan and for the consultant to keep abreast of these concerns as well as the plan's limitations.

Steps in Establishing Coordination of Efforts

We have also mentioned that it is imperative that different service providers coordinate their services for efficient and effective treatment planning and implementation. How does this coordination of services actually take place? Typically a psychologist, special educator or other professional assumes the role of behavioral consultant. Behavioral consultation is typically regarded in terms of a means for problem solving in which the consultant helps the consultee (e.g., parents, teachers, institutional staff) to define and assess the attainment of various goals. Whatever the setting or purpose, however, consultative services typically progress through four stages— problem identification, problem analysis, plan implementation, and problem evaluation—requiring varying amounts of participation across disciplines at different points in time (Kratochwill & Bergan, 1978).

In the problem identification stage, a clear specification of the program and problems to be addressed should be outlined (Kratochwill & Bergan, 1978). To achieve this goal, the consultant must be efficient and use good interviewing skills in order to identify consultee problems (Bergan & Tombari, 1976). Identifying the problem is achieved mainly through an interview in which the consultant asks questions to elicit a fairly precise description of the problems of interest and the desired outcomes. The problem identification interview should further allow for the specification of the particular procedures to be utilized in evaluating treatment outcome (Kratochwill & Bergan, 1978). Whatever problems are identified should be discussed in detail with all team members to determine whether these indeed are the problems of interest and whether consensual agreement on procedures occurs.

In the problem analysis stage, the consultant and consultee(s) discuss and plan an intervention to produce the decided-upon criterion for performance. It is at this point that the behavioral consultant utilizes his or her knowledge of behavioral principles and of the research literature to devise a workable treatment plan that is socially valid and otherwise acceptable to the consultee and the rest of the treatment team (Kratochwill & Bergan, 1978).

During the plan implementation phase, the intervention designed in the previous stage is carried out by the consultee/behavioral manager and is supervised by the consultant and/or the consultee's immediate supervisors. During this phase, the consultant ensures that the treatment is being carried out with integrity. Outside observers may be trained in recording procedures to collect data to identify problem areas. Should problematic areas in the treatment implementation process occur, the consultant should address them in an individual meeting with the behavior manager or in a team meeting (Kratochwill & Bergan, 1978).

Finally, during the evaluation phase of problem solving, the consultant and other team members individually or as a whole frequently evaluate the extent to which the treatment is promoting the achievement of program objectives. In addition, discussion during this phase often centers around the options of retraining, altering, or discarding the existing plan (Kratochwill & Bergan, 1978).

From the above information on the how-to aspects of coordinating treatment services, it is obvious that frequent communication between individual team members and the treatment team is essential. It is important that the consultant present enough information for the other team members to decide on an effective intervention, carry it out, and decide on its impact in the achievement of the treatment goals (Kratochwill & Bergan, 1978). In addition, other team members must communicate their questions and practical concerns that relate to their various areas of expertise (e.g., law). Once a treatment team decision is achieved, however, it is important that the team members back each other up to ensure treatment integrity and consistency in carrying out the plans across persons and settings.

Finally, consultation may be on a long-term basis or center on specific problem behaviors of immediate concern. The duration of the consultative process and of team involvement depends on various factors, including problem severity, the familiarity of the behavior manager with learning principles, and the complexity of the behavioral contingencies maintaining the behavior. In the case of aversives, for example, the consultant will be required to monitor the treatment implementation and progress carefully to minimize the potential for abuse. The consultant might be involved in treatment more intensely and for a longer time period than usual in order to ensure patient safety.

SUMMARY

This chapter has concerned the coordination of treatment across various disciplines, particularly as it relates to the use of aversives. It is evident from the discussion that without good working relationships and a division of responsibility among professionals, treatment development, implementation, and evaluation would not be effective. A multidisciplinary approach enables individuals of various specialty areas to coordinate their services throughout treatment.

As mentioned previously, with a change to a multidisciplinary approach to treatment has come a change in treatment goals to include an emphasis on implementing the most effective treatment, encouraging early detection and intervention, ensuring treatment acceptability, minimizing side effects, and programming maintenance and generalization. In addition, the target of intervention has changed from direct intervention of the clinician with the target individual to indirect intervention through consultation and training of parents, teachers, inpatient staff, peers, and other individuals in treatment implementation. Finally, the methods used in providing this training and in coordinating among disciplines to establish a team approach were detailed.

REFERENCES

Abidin, R. (1971). What's wrong with behavior modification. *Journal of School Psychology, 9*, 38–42.

Alexander, D. F. (1985). The effect of study skill training on learning disabled students' retelling of expository material. *Journal of Applied Behavior Analysis, 18*, 263–267.

Allen, C. T., & Forman, S. G. (1984). Efficacy of methods of training teachers in behavioral modification. *School Psychology Review, 13*(1), 26–31.

Baer, A., Rowbury, T., & Baer, D. (1973). The development of instructional control over classroom activities of deviant preschool children. *Journal of Applied Behavior Analysis, 6*, 289–298.

Benberich, J. P. (1971). Do the child's responses shape the teaching behavior of adults: *Journal of Experimental Research in Personality, 5*, 92–97.

Bergan, J. R., & Tombari, M. L. (1976). Consultant skill and efficiency and the implementation and outcomes of consultation. *Journal of School Psychology, 14*, 3–14.

Blechman, E. A. (1984). Competent parents, competent children: Behavioral objectives of parent training. In R. F. Dangel & R. A. Polster (Eds.), *Parent training: Foundations of research and practice* (pp. 34–63). New York: Guilford.

Bornstein, P. H. (1985). Self-instructional training: A commentary and state-of-the-art. *Journal of Applied Behavior Analysis, 18*, 69–72.

Bornstein, P. H., Hamilton, S. B., & Quevillon, P. R. (1977). Behavior modification by long distance: Demonstration of functional control over disruptive behavior in a rural classroom setting. *Behavior Modification, 1*, 369–394.

Bornstein, P. H., & Quevillon, R. P. (1976). The effects of a self-instructional package on overactive preschool boys. *Journal of Applied Behavior Analysis, 9*, 179–188.

Budd, K. S., & Fabry, P. L. (1984). Behavioral assessment in applied parent training: Use of a structured observation system. In R. F. Dangel & R. A. Polster (Eds.), *Parent training: Foundations of research and practice* (pp. 417–442). New York: Guilford.

Budd, K. S., Riner, T. S., & Brockman, M. P. (1983). A structured observation system for clinical evaluation of parent training. *Behavioral Assessment, 5*, 373–393.

Bugental, D. B., Whalen, C. K., & Henker, B. (1977). Causal attributions of hyperactive children and motivational assumptions of two behavior-change approaches: Evidence for an interactionist position. *Child Development, 48*, 874–884.

Burgio, L. D., Whitman, T. L., & Johnson, M. R. (1980). A self-instructional package for increasing attending behavior in educable mentally retarded children. *Journal of Applied Behavior Analysis, 13*, 443–459.

Cheek, F. E., Laucius, J., Mahncke, M., & Beck, R. (1971). A behavior modification training program for parents of convalescent schizophrenics. In R. D. Rubin, H. Fersterheim, A. A. Lazarus & C. M. Franks (Eds.), *Advances in behavior therapy*. New York: Academic Press.

Clark, D. B., & Baker, B. L. (1983). Predicting outcome in parent training. *Journal of Consulting and Clinical Psychology, 51*(2), 309–311.

Dadds, M. R., Schwartz, S., & Sanders, M. R. (1987). Marital discord and treatment outcome in behavioral treatment of child conduct disorders. *Journal of Consulting and Clinical Psychology, 55*(3), 396–403.

Dangel, R. F., & Polster, R. A. (Eds.). (1984). *Parent training: Foundations of research and practice.* New York: Guilford.

Denney, D. R. (1975). The effects of exemplary and cognitive models and self-rehearsal on children's interrogative strategies. *Journal of Experimental Child Psychology, 19,* 467–488.

Dumas, J. E., & Wahler, R. G. (1983). Predictors of treatment outcome in past training: Mother insularity and socioeconomic disadvantages. *Behavioral Assessment, 5,* 301–313.

Dyer, K., Schwartz, I. S., & Luce, S. C. (1984). A supervision program for increasing functional activities for severely handicapped students in residential setting. *Journal of Applied Behavior Analysis, 17,* 249–259.

Favell, J. E. (1990). Issues in the use of nonaversive and aversive interventions. In S. L. Harris & J. S. Handelman (Eds.), *Aversive and nonaversive interventions: Controlling life-threatening behavior by the developmentally disabled* (pp. 36–56). New York: Springer.

Forehand, R., & King, H. E. (1977). Noncompliant children: Effects of parent training on behavior and attitude change. *Behavior Modification, 1,* 93–108.

Forman, S. G. (1980). A comparison of cognitive training and response cost procedures in modifying aggressive behavior of elementary school children. *Behavior Therapy, 11,* 594–600.

Foxx, R. M., Bittle, R. G., & Faw, C. D. (1989). A maintenance strategy for discontinuing aversive procedures: A 52-month follow-up of the treatment of aggression. *American Journal of Mental Retardation, 94,* 27–36.

Friedling, C., & O'Leary, S. G. (1979). Effects of self-instructional training on second- and third-grade hyperactive children: A failure to replicate. *Journal of Applied Behavior Analysis, 12,* 211–219.

Gottman, J., Gonso, J., & Schuler, P. (1976). Teaching social skills to isolated children. *Journal of Abnormal Child Psychology, 4,* 79–197.

Grabowski, J., & Thompson, T. (1972). A behavior modification program for behaviorally retarded institutionalized males. In T. Thompson & J. Grabowski (Eds.), *Behavior modification of the mentally retarded.* New York: Oxford University Press.

Greenwood, C. R., Carta, J. J., & Hall, R. V. (1988). The use of peer tutoring strategies in classroom management and educational instruction. *School Psychology Review, 17,* 258–275.

Greenwood, C. R., Dinwiddie, G., Terry, B., Wade, L., Stanley, S., Thibadeaux, S., & Delquadri, J. (1984). Teacher- versus peer-mediated instruction: An ecobehavioral analysis of achievement outcomes. *Journal of Applied Behavior Analysis, 17,* 521–538.

Hall, R. V. (1971). Training teachers in classroom use of contingency management. *Education Technology, 4,* 31–38.

Hall, J., & Baker, R. (1973). Token economy systems, breakdown and control. *Behavior Research and Therapy, 11,* 253–267.

Hall, R. V., Fox, R., Willard, D., Goldsmith, L., Emerson, M., Owen, M., Davis, F., & Porcia, E. (1971). The teacher as observer and experimenter in the modification of disputing and talking-out behavior. *Journal of Applied Behavior Analysis, 4,* 141–149.

Harris, V., & Sherman, J. (1973). Use and analysis of the "good behavior game" to reduce disruptive classroom behavior. *Journal of Applied Behavior Analysis, 6,* 405–417.

Heffer, R. W., & Kelley, M. L. (1987). Mothers' acceptance of behavioral interventions for children: The influence of parent race and income. *Behavior Therapy, 2,* 153–163.

Herr, S. S. (1990). The law on aversive and nonaversive behavioral intervention. In S. L. Harris & J. S. Handelman (Eds.), *Aversive and nonaversive interactions: Controlling life-threatening behavior by the developmentally disabled* (pp. 80–118). New York: Springer.

Hughes, J. N. (1985). Parents as cotherapists in think aloud. *Psychology in the Schools, 22,* 436–443.

Iwata, B. A., Dorsey, M. F., Slifer, K. J., Bauman, K. E., & Richman, G. S. (1982). Toward a functional analysis of self-injury. *Analysis and Intervention in Developmental Disabilities, 2,* 3–20.

Johnson, D. W., & Johnson, R. T. (1983). Effects of cooperative, competitive, and individualistic learning experiences on social development. *Exceptional Children, 49,* 323–329.

Johnson, D. W., Johnson, R. T., Warring, D., & Maruyama, G. (1986). Different cooperative learning procedures and cross-handicap relationships. *Exceptional Children, 53,* 247–252.

Kanfer, F. H. (1975). Self-management methods. In F. H. Kanfer & A. P. Goldstein (Eds.), *Helping people change: A textbook of methods.* New York: Pergamon.

Kapadia, E. S., & Fantuzzo, J. W. (1988). Effects of teacher- and self-administered procedures on the spelling performance of learning-handicapped children. *Journal of School Psychology, 26,* 49–58.

Karoly, P. (1980). Operant methods. In F. H. Kanfer & A. P. Goldstein (Eds.), *Helping people change: A textbook of methods.* New York: Pergamon.

Kazdin. A. E. (1974). Assessment of teacher training in a reinforcement program. *Journal of Teacher Education, 25,* 266–270.

Kazdin, A. E. (1984). *Behavior modification in applied settings* (3rd ed.). Homewood, IL: Dorsey.

Kazdin, A. E., & Esveldt-Dawson, K. (1981). *How to maintain behavior.* Austin, TX: Pro-Ed.

Kazdin, A. E., & Polster, R. (1973). Intermittent token reinforcement and response maintenance in extinction. *Behavior Therapy, 4,* 386–391.

Kendall, P. C., & Finch, A. J., Jr. (1978). A cognitive-behavioral treatment for impulsivity: A group comparison study. *Journal of Consulting and Clinical Psychology, 46,* 110–118.

Klingman, A., Melamed, B. G., Cuthbert, M. I., & Hermecz, D. A. (1984). Effects of participant modeling on information acquisition and skill utilization. *Journal of Consulting and Clinical Psychology, 52,* 414–422.

Koegel, R., Glahn, T. J., & Nieminen, G. S. (1978). Generalization of parent-training results. *Journal of Applied Behavior Analysis, 11,* 95–109.

Kratochwill, T. R., & Bergan, J. R. (1978). Evaluating programs in applied settings through behavioral consultation. *Journal of School Psychology, 16,* 375-386.

Lahey, B. B., Gendrich, J. G., Gendrich, S. I., Schnelle, J. F., Gant, D. S., & McNees, M. P. (1977). An evaluation of daily report cards with minimal teacher and parent contacts as an efficient method of classroom intervention. *Behavior Modification, 1,* 381–394.

LaVigna, G. W., & Donnellan, A. M. (1986). *Alternatives to punishment: Solving behavior problems with nonaversive strategies.* New York: Irvington.

Lentz, F. E. (1988). Reductive procedures. In C. Witt, S. N. Elliott, & F. M. Gresham (Eds.), *Handbook of behavior therapy in education.* New York: Plenum.

Lichstein, K. L., & Shreibman, L. (1976). Employing electric shock with autistic children: A review of the side effects. *Journal of Autism and Childhood Schizophrenia, 6,* 163–173.

Loeber, R., & Weisman, R. G. (1975). Contingencies of therapist and trainer performance: A review. *Psychological Bulletin, 82,* 660–688.

Lovaas, O. I. (1987). Behavioral treatment and normal education and intellectual functioning in young autistic children. *Journal of Consulting and Clinical Psychology, 55,* 3–9.

Lovaas, O. I., & Favell, J. E. (1987). Protection for clients undergoing aversive/restrictive interventions. *Education and Treatment of Children, 10,* 311–325.

Maheady, L., & Sainato, O. (1985). The effects of peer tutoring upon the social status and social interaction patterns of high and low status elementary students. *Education and Treatment of Children, 8,* 51–56.

Marchetti, A. G. (1987). Wyatt vs. Stickney: A consent decree. *Research in Developmental Disabilities, 8,* 249–260.

Marholin, D., & Steinman, W. (1977). Stimulus control in the classroom as a function of the behavior reinforced. *Journal of Applied Behavior Analysis, 5,* 465–478.

Martin, G., Pallotta-Cornick, A., Johnstone, G., & Goyos, A. C. (1980). A supervisory strategy to improve work performance for lower functioning retarded clients in a sheltered workshop. *Journal of Applied Behavior Analysis, 13,*183–190.

Matson, J. L., & DiLorenzo, T. (1983). *Punishment and its alternatives: A new perspective for behavior modification.* New York: Springer.

Matson, J. L., & Gorman-Smith, D. (1986). A review of treatment research for aggressive and disruptive behavior in the mentally retarded. *Applied Research in Mental Retardation, 7,* 95–103.

Matson, J. L., & Ollendick, T. H. (1977). Issues in toilet training. *Behavior Therapy, 8,* 549–553.

Matson, J. L., & Swiezy, N. B. (1990). The aversives controversy: Policy issues in behavior modification and therapy. *Scandinavian Journal of Behavior Therapy, 19,* 25–31.

Matson, J. L., & Taras, M. E. (1989). A 20 year review of punishment and alternative methods to treat problem behaviors in developmentally delayed persons. *Research in Developmental Disabilities, 10,* 85–104.

Matson, J. L., & Zeiss, R. A. (1979). The buddy system: A method for generalized reduction of inappropriate interpersonal behavior of retarded psychiatric patients. *British Journal of Social and Clinical Psychology, 18,* 401–405.

Meichenbaum, D., & Goodman, J. (1971). Training impulsive children to talk to themselves: A means of developing self-control. *Journal of Abnormal Psychology, 77,* 154–126.

Monahan, J., & O'Leary, K. D. (1971). Effects of self-instruction on rule-breaking behavior. *Psychological Reports, 29,* 1059–1066.

Mulick, J. A., & Linscheid, T. R. (1988). [Review of *Alternatives to punishment: Solving behavior problems with non-aversive strategies.*] *Research in Developmental Disabilities, 1*(1), 3.

Nay, W. R. (1979). Parents as real life reinforcers: The enhancement of parent training effects across conditions other than training. In A. P. Goldstein & F. H. Kanfer (Eds.), *Maximizing treatment gains: Transfer enhancement in psychotherapy.* New York: Academic Press.

Newsom, C., Favell, J. E., & Rincover, A. (1983). In S. Axelrod & L. Apsche (Eds.), *The effects of punishment on human behavior* (pp. 285–311). New York: Academic Press.

Newsom, C., & Rincover, A. (1989). Autism. In E. J. Mash & R. A. Barkley (Eds.), *Treatment of childhood disorders.* New York: Guilford.

O'Dell, S. (1985). Progress in parent training. In M. Hersen, R. M. Eisler, & P. M. Miller (Eds.), *Progress in behavior modification, vol. 19* (pp. 57–108). New York: Academic Press.

O'Leary, K. D., Poulus, R. W., & Devine, V. T. (1972). Tangible reinforcers: Bonuses or bribes. *Journal of Consulting and Clinical Psychology, 38,* 1–8.

Ollendick, T. H. (1981). Self-monitoring and self-administered overcorrection: The modification of nervous tics in children. *Behavior Modification, 5,* 75–84.

Panyan, M. C., & Patterson, E. T. (1974). Teaching attendants the applied aspects of behavior modification. *Mental Retardation, 12,* 30–32.

Patterson, G. R. (1974). Interventions for boys with conduct problems. Multiple settings, treatment and criteria. *Journal of Consulting and Clinical Psychology, 42,* 471–481.

Patterson, G. R. (1982). *Coercive family process.* Eugene, OR: Castalia.

Patterson, G. R., Chamberlain, P., & Reid, J. B. (1982). A comparative evaluation of a parent training program. *Behavior Therapy, 13,* 638–650.

Pigott, H. E., & Heggie, D. L. (1986). Interpreting the conflicting results of individual versus group contingencies in classrooms: The targeted behavior as a mediating variable. *Child and Family Behavior Therapy, 7,* 1–15.

Pizzat, F. J. (1974). *Behavior modification in residential treatment for children: Model of a program.* New York: Behavioral Publications.

Pomerleau, O. F., Bobrove, P. H., & Smith, R. H. (1973). Rewarding psychiatric aides for the behavioral improvement of assigned patients. *Journal of Applied Behavior Analysis, 6,* 383–390.

Quilitch, H. R. (1975). A comparison of three staff-management procedures. *Journal of Applied Behavior Analysis, 8,* 59–66.

Reid, D. H., Parsons, M. B., & Schepis, M. M. (1990). Management practices that affect the relative utility of aversive and nonaversive procedures. In S. L. Harris & J. S. Handelman (Eds.), *Aversive and nonaversive interventions: Controlling life-threatening behavior by the developmentally disabled* (pp. 144–162). New York: Springer.

Repp, A. C., Barton, L. E., & Brulle, A. R. (1982). Naturalistic studies of mentally retarded persons: The effect of staff instructions on student responding. *Applied Research in Mental Retardation, 3,* 55–65.

Repp, A. C., & Deitz, D. E. E. (1978). Ethical issues in reducing responding of institutionalized mentally retarded persons. *Mental Retardation, 16,* 45–46.

Rickert, V. I., Sottolano, D. C., Parrish, J. M., Riley, A. W., Hunt, F. M., & Pelco, L. E. (1988). Training parents to become better behavior managers: The need for a competency-based approach. *Behavior Modification, 12,* 475–496.

Rimland, B. (1978). Risks and benefits in the treatment of autistic children: A risk/benefit perspective on the use of aversives. *Journal of Autism and Child Schizophrenia, 8,* 100–104.

Saigh, P. A., & Umar, A. M. (1983). The effects of a good behavior game on the disruptive behavior of Sudanese elementary school students. *Journal of Applied Behavior Analysis, 16,* 339–344.

Sanders, M. R., & James, J. E. (1983). The modification of parent behavior: A review of generalization and maintenance. *Behavior Modification, 7,* 3–27.

Schmidt, G. W., & Ulrich, R. E. (1969). Effects of group contingent events on classroom noise. *Journal of Applied Behavior Analysis, 2,* 171–179.

Schmitt, B. D. (1985). When baby just won't sleep. *Contemporary Pediatrics,* 38–52.

Schinke, S. P., & Wong, S. E. (1977). Evaluation of staff training in group homes for retarded persons. *American Journal of Mental Deficiency, 82,* 130–136.

Schinke, S. P., & Wong, S. E. (1978). Teaching child care workers: A behavioral approach. *Child Care Quarterly, 7,* 45–61.

Skinner, B. F. (1988). A statement on punishment. *IARET Newsletter, 1*(1), 3.

Skinner, C. H., Turco, T. L., Beatty, K. L., & Rasavage, C. (1989). Cover, copy, and compare: A method for increasing multiplication performance. *School Psychology Review, 18,* 412–420.

Sobey, F. (1970). *The nonprofessional revolution in mental health.* New York: Columbia University Press.

Stokes, T. F., & Baer, D. M. (1977). An implicit technology of generalization. *Journal of Applied Behavior Analysis, 10,* 349–367.

Touchette, P. E., MacDonald, R. F., & Langer, S. N. (1985). A scatterplot for identifying stimulus control of problem behavior. *Journal of Applied Behavior Analysis, 18,* 343–351.

Van Houten, R., Axelrod, S., Bailey, J. S., Favell, J. E., Foxx, R. M., Iwata, B. A., & Lovaas, O. I. (1988). The right to effective treatment. *Journal of Applied Behavior Analysis, 21,* 381–384.

Wahler, R. G. (1976). Deviant child behavior within the family: Developmental speculations and behavior change strategies. In H. Leitenberg (Ed.), *Handbook of behavior modification and behavior therapy.* Englewood Cliffs, NJ: Prentice-Hall.

Watson, L. S., Gardner, J. M., & Sanders, C. (1971). Shaping and maintaining behavior modification skills in staff members in a mental retardation institution: Columbus State University behavior modification program. *Mental Retardation, 9,* 39–42.

Webster-Stratton, C. (1985). Predictors of treatment outcome in parent training for conduct disordered children. *Behavior Therapy, 16,* 223–243.

Wells, K. C., Griest, D. L., & Forehand, R. (1980). The use of a self-control package to enhance temporal generality of a parent training program. *Behaviour Research and Therapy, 18,* 347–354.

Witt, J. C., & Elliott, S. N. (1982). The response cost lottery: A time efficient and effective classroom intervention. *Journal of School Psychology, 20,* 155–161.

Witt, J. C., Hannafin, M., & Martens, B. (1983). Home based reinforcement: Behavioral covariation between academic performance and inappropriate behavior. *Journal of School Psychology, 21,* 337–348.

Ziarnik, J. R., & Bernstein, G. S. (1982). A critical examination of the effect of inservice training on staff performance. *Mental Retardation, 20,* 109–114.

Promoting Generalization and Maintenance of Treatment Gains

Communication-Based Treatment of Severe Behavior Problems

EDWARD G. CARR, GENE MCCONNACHIE, LEN LEVIN, AND DUANE C. KEMP

The purpose of this chapter is to describe the role of communication training in the reduction or elimination of serious behavior problems in persons with developmental disabilities. We will discuss clinical and conceptual guidelines for implementing a communication-based approach. It is not our intent to provide a treatment manual; such a manual is currently being field tested and will be forthcoming in a separate publication. The material in this chapter does, however, define the major elements of our approach.

CONCEPTUAL AND EMPIRICAL BACKGROUND

We will briefly describe the research and conceptual base from which the communication procedures elaborated on in this chapter were developed. First, we must note that for many years, there have been demonstrations that an inverse relationship exists between the frequency of behavior problems and the level of communicative skill that an individual possesses. Thus, in the child development literature, high levels of communicative competence are often associated with low levels of disturbing behaviors such as crying (Bell & Ainsworth, 1972) and aggression (Brownlee & Bakeman, 1981). In the litera-

EDWARD G. CARR, GENE MCCONNACHIE, LEN LEVIN, AND DUANE C. KEMP • Department of Psychology, State University of New York at Stony Brook, Stony Brook, New York 11794.

Behavior Analysis and Treatment, edited by R. Van Houten & S. Axelrod. Plenum Press, New York, 1993.

ture on developmental disabilities, individuals displaying more advanced verbal skills have been shown to exhibit less aggression (Talkington, Hall, & Altman, 1971) and less self-injury (Shodell & Reiter, 1968) than those who lack such skills.

These observations have led a number of investigators to propose a communication hypothesis of behavior problems. The hypothesis states that many instances of behavior problems can be usefully viewed as a nonverbal form of communication (Carr, 1985; Carr & Durand, 1985a, 1987; Donnellan, Mirenda, Mesaros, & Fassbender, 1984; Neel & Billingsley, 1989; Reichle & Yoder, 1979). The developmental implication, of course, is that as the individual acquires more sophisticated forms of communication (e.g., gesture, speech), primitive forms (e.g., behavior problems) become less effective and therefore drop out of the individual's repertoire or remain only in those situations in which the sophisticated forms are temporarily ineffective.

In lay language, the communication hypothesis implies that behavior problems are not random, bizarre acts but instead are purposeful in nature. There is much evidence in the area of developmental disabilities that supports this assertion. If a behavior is purposeful, then one would expect that specific instances of misbehavior would be reliably associated with specific types of reinforcement. The research literature does indeed demonstrate the existence of three classes of socially mediated reinforcement that are reliable consequences of misbehavior: attention, escape, and tangibles. Some instances of behavior problems are maintained by attention (Carr & McDowell, 1980; Lovaas, Freitag, Gold, & Kassorla, 1965; Lovaas & Simmons, 1969; Martin & Foxx, 1973). Metaphorically speaking, the individual in such cases uses aggression and self-injury in a manner analogous to communicating the request, "Pay attention to me." Other instances of behavior problems are maintained by escape (negative reinforcement) variables (Carr & Newsom, 1985; Carr, Newsom, & Binkoff, 1976, 1980; Iwata, Dorsey, Slifer, Bauman, & Richman, 1982; Plummer, Baer, & LeBlanc, 1977; Sailor, Guess, Rutherford, & Baer, 1968; Weeks & Gaylord-Ross, 1981), in which the individual uses behavior problems to communicate the request, "I don't want to do this activity any more." Finally, still other instances of misbehavior are maintained by tangible stimuli (Durand & Crimmins, 1988; Edelson, Taubman, & Lovaas, 1983), in which the individual uses behavior problems to communicate the request, "I want food" (or to engage in a particular activity).

We have stressed that we use the communication concept as a metaphor. From a methodological standpoint, it is doubtful that one could ever demonstrate definitively what the intent or purpose of a given communicative act is. That being the case, the issue can be raised as to whether it would be preferable to state simply that a problem behavior was, for example, reinforced by food consequences rather than saying that the problem behavior represents a request for food. We would argue that the communication metaphor is heuristic and serves as a prompt for the teacher or parent to engage in skill building. In contrast, stressing the idea that a behavior problem is maintained by food leads too readily, in our opinion, to the practice of providing such consequences without requiring specific socially desirable behaviors on the part of the individual receiving them. For example, reinforcers may be provided in a differential reinforcement of other behavior (DRO) format in which the individual receives food contingent on not performing the behavior for a period of time. Though DRO may be effective in selective cases, it does not emphasize the teaching of replacement behaviors. Of equal importance, it places individuals who have disabilities in a passive role, a role that they already play too often.

The communication notion, however metaphorical, acts as a prompt for teachers and parents to consider what alternative forms of communication could be taught to replace the objectionable behavior. In other words, skill building and educational considerations become the major focus. Further, these skills, once taught, put individuals in the position of being able to initiate specific interactions with others that eventually lead to preferred reinforcers. Thus, the individual with disabilities assumes an active role in the treatment process.

The purposive nature of behavior problems is also illustrated by studies of how children affect adults through misbehavior (child effects). Recently, we completed a study of the impact of escape-motivated behavior problems on the teaching behavior of adults (Carr, Taylor, & Robinson, 1991). We found that children selectively misbehave when adults try to teach them. Thus, when the teacher tried to give vocabulary instruction, a child might engage in self-injury or aggression, but when the teacher did not attempt instruction, the child was well behaved. Importantly, as a consequence of this interaction, teachers tended to distribute their instructional time so as to minimize contact with those children whose behavior problems were escape moti- vated. Of equal interest, if a teacher did instruct the problem child, the teacher tended to focus on those tasks that were associated with low levels of behavior problems and to avoid those tasks associated with high levels of behavior problems. What we have been describing, of course, is the shaping of a teacher's behavior by a child. In a sense, by means of behavior problems, the child controls what and how much he or she is taught. In short, the effects of behavior problems are not random but rather systematic and reliable, exactly the pattern from which one would infer that they serve an adaptive function for the individual displaying them.

If the communication hypothesis has merit, then one would expect that teaching an individual some form of language (e.g., speech, sign, gesture, or symbol) that accesses the same reinforcers as those maintaining the problem behavior should make the problem behavior unnecessary, thereby leading to its reduction or elimination. There is a growing research base supporting this prediction. A number of studies demonstrate that systematically teaching an individual communicative forms that are functionally equivalent to behavior problems (i.e., that are maintained by the same reinforcers) results in dramatic decreases—and sometimes elimination—of the problems (Billingsley & Neel, 1985; Bird, Dores, Moniz, & Robinson, 1989; Carr & Durand, 1985b; Carr et al., 1980; Day, Rea, Schussler, Larsen, & Johnson, 1988; Durand & Kishi, 1987; Horner & Budd, 1985). Further, treatment gains appear to generalize across settings and people (Bird et al., 1989; Durand & Carr, in press) and maintain over periods extending from several months to several years (Bird et al., 1989; Durand & Carr, 1991; Durand & Kishi, 1987; Levin et al., 1990). Finally, several studies demonstrate that multifaceted communication approaches (not restricted to teaching functionally equivalent responses) may also have an ameliorative effect on the incidence of behavior problems (Hunt, Alwell, & Goetz, 1988; Koegel, Koegel, Murphy, & Ryan, 1989). In sum, there is a research base for the proposition that training communication skills can be an effective method for treating severe behavior problems.

DESCRIPTION OF PARTICIPANTS

The intervention model that we will describe is based on our observations of more than 30 individuals who have participated in our research on communication-based treatment of severe behavior problems over the years. For purposes of illustration, however, we will frequently allude to three individuals who are the focus of a longitudinal study currently in progress (Levin et al., 1990). At the start of treatment, Val was 15 years old, Gary was 18, and Jim was 39. Val and Gary lived at home with their parents, and Jim resided in a group home. Val was diagnosed as severely retarded with cerebral palsy. Gary and Jim were both diagnosed as having autism with profound mental retardation. All three individuals displayed varying amounts of self-injury, tantrums, aggression, and property destruction. In short, we were dealing with people who posed serious threats to themselves and/or others and who frequently were involved in crises in the home, school, or community. For that reason, we will begin with the issue of crisis management.

CRISIS MANAGEMENT

It takes time to implement fully a communication-based intervention for severe behavior problems. Therefore, at the beginning of treatment and even after treatment effects have been well established, occasions may arise in which an individual displays dangerous behaviors that pose safety risks to self and others. On those occasions, some form of crisis management will be necessary. The purpose of such procedures is to reduce the frequency and intensity of dangerous behavior quickly. We have found the crisis strategies that we will describe to be clinically useful; however, the exact role of these strategies in intervention awaits empirical analysis. It is worthwhile to emphasize at this point that although crisis strategies may be a useful part of an overall treatment plan, no such plan is complete unless there is a constructive component that focuses on building new skills that make the future performance of severe behavior problems unnecessary (Carr, Robinson, & Palumbo, 1990).

What are some of the clinical considerations in managing crises within the context of a communication-based program? First, one must identify the type of situation in which the crisis arises. Second, one must choose a management strategy that is appropriate to the situation but does not seriously interfere with the treatment (skill-building) effort. With respect to the first consideration, we have encountered five generic types of situations in which crises are likely to arise: before the communicative response is strongly developed; when the delay between a communicative request for a reinforcer and the receipt of the reinforcer is too long; in new situations, before generalization has been achieved; when the initial assessment of motivation was wrong; and when we have been unable to assess the motivation of a behavior problem. With respect to the second consideration, we have used five categories of procedures to manage crises: *ignore* the behavior problem; *protect* the individual or others from the physical consequences of the behavior problem; momentarily *restrain* the individual during episodes of behavior problems; *remove* anyone whom the behavior problem endangers from the vicinity in which the crisis episode is occurring; and *introduce* discriminative stimuli that evoke nonproblem behavior.

How are the above two considerations combined to produce effective management? In the most severe instances of behavior problems, our options frequently centered on protecting, restraining, or removing. Thus, if Jim slapped or kicked us, we deflected his blows (protect). If Gary punched us, we backed off beyond the reach of his fist (remove), but if he attempted to bite himself on the hand, we blocked his hand before he could put it in his mouth (protect). If Val hit another child, we immediately put ourselves between her and the victim (protect) and then, while attending to the victim, escorted that individual from the vicinity (remove). If Val grabbed the hair of another person and began to pull vigorously, we unclenched her fingers to release her grip (protect) and continued to hold her arms momentarily (restrain) until we could get the person in danger out of the area (remove). Restraint proved to be the least desirable tactic, because attention-seeking individuals such as Val sometimes responded to restraint as a form of positive social reinforcement, and other individuals such as Gary responded to restraint as an aversive tactile stimulus necessitating an escape response. In both cases, momentary restraint would intermittently escalate the level of aggression. In spite of this clear disadvantage, restraint was sometimes used to provide a few extra seconds for the intervention agent to implement remove and protect strategies.

Ignoring was a fourth tactic that we occasionally used. The crisis strategy of ignoring a behavior problem is not the same as the treatment strategy of extinction. Extinction involves the systematic and consistent removal of those reinforcers that maintain a behavior problem each time that the problem occurs. Ignoring, in contrast, is applied only to those instances of the behavior problem that are not perceived as dangerous, although they may have the potential to become dangerous if they are treated inappropriately. Thus, if Val threw her cosmetics at the wall, or Jim screamed, or Gary bit himself very lightly on the hand, we took no action and continued to carry out whatever activity was ongoing.

Our experience has been that parents and staff find it difficult to ignore these misbehaviors and frequently resort to berating the individuals involved or, at the other extreme, cajoling them to behave appropriately. Almost invariably, this strategy leads to an escalation of the problem, requiring protect, remove, and restrain tactics. Through modeling and instruction, it is necessary to teach treatment agents how to ignore nonthreatening problem behavior and focus instead on treatment intervention (described later) as the main vehicle for long-term amelioration of crisis episodes. In sum, attending to crises appears to perpetuate crises.

It is sometimes possible to employ an additional strategy to manage crises, namely, to introduce discriminative stimuli that evoke nonproblem behavior. For example, even while Gary was biting his hand and attempting to punch others, it was frequently possible to interrupt the crisis by asking him the question, "What do you want?" Through training, this question had acquired powerful discriminative stimulus control over a variety of Gary's requests, and he often broke off his attacks to ask for a break from work or specific tangible items. Clearly this strategy would be available only after some communication training had been carried out, but it is a useful strategy because Gary and other individuals invariably show brief relapses even well into training. Therefore, some form of crisis management remains necessary.

Sometimes a discriminative stimulus strategy can be useful even prior to the development of communication skills. Val, for instance, showed few behavior problems in the presence of one or two individuals even prior to treatment. For reasons that were unclear, these individuals exerted strong discriminative control over nonproblem behavior. Thus, if a crisis arose, it was sometimes possible to introduce these individuals into the problem situation and produce a rapid decrease in aggressive behavior. This procedure parallels the one developed by Touchette and his colleagues (Touchette, MacDonald, & Langer, 1985); these and other stimulus control strategies have been discussed in detail elsewhere (Carr, Robinson, Taylor, & Carlson, 1990) and represent an emerging set of tactics for dealing with severe behavior problems in a crisis situation.

We have outlined several strategies that we have used to deal with crises. No clinical protocol has credibility unless it can articulate a set of procedures for dealing with the almost inevitable occurrence of dangerous behavior in individuals who are known for such behavior. Having made this point, we would also like to say that the virtual obsession of the field with crisis management over the past 25 years has been a mistaken emphasis (Carr, Robinson, & Palumbo, 1990). The ultimate solution to crises is to develop new treatments (e.g., skill building), not more methods of crisis management.

Although we have had to make use of the crisis strategies described, our focus in dealing with problematic situations in the long run was to build appropriate functional behaviors to replace the undesirable behaviors. We will describe this process in detail later. For the moment, we may briefly note the following with respect to the list of five crisis situations mentioned at the beginning of this section. If crises arise because a communicative response is not yet strongly developed, the long-term treatment strategy is to continue to strengthen and broaden the individual's communicative repertoire. If crises arise because the delay between a communicative request and receipt of the object of that request is too great, the long-term treatment strategy is to restructure the situation so that the individual learns to tolerate delays by engaging in interpolated periods of work (or some other functional activity that bridges the delay). If crises arise in new situations because generalization has not yet been achieved in those situations, the long-term treatment strategy is to program generalization into those situations in a systematic and comprehensive manner. If crises arise because the initial assessment of motivation was wrong, then the assessment must be redone so as to incorporate the information (negative data) garnered from the first attempt at treatment. Finally, if crises continue to arise because repeated attempts at motivational assessment do not yield systematic information about relevant controlling variables, then one may have to rely intermittently on the crisis procedures already described.

Our experience has been that only a very small percentage of behavior problems encountered are resistant to the use of functional analysis as a treatment planning guide. Nonetheless, their existence must be frankly acknowledged and is reason for humility and openness to the development of new research strategies and concepts, a posture that stands in contrast to bold assertions of effectiveness that are occasionally forthcoming in some quarters of the field.

FUNCTIONAL ANALYSIS

Ultimately, the most important question is not how to deal with a crisis but rather why the crisis arose in the first place. To answer this question, we have to identify the variables of which the behavior problems are a function; that is, we must carry out a functional analysis. In lay terms, the underlying assumption is that behavior problems serve a purpose for the individual displaying them. Therefore, if we identify what that purpose is, we will be in a position to provide the individual with new means (behaviors) for achieving that purpose. Thus, problem behaviors will be unnecessary and further crises will be averted.

A literature is emerging concerning the practical assessment of the variables controlling severe behavior problems. This literature includes the use of questionnaires, interviews, and direct observation to identify relevant variables (Durand & Crimmins, 1988; Groden, 1989; O'Neill, Horner, Albin, Storey, & Sprague, 1989). Our assessment strategy parallels these developments and is specifically focused on analyzing those behavior problems whose reinforcers are socially mediated. Attention, escape, and tangible/activity reinforcers all fall in this category, because access to these events is typically dependent on an individual's ability to influence others, frequently (and unfortunately) through misbehavior. Our assessment strategy, designed to identify the multiple functions of behavior, is carried out in three stages that can be summarized as follows: describe, categorize, and verify.

Describe

The purpose of this stage is to establish that a particular individual does indeed exhibit serious behavior problems and, further, that these problems are likely mediated socially rather than being a function of organic or self-stimulatory variables. This stage consists of two components. The first component involves the use of interview; the second, direct observation.

In the interview component, classroom staff, group home staff, and parents are asked to describe the behavior problem and the circumstances in which it occurs, as well as the reaction the problem evokes from others. The following two vignettes illustrate material generated from our interviews, one with a classroom teacher and the other with a member of the group home staff:

> When I'm doing individual work with Val, she does very well, but when I move on to work with other children, she becomes disruptive and may strike another child. Also, I noticed that when the speech pathologist comes in to talk to me or to observe the class, Val puts on quite a show. She'll spit or swear or grab things off the table and throw them. When she's acting like this, we'll lay down the law and tell her that we don't allow this kind of thing in our classroom and that she'd better start to act more like a young lady.
>
> When we're having break time, Jim is quiet and happy, but when I ask him to go back to work, he yells and pushes me out of the way. When we're doing [physical] exercises, I never get through more than one or two sit-ups before Jim runs away. If I ask him to come back, he tries to kick me. After a while, it's just not worth it for me to force him. When we start folding his laundry and I tell him we'll all have a snack when we're done, he'll fold one shirt and ask for the snack. If I say 'we have to fold more,' Jim will have a tantrum. When he gets really bad, it's easier to finish folding the laundry myself.

The descriptive material provided by the interviewees suggests that Val's aggressive behavior is attention seeking, whereas Jim's is motivated by escape from work. Our experience has been that interview data may sometimes overestimate the severity and/or frequency of the behavior problem. Therefore, we have learned to follow up our interviews with direct observation.

In the direct observation component, we follow the student or resident around for a period of 2 weeks. During this time, we sample the various situations that the individual encounters as part of his or her daily routine (including the problematic situations identified from the interview process). Each problem behavior incident is recorded on an index card. The card uses a variant of the A-B-C (antecedents-behavior-consequences) format that focuses on the social context of the problem. This format is illustrated in Figure 1.

Consider the index card at the top of the figure, which describes an incident involving Val. In addition to listing the name of the person being observed (Val), the card lists the name of the person making the observation (Len) and the date of the observation (11/12/87). Each episode is described in terms of a general context (in this case, lunch at 12:30 p.m.) and a specific interpersonal context that is correlated with the behavior problem. Ultimately, we find that the interpersonal context is the most informative piece of information. Thus, in the example given, the general context (lunch) is not strongly correlated with behavior problems unless a more specific set of circumstances occurs in which the teacher has to reduce the amount of attention she is paying to Val.

Interestingly, the index card data confirm some information obtained from the earlier interview. Specifically, in the interview it was noted that when the speech pathologist engaged the teacher in conversation, thereby taking attention away from Val, Val exhibited behavior problems. The direct observation material thus parallels the interview material. The index card also contains information describing the nature of the behavior problem (in this case, yelling and grabbing) and the nature of the reaction to that problem (the teacher responds by angrily berating Val). Again, the index card information corroborates the interview data described earlier. Figure 1 also provides two additional examples of the assessment format, one for Gary and one for Jim.

Several points are worth mentioning with respect to the use of the index cards. Our experience has been that observers find this system easy to work with, because the narrative format resembles teacher notes or parent diaries (i.e., a familiar system of coding information). Direct observation for protracted periods of time appears to be crucial for three reasons. First, there is often an overshadowing effect in which severe and/or frequent behavior problems are mentioned in the interview at the expense of noting less severe or relatively infrequent problems. These latter problems typically have to be dealt with as well; therefore, their possible omission from the interview data needs to be compensated for through direct observation. Second, child

```
┌─────────────────────────────────────────────────────────────────┐
│ NAME: Val              OBSERVER: Len            DATE: 11/12/87    │
├─────────────────────────────────────────────────────────────────┤
│ GENERAL CONTEXT: lunch                       TIME: 12:30 p.m.     │
├─────────────────────────────────────────────────────────────────┤
│ INTERPERSONAL CONTEXT: Teacher attending (talking to) another    │
│    adult.  Val and others sitting at table.                      │
│                                                                  │
│ BEHAVIOR PROBLEM: Val yelled at the teacher telling her to get   │
│    her some magazines to read.  Val grabbed the teacher's arm    │
│    and shook her.                                                │
│                                                                  │
│ SOCIAL REACTION: The teacher angrily told Val to let go of her   │
│    arm and continued to berate her for approximately two         │
│    minutes.                                                      │
└─────────────────────────────────────────────────────────────────┘


┌─────────────────────────────────────────────────────────────────┐
│ NAME: Gary             OBSERVER: Gene           DATE: 12/10/87   │
├─────────────────────────────────────────────────────────────────┤
│ GENERAL CONTEXT: gym                         TIME: 10:30 a.m.    │
├─────────────────────────────────────────────────────────────────┤
│ INTERPERSONAL CONTEXT: Gary was rollerskating by himself but     │
│    there were a lot of people near him.                          │
│                                                                  │
│ BEHAVIOR PROBLEM: He looked at the teacher and when the teacher  │
│    looked back, Gary hit a nearby child and bolted for the       │
│    gymnasium exit.                                               │
│                                                                  │
│ SOCIAL REACTION: The teacher shouted at Gary to stop and         │
│    pursued him to the exit.                                      │
└─────────────────────────────────────────────────────────────────┘


┌─────────────────────────────────────────────────────────────────┐
│ NAME: Jim              OBSERVER: Duane          DATE: 1/5/88     │
├─────────────────────────────────────────────────────────────────┤
│ GENERAL CONTEXT: cleaning bathroom           TIME: 4:30 p.m.     │
├─────────────────────────────────────────────────────────────────┤
│ INTERPERSONAL CONTEXT: A member of the group home staff          │
│    accompanied Jim to the bathroom and supplied him with         │
│    cleaning materials.  Jim was asked to wipe down the counter.  │
│                                                                  │
│ BEHAVIOR PROBLEM: After wiping with sponge for two swipes,       │
│    Jim threw the cleaning materials against the wall and         │
│    ran out of the bathroom screaming.                            │
│                                                                  │
│ SOCIAL REACTION: Staff member watched Jim as he sat in the       │
│    corner of the living room but made no attempt to resume       │
│    the cleaning task.                                            │
└─────────────────────────────────────────────────────────────────┘
```

FIGURE 1. Index card format used in functional analysis of socially motivated behavior problems.

effects (discussed earlier) may have caused intervention agents to avoid certain situations that evoke problem behavior, and thus these situations tend not to be reported during the interview process. Protracted direct observation, however, generally reveals that these situations still occur (albeit at a very low rate) and still evoke serious behavior problems. Third, there is sometimes a discrepancy between how intervention agents say they respond to misbehavior (i.e., information gathered during the interview process) and how they actually do respond in live situations. Thus, agents may say that they ignore attention-seeking misbehavior, whereas in reality they shout at the individual; or they may say that they never permit misbehavior to terminate a work session, whereas in reality they radically alter the work session following misbehavior so that the session is mostly free time and no pressure is put on the individual to perform adequately.

Direct observation is also necessary in order to confirm that the reaction to a given behavior problem is indeed socially mediated. If a behavior problem fails to evoke a consistent reaction from others but the problem nonetheless persists, then the behavior may be self-stimulatory in nature, or it may be maintained by its direct physical effect on the environment (e.g., breaking open a cabinet in order to access preferred toys). In these instances, social mediation of reinforcers may be irrelevant to the maintenance of the misbehavior, and therefore a communication-based approach that stresses such social mediation would likely prove ineffective.

Categorize

The descriptive process just outlined typically results in a large number of index cards. For the three cases on which we have been focusing, we generated more than 100 cards per individual. Once the descriptive stage is over, a way must be found to group the index cards so that treatment planning can proceed. Our method of achieving this goal was to have the observer read each card and develop an hypothesis in response to the question, "What did the student or resident want to happen as a consequence of engaging in the behavior problem?" When two or more observers agreed on what the individual "wanted" to achieve with his or her misbehavior, the interpretation was recorded on the index card. Cards lacking reliability were eliminated from further consideration. Thus, for Val in Figure 1, the observers agreed that the purpose of her aggression was to reinstate the teacher's attention (in the form of conversation). For Gary, the purpose was to obtain teacher attention (in the form of eliciting a chase). For Jim, the purpose was to get out of doing work (in the form of avoiding having to clean the bathroom). All of the remaining cards were dealt with in the manner just outlined.

The next step was to post each of the cards on a bulletin board under one of four categories: attention seeking, escape, tangible seeking, and other. The first three categories concern hypotheses that are clearly related to the specific classes of reinforcers, all socially mediated, thought to be maintaining the identified behavior problems. The fourth category requires some explanation. The term *other* generally referred to behaviors that appeared to be self-stimulatory and thus not under social control. Alternatively, a behavior could also be categorized under "other" if it were tangible seeking but not under social control. Specifically, if the individual broke a cabinet in order to access food and there was no one around when the behavior occurred, then the aggressive act would be categorized as "other" because social mediation of reinforcement was not involved. In contrast, if the same individual screamed and hit the teacher while pointing to food in the cabinet, and the teacher responded by providing the food, then the behavior would be categorized as tangible seeking because receipt of the reinforcer depended on the teacher's cooperation (i.e., reinforcer access was socially mediated).

The term *other* also referred to certain classes of idiosyncratic behaviors for which a socially mediated reinforcer was not apparent. Jim, for example, sometimes became aggressive if people stood in an open doorway. Such idiosyncratic behavior is often seen in individuals diagnosed as autistic, but the maintaining variables are unclear. Generally, in these situations, one is forced to use one or more of the crisis management strategies described earlier. In sum, the category of "other" was one that did not lend itself to a communication-based approach. Fortunately, with respect to severe behavior problems, this category constituted only a very small percentage of the problem episodes observed.

Our method of interpreting the motivation of misbehavior from the index cards was subjective. Two points, however, are worth making. First, the attention-seeking, escape, and tangible-seeking classes of situations that were represented by the descriptions on the index cards were similar to those situations analyzed in the research literature reviewed at the beginning of this chapter. Thus, the interpretations derive some plausibility from their similarity to situations analyzed more formally. Second, the interpretations allow us to design specific treatments, and the success or failure of these treatments becomes, in a sense, a test of the hypotheses on which they were grounded. This notion of hypothesis-driven treatment is also based on the research literature (Repp, Felce, & Barton, 1988) and represents a systematic means for deriving treatments in a rational manner.

Typically, when the index cards were categorized in the way we have been describing, we found that the behavior problems for each individual were multiply motivated. Thus, a single behavior such as aggression could be motivated by attention seeking, escape, and tangible seeking, depending on the specific context. This fact is a further demonstration that behavior topography per se is a poor guide for treatment planning, because a given topography is usually controlled by several different classes of variables. It was common, however, to find that these classes of variables were not equally probable for a given individual. Thus, for Val, we found that attention seeking was the most common motivation, followed by tangibles and escape, respectively. Once a motivational hierarchy had been identified, we continued our analysis by focusing on the highest probability category first, followed by the others in descending order.

Attention was Val's highest probability motivational category. Therefore, we proceeded to categorize further the index cards representing attention seeking. At this stage, the goal was to categorize emergent *themes* around which groups of index cards clustered. In Val's case, most of her attention cards clustered into three generic themes: The first consisted of situations in which she was required to do independent work; the second involved situations in which the teacher was working with other children; and the third consisted of instances in which the teacher was called away to talk with another adult who had entered the classroom. Val responded to all three types of situations with outbursts of behavior problems, and these displays generally evoked various forms of teacher attention. It should be clear from this description that although all these situations involved attention-seeking misbehavior, the social context represented by the three themes differed. We have found that the identification of subcategories within a given type of motivation is important in designing treatment, as each subcategory calls for a unique set of communication skills. In short, there is no general attention-seeking response that can be taught, because there is no general attention-seeking situation. Treatment must be tailored to fit the thematic clusters that emerge from the analysis of the index cards constituting each motivational category.

Verify

It is possible that the situations identified in the describe and categorize stages of the functional analysis were spuriously correlated with the display of behavior problems and that in fact other variables, not identified, were the true controlling factors. To rule out this possibility and to demonstrate causal relationships, we carried out a final stage of analysis in which we systematically constructed and repeated those situations hypothesized to be causal based on the earlier stages of our analyses. Because this final stage involved a direct manipulation of relevant variables, it represented the most conservative level of our analysis. Situations that reliably evoked behavior problems would thus be verified as likely to be causal in nature.

Our method of verification involved constructing several situations that were examples of each particular theme. Recall that Val's first theme involved independent work; typically, we constructed several scenarios reflecting this theme. For example, Val might be asked to sort laundry by herself, or to wash up, or to prepare her lunch. Recall that her second theme involved situations in which the teacher was working with other children. Relevant scenarios might include working with these children on a workshop task, or getting them dressed to go outside, or preparing them to board the bus. The third theme centered on situations in which the teacher became involved talking with another adult. Relevant scenarios could include conversations with the assistant teacher, or the speech pathologist, or the gym teacher. Because Val's misbehavior was also controlled by tangible-seeking and escape variables, additional scenarios would be constructed to verify the impact of these variables as well. It should be noted that, in all cases, the particulars of the scenarios were based on information derived from the index cards.

The final step involved exposing each individual to the array of scenarios created for him or her. Each scenario was presented several times across a number of days in order to determine how consistently behavior problems were evoked. Because the array of scenarios involved many settings and many different people, the generality of behavior problems with respect to situations commonly encountered in the daily living environment could also be assessed. If the various scenarios reliably evoked behavior problems (as they in fact did) and, in contrast, the individual behaved relatively well during periods of time during which the scenarios were not presented, then we could be reasonably sure that it was the scenarios that were the proximal cause of misbehavior. It is worth noting that the frequency of behavior problems occurring during the scenarios constituted a baseline against which future treatment effects could be assessed. Further, as will be noted later, the scenarios themselves became the vehicle for designing specific treatment strategies and a major locus for the implementation of those strategies.

COMMUNICATION-BASED TREATMENT

As noted previously, individuals can be taught specific communicative forms that serve the same function (i.e., are maintained by the same rein-forcers) as severe behavior problems. The result of such training is that behavior problems are greatly reduced and sometimes eliminated altogether. Technically speaking, treatment per se is not the most difficult part of our protocol. Prompting specific communicative forms is not a complex matter, and procedures for doing so have been reported in the literature for years (e.g., Carr & Kologinsky, 1983; Hart & Risley, 1978; Lovaas, 1977). What is complex is the functional analysis leading up to the design of treatment. It is the complexity of functional analysis that led us to discuss this process at length in the preceding section. If the functional analysis is carried out competently, then the selection of specific communicative forms to replace misbehavior may be a relatively straightforward matter. If the functional analysis is carried out poorly or not at all, then treatment can become a frustrating and directionless activity in which procedures are changed fre-quently and without effect, and more intrusive interventions begin to appear as an attractive possibility to pressured and anxious staff. In sum, the ultimate success or failure of communication-based treatment depends on whether a thorough and revealing functional analysis has been conducted and whether treatment planning is based on a rational and systematic extension of the results of this analysis. Now we may turn to a description of the intervention model itself, beginning with the issue of building rapport.

Building Rapport

In everyday language, *rapport* refers to a relationship existing between two people that is characterized by closeness, empathy, and general liking. Although the notion of rapport has been a mainstay of clinical and counseling psychology for years (Egan, 1975), it has not penetrated the field of applied behavior analysis in a systematic manner. It is true that the notion of building rapport lacks the objectivity and rigor that are the ideals of behaviorism. Nonetheless, there are substantive reasons, both clinical and theoretical, for focusing on this concept and attempting to operationalize it so that it can be understood empirically and applied effectively. What we have to say on this topic derives from our clinical experiences in implementing communication-based treatment, as well as from some extrapolations that can be made from the nonbehavioral literature. Our comments are meant to be heuristic rather than definitive and should be read in that spirit.

Rapport is an inherent notion in a communication model of intervention, because the model involves a speaker and a listener and the face-valid assumption that the two want to communicate with one another. In operant terms, we mean that the speaker and listener provide an array of reinforcers for one another and that the dispensation of such reinforcers is contingent on the emission of various communicative acts. If the behavior of either party in the exchange constitutes an aversive or neutral stimulus for the other party, then the presence of one of the individuals may not be a discriminative stimulus for the communicative behavior of the other. The most common example of this problem that we have seen is in the case of teacher-student interaction. A teacher may have a long history with a particular student in which most interactions center on providing discipline. That is, the teacher may frequently shout at, reprimand, and physically restrain a student who is severely aggressive and self-injurious. The presence of the teacher is thus highly correlated with a variety of presumably aversive stimuli. When the student is occasionally well behaved, the teacher consistently ignores him or her and may even verbalize a sense of relief at not having to interact with the student. In this case, the presence of the teacher is correlated with extinction of appropriate behavior.

Clearly, a teacher who has this history of interaction with a student is not likely to be a discriminative stimulus for approach and communicative behavior on the part of the student. Outside observers would make the subjective judgment that the teacher lacked rapport with the student. Like-wise, one finds that when an unfamiliar adult attempts to work with an individual who has severe behavior problems, the individual may initially be quite unresponsive to the stranger. In this case, it seems that the presence of the adult constitutes a neutral stimulus for approach and communicative behavior, because these behaviors have no history of being reinforced in the presence of the new adult. Again, observers might make the judgment that the adult had not yet established rapport with the individual who was the focus of intervention.

Although the descriptions we have offered are anecdotal and subjective, we have observed the scenarios described on countless occasions during the course of our clinical research. We can summarize what we have been trying to say by noting that individuals who have a negative or neutral history of interaction with a person who displays severe behavior problems are not likely to succeed within a communication model of treatment until they establish rapport with the person who is the focus of treatment. Another way of expressing this notion is to say that both the treatment agent and the individual who is being treated must like each other. Having made this subjective statement, we will try to provide some guidelines for approaching this problem from a behavioral perspective. At the outset, we must admit that the conceptual framework of applied behavior analysis may ultimately have to evolve further in order to capture fully the nuances and subtleties inherent in relationship notions such as rapport.

We have typically begun the process of building rapport with people who have handicaps by trying to establish ourselves as generalized rein-forcers in the manner discussed by Skinner (1953). Specifically, we attempted to pair our presence with the dispensation of frequent and varied types of reinforcers. At first, we simply offered the reinforcers directly to the individ-ual and had other treatment agents do the same without requiring that a particular behavior occur (i.e., reinforcers were dispensed noncontingently). In the case of Val, who was socially oriented, we spent a great deal of time talking to her, conversing about activities and events that she was interested in, and generally joking with her and making her laugh. In the case of Gary and Jim, who were less socially oriented, we provided a variety of tangible reinforcers (foods) as well as entertaining activities (e.g., listening to rock and roll music). Whenever possible, we attempted to intersperse social reinforcers (conversation, jokes) among the tangible and activity reinforcers, as rapport building is fundamentally a social interaction process.

The purpose of this phase of rapport building was to associate individ-uals (future treatment agents) with a sustained, consistent, and varied array of positive reinforcers. Once this goal was achieved (typically after 2 to 3 days), we added a contingency. Specifically, we required that the individual approach us in order to receive the array of reinforcers. Once approach behavior was well established (after 1 or 2 more days), we added another contingency by requiring (sometimes prompting) individuals to display any preexisting communicative behavior in their repertoire that was relevant to the identified reinforcers we were using. These communicative acts were often quite unsophisticated in nature (e.g., grunting, leading the treatment agent by the hand over to the reinforcer), but sometimes were more developmentally advanced (e.g., pointing, saying "Hey," using a specific word such as "Cookie" to make a request). This stage continued for 2 or 3 more days; thus, after a week or so, each individual was reliably approaching one or more of the treatment agents and making a variety of rudimentary requests or bids for attention. The purpose of this phase was to establish a number of treatment agents as discriminative stimuli for approach and simple communicative behaviors. Essentially, this outcome represents the first step in ensuring that nonproblem behavior becomes a reliable and consistent way of influencing others.

Building rapport involves more than a series of mechanical steps designed to establish the presence of treatment agents as generalized reinforcers, and this idea poses great difficulty for those operating within a strictly behavioral framework (Evans, 1990). Recently, there have been calls for practitioners to adopt a less controlling stance with respect to persons displaying severe behavior problems. More specifically, there have been suggestions to focus on interpersonal styles that emphasize caring, friendship, and warmth (McGee, Menolascino, Hobbs, & Menousek, 1987). Unfortunately, these ideas have been expressed in a manner that casts the issue in terms of behaviorism versus humanism. The polemical and mostly subjective style in which these ideas are presented has made it easy for behaviorists to reject the arguments set forth, but it is a mistake not to challenge the idea that behaviorism cannot also be humanistic. It is also a mistake not to examine some implicit values that exist in the current practice of behaviorism with a view to reforming those values. One implicit value is the notion that treatment agents should control the behavior of individuals who have problems (i.e., that a unidirectional model of control is desirable). As our earlier review of child effects made clear, however, a communication-based model is predicated on an assumption of reciprocity rather than unidirectional control.

Another implicit value that is reflected in current behavioral practice is the notion that it is desirable to focus one's interactions with people who have handicaps on helping them to acquire new skills and to solve problems with which they are confronted. These goals are in fact desirable, but there are other useful goals, especially with respect to issues of establishing rapport and facilitating communicative interaction. These other goals are reflected by the fact that few of us who are putatively without handicaps structure every day of our lives into a series of time periods in which skills are learned and problems are solved. If we did so, we would shortly complain that life was too task oriented and boring, and we might well take steps to avoid interacting with people who continuously stressed such a structured life-style. Yet behavior modification programs are frequently structured in such a manner, leaving the impression (particularly among those who are critical of behaviorism) that there is no time for personal enjoyment per se.

We have found, clinically, that in building rapport it is necessary to ensure that there are periods of time available every day in which the treatment agent and the individual displaying behavior problems can interact with each other within a context of playing games, sharing entertaining activities, and generally enjoying each other's company. These interactions may not be educational in themselves and may in fact be labeled by others as "being silly" or "goofing off." Nonetheless, they may be related to establishing oneself as a generalized reinforcer. More likely, they are related to broader issues of friendship formation that have yet to be explored within a behavioral framework. In any case, our clinical effectiveness appears to be partly related to our ability and willingness to schedule the types of activities just mentioned purposely into daily interactions with people who have handicaps.

A communication model requires that the treatment agent be responsive to the communicative attempts of the person exhibiting behavior problems. So far, we have stressed general guidelines for making the treatment agent more "likable" to the person with handicaps. There is a related point that is seldom discussed—namely, how to make the person with handicaps more likable to the treatment agent. To some extent there is an implicit assumption in the field that each of us who works with people having developmental disabilities *ought* to like such people, and that it borders on heresy to admit any other feeling. In truth, each of us has to examine the possibility that we may find particular individuals physically unattractive, uninteresting, and fear provoking. An honest examination of such feelings is the first step in attempting to overcome these feelings and enhancing rapport. A denial of these feelings, on the other hand, may lead to continuation of a pattern of interaction characterized by avoidance and rejection. Indeed, in moments of desperation, both parents and treatment staff have confided to us their negative feelings about certain individuals and their desire to distance themselves from these same individuals. Clearly, any pattern of interaction characterized by distancing, avoidance, and rejection is fundamentally incompatible with being a responsive listener and a promoter of communicative skills.

It is difficult to know how to overcome these impediments to rapport building; however, one possibility may lie in the social psychology literature as it pertains to the development of liking. There is a large experimental literature demonstrating that whether or not we like another person depends on variables such as the social competence, physical attractiveness, and interests of the other person (Aronson, 1984). The implication of this research is that part of rapport building should address some of the issues implied by these variables. For example, with respect to physical attractiveness, attention should be paid to clothing style, grooming, and table manners. Some may reject this notion as superficial. If one reflects for a moment, however, on the desirability of interacting with a person who consistently has food in his or her hair, whose clothes are torn and dirty as well as poorly fitted, and who smears his or her food during dinner, then it will be clear that many people may choose to distance themselves, when they can, from such an individual. To consider common interests, if the individual with disabilities is interested in rock music, enjoys jogging, and likes to go for pizza, then it seems possible that a treatment agent having the same profile of interests would be predisposed to interact with such an individual and that rapport could be quickly established. There is much valuable research to be done on this topic. The fact that the social psychology literature is generally nonbehavioral should be seen as an irrelevant consideration, as many of its findings and ideas could be translated into the language of applied behavior analysis in order to facilitate rapport building within a communication-based model of treatment.

We have deliberately explored the issue of rapport building in some detail because it is not a popular issue with researchers operating within the behavioral tradition. We feel, however, that concepts such as rapport and friendship have great relevance to a communication model of treatment. In lay language, you are more apt to be socially responsive to the communicative attempts of a person whom you like than one whom you do not like. Social responsiveness is measurable, and with some creativity, it is possible to operationalize rapport and related concepts so that their effects on responsivity can be analyzed. In other words, the ideas we have been discussing are potentially testable and, in this sense, congruent with behavioral tradition.

Appropriate Use of the Communication Model

It is important to place the communication model for the treatment of severe behavior problems in an appropriate clinical and educational context. First and foremost, it is worth stressing that the model that we have been describing represents only a small fraction of what a general communication curriculum should look like. The model is not meant to replace a general curriculum, although it may be a useful part of such a curriculum. A general curriculum must attend to a large number of issues involving expressive and receptive language skills applied across a wide variety of social contexts. These issues have been ably discussed elsewhere (Goetz, Schuler, & Sailor, 1981; Hart & Risley, 1978; Lovaas, 1981; Mirenda, Iacono, & Williams, 1990; Musselwhite & St. Louis, 1988). The communication model, in contrast, has more modest goals, namely, training specific skills that are focused on replacing serious behavior problems.

Second, as emphasized previously, our model is not relevant to treating behavior problems that are likely controlled by sensory, homeostatic, or organic factors. Data suggest that some instances of behavior problems are maintained by sensory reinforcers, and therefore treatment must focus on eliminating or competing with these sources of reinforcement (Favell, McGimsey, & Schell, 1982; Rincover, Cook, Peoples, & Packard, 1979). Other data suggest that behavior problems, particularly those involving stereo-typed motor acts, can serve a homeostatic function whose purpose is to regulate arousal level (Hutt & Hutt, 1970). Therefore, treatment must consider variables related to state of arousal (Guess et al., 1988). There is also literature documenting the association of organic factors with specific behavior prob-lems (Carr, 1977; Cataldo & Harris, 1982; Schroeder, Rojahn, Mulick, & Schroeder, 1990) and several demonstrations of the role that biochemical interventions may play (Barrett, Feinstein, & Hole, 1989; Herman et al., 1987).

Finally, we must clarify what we mean by communication-based treat-ment. We believe that even when communication training is an appropriate intervention for severe behavior problems, it is very unlikely that a focus on communication alone will suffice. Instead, a variety of other procedures must accompany the communication training effort. It is beyond the scope of this chapter to review all of the relevant procedures; however, many of these have been discussed elsewhere (Carr, Robinson, Taylor, & Carlson, 1990). For the present, we may note that rapport building (already described), embedding, building tolerance for reinforcement delay, and provision of choices (to be described later) constitute additional procedures that must typically be integrated into a communication-based model if treatment is to be effective.

Choosing Communicative Forms

Our conceptual model is based on the hypothesis that most individuals who exhibit severe behavior problems already possess a variety of communi-cative forms in their repertoires—specifically, the behavior problems them-selves. Thus, aggression, self-injury, and tantrums may function as primitive forms of communication to secure attention, tangibles, or escape from aver-sive situations. There are no data in the literature demonstrating that the *functions* that behavior problems serve can be eliminated. If one employs extinction as an intervention, then the research literature demonstrates that specific forms of behavior problems may be eliminated, but the functions that those forms serve are not. Extinction may eliminate aggression that is motivated by attention seeking, but it does not change the fact that attention per se remains reinforcing. We have stated this idea elsewhere by noting, more poetically, that whereas behavior forms may come and go, functions are forever (Carr, 1988).

That being the case, the most we can hope to achieve is to teach an individual new, socially acceptable forms for accessing reinforcers that are currently obtained following the emission of severe behavior problems. The new form (communicative responding through speech, sign, or some other modality) must be a function of the same variables (reinforcers) as the old form (behavior problems); in short, the new and old forms must be functionally equivalent (Carr & Durand, 1985a, b). Functional equivalence is the cornerstone of our model, and that is why the functional analysis that is the basis for choosing communicative forms must be carefully done. Knowing, for example, that escape was a major variable controlling Jim's aggression in a wide variety of contexts forced us to focus on choosing a communicative form that was effective in extricating Jim from presumably aversive situations without compromising broader habilitative efforts. At the same time, the functional analysis suggested the futility of teaching Jim to ask for attention in those contexts since attention was not the variable controlling his behavior problems.

Functional equivalence is not the only consideration in choosing communicative forms. It is also necessary that the new communicative form be more efficient than the problem behavior that it is to replace. That is, the new response should access the relevant reinforcers with a shorter delay, greater consistency, and less effort than the problem behavior (Billingsley & Neel, 1985; Carr & Kemp, 1989; Carr & Lindquist, 1987; Horner & Billingsley, 1988). There are at least two major classes of variables that influence response efficiency: ease of performance and ease of interpretability. If the new communicative response is difficult to perform, then the delay between performance of this response and receipt of the reinforcer may be greater than the delay between performance of the problem behavior and receipt of the reinforcer. This means that the behavior problem is likely to persist, as it is the more efficient of the two types of responses. For example, if a girl bites herself consistently in the presence of juice, a teacher might learn to give the girl juice immediately, because doing so brings about an abrupt termination of self-biting. In contrast, a teacher may have instructed the child to say "Juice, please," but because of articulation problems and insufficient training, the girl may stumble over the phrase and experience repeated correction and prompting that results in considerable delay in obtaining the juice. In this case, the phrase is associated with great effort and long reinforcer delay, whereas self-biting is associated with little effort and no reinforcer delay. The inefficiency of the phrase, generated by performance difficulty, may well ensure perpetuation of self-biting in spite of the functional equivalence existing between the phrase and the problem behavior. The solution, at least initially, would be to provide reinforcement contingent on any reasonable approximation of the phrase, thereby reducing both effort and reinforcer delay.

The second class of variables affecting response efficiency relates to ease of interpretability. In cognitive terms, people must be able to understand (interpret) the message in the communicative form in order to respond appropriately (Mirenda et al., 1990). In operant terms, the communicative form must be a discriminative stimulus for the listener to dispense a specific reinforcer. Interpretability becomes an issue whenever the communication modality is unfamiliar to the listener. For example, if a boy asks for a break from work using poorly articulated speech (e.g., saying "ake" rather than "break"), individuals who do not know the boy well (e.g., substitute teachers, new group home staff) may not respond at all to the request, or may offer the wrong reinforcer. In other words, interpretability problems could produce a long delay of reinforcement or inconsistent reinforcement. If the boy aggresses, however, all work stops immediately and reliably (i.e., there is little delay of reinforcement and high consistency of reinforcement). Again, although the verbal request and the aggression are functionally equivalent, the aggression persists because of its greater efficiency. The solution would be to choose an unambiguous (easily interpretable) communicative form (e.g., a card with the word *break* on it) or to take steps to ensure that all relevant people who interact with the boy know that the word *ake* uttered in a work context is a request for a break.

Efficiency notions may also help explain why some individuals who have reasonably good communication skills nonetheless periodically engage in severe behavior problems. For example, an individual may be able to request an item (e.g., saying, "I want juice") but nonetheless exhibit aggressive behavior in the presence of the item. Clinically, we have seen this situation arise most commonly in those contexts in which other people are periodically unresponsive to the request. The individual may request the item repeatedly and, when no response from others is forthcoming, then become aggressive. A lack of consistent responsivity from others ensures that verbal communication is inefficient, and therefore the individual reverts to previously learned responses (behavior problems) that have been associated with reliably obtaining the reinforcer. It is thus important to make sure that a reasonable level of responsivity is maintained with respect to the communicative response. We would like to point out that the process just described is not unique to people with developmental disabilities. For example, in marital therapy, one often deals with people who have well-developed communicative repertoires; yet in some situations, these repertoires become inefficient means for obtaining reinforcers, and the individuals resort to aggressive behavior (Jacobson & Margolin, 1979).

Many communication modalities can be used within the context of the treatment procedures we have been describing. Clearly speech, because of its universality, is the modality of choice. Because not everyone can talk or talk well, however, other modalities (including sign language, gesture, and visual symbols) are also possible. Within each modality, there is still the question of whether one form may be better to begin with than another. Our initial strategy was always to select those communicative forms that could be used in a general manner across a wide variety of situations. Because Val, for example, had very poor articulation, and because her behavior problems were mostly attention seeking, we initially taught her to tap people on the shoulder when she wanted their attention. This response could be used in virtually any situation in which attention was implicated, and further, it was not dependent on articulation skill. Later, after Val had mastered this response, we began to teach her a variety of more specific ways of getting attention by using speech, but even then she always had the tapping response to fall back on if people failed to respond.

Likewise, Gary and Jim were initially taught communicative forms that could be effective in a wide variety of contexts. Thus, Jim, who was without speech, was taught to display the word *break* (printed on a label on a key chain attached to his belt) whenever he was in a work situation that was presumably aversive for him. This response was thus available as a general substitute for his escape-motivated aggression and tantrums. Gary, also typically escape motivated, was verbal, and therefore he was taught to give the general response "Help me, please" in any of the numerous situations in which his performance was inadequate. Eventually, all individuals may be taught a variety of communicative forms to deal with unique social contexts. We have found, however, that it is better initially to choose forms that can be used more generally. In this manner, individuals can learn that communication is a powerful way of altering a variety of social contexts in a desirable direction resulting in the efficient and reliable receipt of reinforcers.

Creating Communication Opportunities

Once communicative forms have been chosen, the next step is to provide opportunities for those forms to be taught, displayed, and reinforced. At the outset, we must stress that in the absence of an appropriate educational context, none of the procedures that we have been describing is likely to be effective. To begin, what is an *inappropriate* context? First, a very low staff-student ratio is inappropriate. When we conduct in-service training, we are sometimes confronted by staff who tell us that they must be responsible for 30 or more individuals and cannot possibly attend consistently to the communicative acts of a single person. They are probably right, and treatment will certainly fail. Second, uncooperative and/or unmotivated staff constitute an inappropriate context. During presentations to parent groups, we are sometimes approached by people who tell us that they are enthusiastic about a communication approach for their children, but that they are pessimistic about whether they can convince members of the school staff to support them with respect to this approach. A lack of cooperation will sharply limit treatment efficacy.

Third, a barren, segregated environment also constitutes an inappropriate context. Teachers sometimes tell us that there are few things in their classroom that students find worth communicating about and that the separation of the classroom from the community reduces the richness of the teaching environment, thereby further limiting communication opportunities. These teachers are prophetic, as our treatment protocol will probably fail in the environment described. Fourth, a program in which functional education is not the priority constitutes an inappropriate context. One danger signal is to be told that a student cannot participate in the communication protocol on a regular basis because such participation may interfere with scheduled dance therapy involving the smearing of body lotion on the arms to enhance ego boundaries, or "vocational" habilitation in which three kinds of plastic spoons are to be sorted into different piles, or field trips in which a 17-year-old man is to be taken to see the Easter bunny. None of the activities described above are educationally functional, and to give them priority over a communication-based treatment for severe behavior problems bodes poorly for the outcome of that treatment.

Over a period of years, we have learned that it is better to work with treatment staff and families who are sensitive to the issues we have outlined than to attempt the impossible, namely, carrying out treatment in an inappropriate context. When confronted with an inappropriate context, each of us has an obligation to try to persuade agencies and families to change the current environment in which they are operating and to be honest about informing all individuals involved that treatment is not possible without basic structural and philosophical changes. In sum, an appropriate context consists of a reasonable staff-student ratio, cooperative and motivated treatment agents, a commitment to community-oriented intervention, and establishing a system in which functional education is the critical priority.

Once an appropriate educational context has been identified, the chief task becomes that of creating communication opportunities. At first it is not wise to wait for such opportunities to occur naturally, because they may occur too infrequently for meaningful teaching to take place. Instead, as previously mentioned, those scenarios developed during the functional analysis may be used to generate a large number of opportunities across a great variety of situations. Consider Val, for example. Her behavior problems were typically attention seeking. Rather than waiting for difficulties to arise, we would ask the teacher to have Val work independently at a task, a situation that normally evoked screaming and aggression once the teacher reduced her level of attention to Val. This time, however, we prompted Val to tap the teacher on the shoulder after a few seconds of independent work, and we prompted the teacher to respond to Val's new form of attention seeking by cheerfully and enthusiastically acknowledging her ("Yes, Val, what can I do for you?"). The teacher then proceeded to engage Val in some light conversation of Val's choosing.

This tactic was repeated across a large number of scenarios many times each day. There were several outcomes. First, Val accomplished very little work. Second, the teacher accomplished very little work, because Val was constantly nagging her. Third, when Val wanted attention, she tapped the teacher on the shoulder instead of turning the table over, pulling the teacher's hair, and screaming profanities. At least in the short run, most teachers and parents are willing to tolerate low work output and constant nagging in exchange for negligible levels of violent behavior. One must be willing to put up with mildly bothersome behavior in order to firmly establish communication as an alternative to problem behavior. Once communication is firmly established, steps (described later) can be taken to increase work output and decrease nagging. Further, at this later stage, scenarios need no longer be presented at a high rate. Instead, the newly emergent communication skills can be strengthened (reinforced) within the normal sequence of events (natural context) that occur each day.

A second example of using scenarios to create communication opportunities is illustrated in the case of Jim. Because his aggression and tantrums were largely motivated by escape, we challenged him in the group home with a variety of work tasks that he typically tried to avoid (e.g., doing the laundry, cleaning the bathroom, physical exercises). For instance, we asked him to perform a series of stretching exercises. After he did one of them (and before he became aggressive), we prompted him to extend a retractable key chain that we clipped on to his belt. At the end of this key chain, we had attached a laminated piece of paper that read, "May I have a break, please?" We then prompted one of the staff at the group home to respond to requests by letting Jim stop exercising for a few minutes. As was true for Val, Jim made many break requests (i.e., did little work), and staff had to attend to his requests at a high rate. Importantly, however, Jim typically stopped exhibiting behavior problems in the exercise situation.

Gary constitutes a final example of the use of our procedures at this stage of treatment. Because he could speak, his protocol was somewhat different from Jim's. Given that Gary's aggression and self-injury were frequently escape motivated, we began by presenting scenarios that involved work situations. We had Gary's mother ask him to prepare his lunch at home so that he could take it to school the next day. He typically made many errors on this task and responded to negative feedback (e.g., "That's wrong, Gary" or "You made a mistake") with behavior problems. This time, however, we had Gary's mother prompt Gary to say "Help me, please" in response to the negative feedback; in other words, negative feedback became a discriminative stimulus for assistance seeking. The result was that Gary asked for a lot of help and prepared very few lunches, but, most importantly, stopped attacking family members in this situation.

Building Tolerance for Delay of Reinforcement

The main problem at this stage of treatment is to deal with the issues of nagging (i.e., the individual makes too many requests) and low work output (i.e., the individual completes few academic, vocational, or home-related tasks). These issues are, as noted previously, interrelated and can best be addressed by restructuring the social situation so that requests are honored intermittently rather than continuously. Intermittency is assured by requiring that the individual complete gradually increasing amounts of work prior to receiving reinforcers or, more generally, wait for progressively longer periods of time to elapse between reinforcers. Once Jim had learned to extend his key chain to request a break, for example, he began to make this request after completing a single exercise. Because the request was now well established, we acknowledged Jim's response by prompting a member of the group home staff to say, "Sure, Jim, you can have a break, but let's do a few more exercises." A staff member then prompted Jim to complete one or two more exercises, at which point a further prompt was given; specifically, Jim was manually prompted to extend his key chain. At this point, the staff member exclaimed, "OK, Jim, you've done enough for now. Go take a break." Jim was then allowed to leave the exercise area and relax on the living room couch.

As days passed, Jim was required to complete more and more exercises before being given a break. An occasional resurgence of behavior problems was a signal for the staff to reduce temporarily the number of exercises required for a break. Over time, the prompts were faded for both Jim and the staff; in the end, Jim could tolerate a large number of exercises without repeatedly requesting breaks. Here, we may note parenthetically that because Gary's behavior problems were also typically escape motivated, his protocol paralleled that just described for Jim. Thus, in a food preparation situation, Gary was required to work for progressively longer periods of time before being allowed to take a break or move to a different activity. In Gary's case, there was one additional factor: After receiving help a number of times following requests for assistance, Gary became competent at performing the task and made fewer attempts at terminating the hitherto problematic work situation.

Val's treatment represents a more sophisticated version of how to teach individuals to tolerate delay of reinforcement. Val frequently tapped the teacher on the shoulder to get attention, especially when the teacher was engaged in other activities. We therefore decided to teach her to discriminate when it was appropriate to seek attention. One scenario involved having the teacher holding a pad of paper and writing on it. If Val tapped the teacher (Mrs. X) on the shoulder, the assistant teacher told Val, "Not now, Mrs. X is busy." When the teacher put down the pad and stopped writing, the assistant teacher prompted Val again by saying, "Mrs. X is finished. You can talk to her." Now, when Val tapped, the teacher would exclaim, "Yes, Val, you waited until I was finished. What would you like to talk about?" Thus, through differential reinforcement, "busy" behaviors on the part of the teacher were established as discriminative stimuli for waiting, whereas the termination of those same behaviors was established as a discriminative stimulus for attention seeking. Over a period of days, the "busy" periods were lengthened so that Val had to wait increasing amounts of time before tapping. Further, new variants of the "busy" scenarios were introduced to provide a wider range of naturalistic discriminative cues. Concurrently with this training, we had Val engage in various work tasks while waiting for the teacher to finish. Thus, the assistant teacher might tell Val to keep folding laundry, or preparing lunch, while waiting for Mrs. X to be free. In this manner, Val's work output increased while her level of nagging decreased.

A closely related problem concerns the issue of what to do when an individual refuses to stop a reinforcing activity, for example, by becoming disruptive when he or she is told that a break period is over. Our basic strategy, early in training, was to permit the individual to reinstate the break period immediately following a request to do so. The individual was thereby given a history of reinforcement in which preferred activities could be reinstated following appropriate communicative behavior rather than following aggression (for instance). As training progressed, the individual was required to engage in some work, however minimal, before the break could be reinstated with a request. Late in training, the work requirement was increased before break requests would be honored. In sum, termination of reinforcing activities became a discriminative stimulus for the behavior sequence "work, then request break" rather than a discriminative stimulus for problem behavior, as had been the case prior to intervention. A similar strategy was employed to deal with behavior problems maintained by tangibles or attention withdrawal.

Embedding

An additional strategy that we have used within the context of a communication-based approach is a procedure that we have referred to as *embedding* (Carr, Robinson, Taylor, & Carlson, 1990). The essence of this procedure is to embed those stimuli that have been identified as controlling high rates of behavior problems among those stimuli that have been identified as controlling low (or zero) rates of behavior problems. There is a growing literature demonstrating that embedding can be a useful way of controlling behavior problems, particularly those that appear to be escape motivated (Carr et al., 1976; Horner, Day, Sprague, O'Brien, & Heathfield, 1991; Mace et al., 1988; Singer, Singer, & Horner, 1987). Considerable speculation has emerged concerning what processes are responsible for these favorable outcomes. Concepts that have been evoked as explanations include the notion of emergent response classes (Horner et al., 1991; Singer et al., 1987), counterconditioning (Carr et al., 1976), interruption of behavior chains (Carr et al., 1976), stimulus fading (Iwata, 1987), and behavioral momentum (Mace et al., 1988). Any or all of these processes may be involved and are worth systematic exploration within a research framework. At present it is clear that the procedure has clinical merit, and we will therefore illustrate its use for one of the individuals with whom we have worked.

In Val's case, the stimulus that controlled high rates of behavior problems was sometimes a demand to do work. Although most of her behavior problems were attention seeking, she would also become aggressive and throw tantrums even while being attended to, provided that the adult also asked her to perform a nonpreferred task. Thus, if the adult asked her to clean up the kitchen, a task that she was completely competent at performing, she would often respond by yelling "No," spitting at the adult, and throwing objects around the room. The solution to this difficulty was first to identify those stimuli that controlled low rates of problem behavior. From prolonged observation, we had learned that joking with Val and speaking to her in an animated tone of voice were almost invariably associated with good behavior. Therefore, we sought to embed demands within the context of joking and an animated tone of voice. For example, rather than tell Val, "Clean up the kitchen," a stimulus that would evoke aggression and tantrums, we conversed with her as follows: "Boy, does this place stink! Let's get out the gas masks. Val, quick, throw those dirty paper plates in the garbage before they crawl away. Help, there are gross spoons and forks! Val, pick them up and put them in the sink. Don't let them bite you!" Val responded to this conversation with considerable laughter and, most importantly, complied with all the requests while showing no problem behavior.

We do not pretend to know what psychological process underlies the success of this procedure. It is a process that greatly merits systematic experimental analysis. Rapport appears to play a role, as strangers were generally less effective at using the procedure. In all likelihood, what we are dealing with is a complex of procedures that, in lay language, put the individual in a good mood. Because, in behavioral jargon, mood is an example of a setting event, it may be that the time has come to look more systematically at the literature on setting events. This aspect of the applied behavioral literature is grossly underdeveloped, to the detriment of clinical intervention (Wahler & Fox, 1981).

Providing Choices

Earlier, we noted that a unidirectional model of control is implicit in most behavioral treatment approaches. The treatment agent is in charge of what happens, whereas the person being treated is generally accorded a passive role. We questioned this assumption within the context of building both rapport and communication skills. Recently, this assumption has been questioned more broadly still. Clinicians, advocates, and researchers have been converging on the notion that allowing individuals to make choices may be critical from both educational and quality-of-living perspectives (Guess & Siegel-Causey, 1985; Houghton, Bronicki, & Guess, 1987; Shevin & Klein, 1984). Some data now suggest that permitting an individual to make choices may reduce disruptive problem behavior (Dyer, Dunlap, & Winterling, 1990). Keeping these empirical and conceptual points in mind, we have for some time incorporated choice making into our clinical protocol, and we will briefly illustrate its use here.

The goal of this procedure is to provide more opportunities for an individual to influence the environment in a socially appropriate manner through shared control with the treatment agent. If the person is instructed to perform a specific task, then, if possible, he or she should be able to choose where the task is performed, with whom it is performed, and what the consequences (reinforcers) will be upon completion of the task. The person is thus given an alternative to behavior problems as a way of influencing the social environment or exerting control over certain situations. Consider a common problem that Val had, namely, severe behavior problems in transition situations. She was often extremely aggressive when moving from one setting to another (e.g., from the gym to the classroom). Typically, several staff members came to talk to Val as she fell to the ground screaming and flailing, an unwise strategy given her attention-seeking motivational profile. We implemented a different strategy. Specifically, we instructed staff not to plead with her; instead, they were to offer her a choice of people whom she would like to accompany her to the designated area (e.g., "Do you want to go back to the classroom with Sandi or with Karen?"). Frequently, when given such a choice, Val would return, without problems, to the classroom. Occasionally, she had to be escorted back against her will because she failed to make a choice and became disruptive. Importantly, however, as her choice-making behavior became more firmly established over time, forced escorts became rare.

In general, we characterized this intervention as "walk and talk," by which we meant that Val could choose the person who would pay attention (talk) to her as she walked from one setting to the next. In a sense, Val was choosing her reinforcer (i.e., source of attention) by verbally indicating her preferences. In a similar manner, we permitted Gary to select the task on which he wished to work, and both Gary and Jim to select the reinforcers for which they wished to work. We must note, however, that choices were not unlimited; we defined a pool of educationally beneficial and socially appropriate items from which individuals were allowed to choose. Thus, choice making involved shared control.

EXTENDING TREATMENT GAINS:
GENERALIZATION AND MAINTENANCE

The issues of generalization and maintenance are complex and merit chapter-length treatment in themselves. It is worthwhile, however, to highlight briefly some of the major considerations that we have confronted.

Generalization

Procedurally, our approach to promoting generalization has two major elements: We begin in a controlled setting and then move to a less controlled setting; and we train sufficient naturalistic exemplars. With respect to the first element, though it may be commendable from a naturalistic standpoint to begin communication training in the middle of a shopping mall during the busy holiday season, it is not advisable. There are too many competing stimuli, and an outburst of behavior problems could produce major difficulties with crisis management. Instead, we begin with a more controlled setting.

For example, at first we engaged Gary in a tutorial situation comprised of himself and one treatment agent in a small, quiet room in the school. The task involved snack preparation, and Gary was taught to influence us by making a variety of requests. Once mastery was achieved in several other controlled situations, we were able to teach communication skills in situations that were more risky as well as more naturalistic. Thus, well into treatment, Gary was participating in scenarios involving group physical exercise and home living skills. These scenarios were much less controlled because of the presence of large numbers of other individuals, activities that were constantly shifting and varied, high ambient noise level, and an array of distracting and potentially desirable (reinforcing) stimuli. Gary's socially appropriate behavior in these scenarios marked the high point of his generalized treatment gains.

We have already alluded to the second element of generalization planning, namely, the use of sufficient, naturalistic exemplars (Stokes & Baer, 1977). Merely training communication skills in a variety of scenarios is not enough. The central concern is that the scenarios chosen are those that the individual is likely to encounter on an ongoing basis in a community (naturalistic) setting. To that end, we made sure that Gary, for instance, was instructed by many natural treatment agents, including his mother, father, siblings, and home respite worker. Likewise, because Gary was eventually to move to a group home, we emphasized settings and tasks that would be directly involved in the success of his future placement, such as meal preparation, laundry, housecleaning, recreational activities, and other community-oriented activities.

We have identified three sets of variables that are commonly associated with generalization failure. First, generalization frequently does not occur in the presence of new treatment agents who have not yet established rapport with an individual. The solution is to use the rapport-building strategies described earlier. Second, generalization failures are observed in new settings in which the controlling variables are different from those operating in the original settings. Thus, an individual's aggression in a classroom setting may be escape motivated, but the same aggressive behavior in a group home setting may be attention seeking. For that reason, a communicative act that may have been effective in the classroom (e.g., asking for a break) will be ineffective in the group home, because the reinforcer in the home is attention and not escape; behavior problems will therefore persist in the new setting. Generalization failures are often soluble in this case when a functional analysis is carried out in the new setting and treatments based on the new analysis are implemented.

Finally, we have seen problems in generalization when the discriminative stimuli that are present in new situations have a long history of powerfully controlling problematic behavior. The effect of these stimuli is to overshadow the effect of the treatment stimuli. For example, Jim became aggressive if raisins were present and visible in any area of his group home, even though the group home had become a setting that occasioned communication rather than behavior problems. Because raisins are not a crucial component of a successful group home environment, the easiest solution was to eliminate them. Once we did so, Jim became communicative again and behavior problems became rare. Sometimes, however, it is not possible or desirable to eliminate the offending discriminative stimuli. For example, some individuals have a long history of coercing their parents via behavior problems, thereby obtaining a variety of reinforcers (e.g., tangibles, attention). Thus, parental presence becomes a discriminative stimulus for immediate aggression or self-injury, even though the individual may have learned to request the same reinforcers from others using speech or sign language. In this case, generalization will have to be carefully programmed rather than confidently expected. The parents will have to be incorporated step-by-step into the entire treatment protocol from the beginning, just as though the individual had not received any prior treatment.

Maintenance

We have found that when the protocol that we have been describing is carefully and systematically implemented, treatment gains are likely to be maintained over a protracted period of time, often measured in years. Our experience has been that there are two factors that act to impede maintenance, and we will briefly describe them.

First, it appears that when the scenarios originally identified as problematic are made the focus of treatment over very long periods of time, a law of diminishing returns seems to set in, and behavior may begin to deteriorate again. Thus, when Val was taught to seek attention and ask for breaks within the context of a laundry task, she performed well for a few months. Over time, however, some of her attention-seeking misbehavior began to return; she seemed to get bored of doing the same tasks with the same people for the same reinforcers at the same time of day. Of course, even a person without disabilities would likely get bored in this situation, and therefore the deterioration in behavior should, in all fairness, be viewed as a normal response rather than as a disorder to be treated. The solution was obvious: Create variations of the scenario. The laundry task could be shared with new people, or alternated among different people so that new tasks could be introduced into the same time period occupied by the laundry task, or the nature of the conversation (attention reinforcer) taking place during the performance of the task could be purposely and systematically changed from day to day. In short, flexibility and variety must be programmed into the daily routine so that maintenance will occur. A too-rigid adherence to the original group of scenarios is a prescription for failure, and it also violates the general principle that people with handicaps ought to be treated whenever possible in the same manner as people without handicaps.

The second problem that we have encountered centers on the fact that maintenance of treatment effects is not possible unless the treatment agents themselves maintain treatment efforts. Treatment agents also appear to get bored once they fall into a routine, and over time, they become less responsive to the communicative efforts of the individuals involved. When this pattern occurs, there tends to be a resurgence in behavior problems. The solution to this difficulty involves elements of systems change, not simply minor adjustments in the treatment protocol per se. Thus, it is not sufficient to tell parents and teachers that they ought to be responsive to communicative attempts because it is their job to do so, and because the data show that this type of intervention is effective. Instead, respite periods and variety must be programmed for treatment agents just as they were for the individual being treated. Staffing patterns may have to be altered; free time (support services) will have to be provided so that parents can carry on with their own lives as well; and daily activities will have to be systematically and intermittently changed to enhance interest. Systems change ought to be a major research priority for applied behavior analysts in the coming decade, for without it, maintenance problems are not likely to be solved.

CONTROL: A SUPERORDINATE CATEGORY

It is clear that teaching communicative forms that access specific reinforcers can be an effective way of reducing the level of behavior problems. We would like to speculate, however, that it may be that communication works not only because it allows an individual to obtain specific reinforcers, but also because it allows the individual to have a more general influence on the environment, thereby rendering other means of influence (i.e., behavior problems) unnecessary. In short, control per se may be a reinforcer (Bijou & Baer, 1965), and we would add that it may be particularly powerful for those individuals who had few socially appropriate means to influence or control their environment prior to treatment. The control notion also appears in the literature on child development, where it is described as "the drive for competence," "mastery motivation," and "effectance motivation" (Harter, 1978; White, 1959). Our point is that whatever label one chooses to use, control over the environment may be reinforcing in and of itself. Therefore, we may reconceptualize communication as being a subcategory of a larger process. Specifically, communication, choice-making procedures, training independence, and various self-management interventions—all of which have recently become popular in the literature—can be seen as exemplars of a single process, namely, gaining control over one's environment. Given the coercive nature of most misbehavior, it is ironic to think that, ultimately, the solution to dealing with severe behavior problems may be to give individuals displaying such problems more control rather than less.

ACKNOWLEDGMENTS. Preparation of this chapter was supported in part by Cooperative Agreement #G0087C0234 from the U.S. Department of Education, "A Rehabilitation Research and Training Center on Community-Referenced Technologies for Nonaversive Behavior Management." We thank Laura Wray Palumbo and Sarah Robinson for their helpful critiques.

REFERENCES

Aronson, E. (1984). *The social animal*. New York: W. H. Freeman.

Barrett, R. P., Feinstein, C., & Hole, W. T. (1989). Effects of naloxone and naltrexone on self-injury: A double-blind, placebo-controlled analysis. *American Journal on Mental Retardation, 93,* 644–651.

Bell, S. M., & Ainsworth, M. D. S. (1972). Infant crying and maternal responsiveness. *Child Development, 43,* 1171–1190.

Bijou, S. W., & Baer, D. M. (1965). *Child development II: Universal stage of infancy*. New York: Appleton-Century-Crofts.

Billingsley, F. F., & Neel, R. S. (1985). Competing behaviors and their effects on skill generalization and maintenance. *Analysis and Intervention in Developmental Disabilities, 5,* 357–372.

Bird, F., Dores, P. A., Moniz, D., & Robinson, J. (1989). Reducing severe aggressive and self-injurious behaviors with functional communication training. *American Journal on Mental Retardation, 94,* 37–48.

Brownlee, J. R., & Bakeman, R. (1981). Hitting in toddler-peer interaction. *Child Development, 52,* 1076–1079.

Carr, E. G. (1977). The motivation of self-injurious behavior: A review of some hypotheses. *Psychological Bulletin, 84,* 800–816.

Carr, E. G. (1985). Behavioral approaches to language and communication. In E. Schopler & G. Mesibov (Eds.), *Current issues in autism; vol. 3: Communication problems in autism* (pp. 37–57). New York: Plenum.

Carr, E. G. (1988). Functional equivalence as a mechanism of response generalization. In R. Horner, R. L. Koegel, & G. Dunlap (Eds.), *Generalization and maintenance: Life-style changes in applied settings* (pp. 194–219). Baltimore: Paul H. Brookes.

Carr, E. G., & Durand, V. M. (1985a). The social-communicative basis of severe behavior problems in children. In S. Reiss & R. Bootzin (Eds.), *Theoretical issues in behavior therapy* (pp. 219–254). New York: Academic Press.

Carr, E. G., & Durand, V. M. (1985b). Reducing behavior problems through functional communication training. *Journal of Applied Behavior Analysis, 18,* 111–126.

Carr, E. G., & Durand, V. M. (1987, November). See me, help me. *Psychology Today*, pp. 62–64.

Carr, E. G., & Kemp, D. C. (1989). Functional equivalence of autistic leading and communicative pointing: Analysis and treatment. *Journal of Autism and Developmental Disorders, 19*, 561–578.

Carr, E. G., & Kologinsky, E. (1983). Acquisition of sign language by autistic children: II. Spontaneity and generalization effects. *Journal of Applied Behavior Analysis, 16*, 297–314.

Carr, E. G., & Lindquist, J. C. (1987). Generalization processes in language acquisition. In T. L. Layton (Ed.), *Language and treatment of autistic and developmentally disordered children* (pp. 129–153). Springfield, IL: Charles C. Thomas.

Carr, E. G., & McDowell, J. J. (1980). Social control of self-injurious behavior of organic etiology. *Behavior Therapy, 11*, 402–409.

Carr, E. G., & Newsom, C. D. (1985). Demand-related tantrums: Conceptualization and treatment. *Behavior Modification, 9*, 403–426.

Carr, E. G., Newsom, C. D., & Binkoff, J. A. (1976). Stimulus control of self-destructive behavior in a psychotic child. *Journal of Abnormal Child Psychology, 4*, 139–153.

Carr, E. G., Newsom, C. D., & Binkoff, J. A. (1980). Escape as a factor in the aggressive behavior of two retarded children. *Journal of Applied Behavior Analysis, 13*, 101–117.

Carr, E. G., Robinson, S., & Palumbo, L. W. (1990). The wrong issue: Aversive versus nonaversive treatment. The right issue: Functional versus nonfunctional treatment. In A. Repp & N. Singh (Eds.), *Perspectives on the use of nonaversive and aversive interventions for persons with developmental disabilities* (pp. 361–379). Sycamore, IL: Sycamore.

Carr, E. G., Robinson, S., Taylor, J. C., & Carlson, J. I. (1990). Positive approaches to the treatment of severe behavior problems in persons with developmental disabilities: A review and analysis of reinforcement and stimulus-based procedures. *Monograph of the Association for Persons With Severe Handicaps, 4*.

Carr, E. G., Taylor, J. C., & Robinson, S. (1991). The effects of severe behavior problems in children on the teaching behavior of adults. *Journal of Applied Behavior Analysis, 24*, 523–535.

Cataldo, M. F., & Harris, J. (1982). The biological basis for self-injury in the mentally retarded. *Analysis and Intervention in Developmental Disabilities, 2*, 21–39.

Day, R. M., Rea, J. A., Schussler, N. G., Larsen, S. E., & Johnson, W. L. (1988). A functionally based approach to the treatment of self-injurious behavior. *Behavior Modification, 12*, 565–589.

Donnellan, A. M., Mirenda, P. L., Mesaros, R. A., & Fassbender, L. L. (1984). Analyzing the communicative functions of aberrant behavior. *Journal of the Association for Persons With Severe Handicaps, 9*, 201–212.

Durand, V. M., & Carr, E. G. (in press). An analysis of maintenance following functional communication training. *Journal of Applied Behavior Analysis*.

Durand, V. M., & Carr, E. G. (1991). Functional communication training to reduce challenging behavior: Maintenance and application in new settings. *Journal of Applied Behavior Analysis, 24*, 251–264.

Durand, V. M., & Crimmins, D. B. (1988). Identifying the variables maintaining self-injurious behavior. *Journal of Autism and Developmental Disorders, 18*, 99–117.

Durand, V. M., & Kishi, G. (1987). Reducing severe behavior problems among persons with dual sensory impairments: An evaluation of a technical assistance model. *Journal of the Association for Persons With Severe Handicaps, 12*, 2–10.

Dyer, K., Dunlap, G., & Winterling, V. (1990). The effects of choice-making on the problem behaviors of students with severe handicaps. *Journal of Applied Behavior Analysis, 23*, 515–524.

Edelson, S. M., Taubman, M. T., & Lovaas, O. I. (1983). Some social contexts of self-destructive behavior. *Journal of Abnormal Child Psychology, 11*, 299–312.

Egan, G. (1975). *The skilled helper: A model for systematic helping and interpersonal relating*. Monterey, CA: Brooks/Cole.

Evans, I. M. (1990). Teaching personnel to use state-of-the-art nonintrusive alternatives for dealing with problem behavior. In A. Kaiser & C. McWhorter (Eds.), *Preparing personnel to work with persons with severe disabilities* (pp. 181–201). Baltimore: Paul H. Brookes.

Favell, J. E., McGimsey, J. F., & Schell, R. M. (1982). Treatment of self-injury by providing alternate sensory activities. *Analysis and Intervention in Developmental Disabilities, 2,* 83–104.

Goetz, L., Schuler, A. L., & Sailor, W. S. (1981). Functional competence as a factor in communication instruction. *Exceptional Education Quarterly, 2,* 51–60.

Groden, G. (1989). A guide for conducting a comprehensive behavioral analysis of a target behavior. *Journal of Behavior Therapy and Experimental Psychiatry, 20,* 163–169.

Guess, D., Mulligan-Ault, M., Roberts, S., Struth, J., Siegel-Causey, E., Thompson, B., Bronicki, G. J., & Guy, B. (1988). Implications of biobehavioral states for the education and treatment of students with the most profoundly handicapping conditions. *Journal of the Association for Persons With Severe Handicaps, 13,* 163–174.

Guess, D., & Siegel-Causey, E. (1985). Behavioral control and education of severely handicapped students: Who's doing what to whom? And why? In D. Bricker & J. Filler (Eds.), *Severe mental retardation: From theory to practice* (pp. 230–244). Reston, VA: Council for Exceptional Children.

Hart, B., & Risley, T. R. (1978). Promoting productive language through incidental teaching. *Education and Urban Society, 10,* 407–429.

Harter, S. (1978). Effectance motivation reconsidered. *Human Development, 21,* 34–64.

Herman, B. H., Hammock, M. K., Arthur-Smith, A., Egan, J., Chatoor, I., Werner, A., & Zelnick, N. (1987). Naltrexone decreases self-injurious behavior. *Annals of Neurology, 22,* 550–552.

Horner, R. H., & Billingsley, F. F. (1988). The effect of competing behavior on the generalization and maintenance of adaptive behavior in applied settings. In R. H. Horner, R. L. Koegel, & G. Dunlap (Eds.), *Generalization and maintenance: Life-style changes in applied settings* (pp. 197–220). Baltimore: Paul H. Brookes.

Horner, R. H., & Budd, C. M. (1985). Acquisition of manual sign use: Collateral reduction of maladaptive behavior and factors limiting generalization. *Education and Training of the Mentally Retarded, 20,* 39–47.

Horner, R. H., Day, H. M., Sprague, J. R., O'Brien, M., & Heathfield, L. T. (1991). Interspersed requests: A nonaversive procedure for decreasing aggression and self-injury during instruction. *Journal of Applied Behavior Analysis, 24,* 265–278.

Houghton, J., Bronicki, G. J. B., & Guess, D. (1987). Opportunities to express preferences and make choices among students with severe disabilities in classroom settings. *Journal of the Association for Persons With Severe Handicaps, 12,* 18–27.

Hunt, P., Alwell, M., & Goetz, L. (1988). Acquisition of conversation skills and the reduction of inappropriate social interaction behaviors. *Journal of the Association for Persons With Severe Handicaps, 13,* 20–27.

Hutt, C., & Hutt, S. J. (1970). Stereotypes and their relation to arousal: A study of autistic children. In S. J. Hutt & C. Hutt (Eds.), *Behavior studies in psychiatry* (pp. 175–204). New York: Pergamon.

Iwata, B. A. (1987). Negative reinforcement in applied behavior analysis: An emerging technology. *Journal of Applied Behavior Analysis, 20,* 361–378.

Iwata, B. A., Dorsey, M. F., Slifer, K. J., Bauman, K. E., & Richman, G. S. (1982). Toward a functional analysis of self-injury. *Analysis and Intervention in Developmental Disabilities, 2,* 3–20.

Jacobson, N. S., & Margolin, G. (1979). *Marital therapy.* New York: Brunner/Mazel.

Koegel, R. L., Koegel, L. K., Murphy, C., & Ryan, C. (1989). *Assessing the effect of two different language teaching paradigms on disruptive behavior.* Unpublished manuscript, Speech and Hearing Center, University of California, Santa Barbara.

Levin, L., McConnachie, G., Carlson, J., Kemp, D., Pancari, J., & Carr, E. G. (1990, May). Multiple criteria evaluation of a communication-based treatment for severe behavior problems. In G. Dunlap (Chair), *Broadened behavioral approaches for managing severe behavior problems.* Symposium presented at the meeting of the Association for Behavior Analysis, Nashville.

Lovaas, O. I. (1977). *The autistic child.* New York: Irvington.

Lovaas, O. I. (1981). *Teaching developmentally disabled children.* Baltimore: University Park Press.

Lovaas, O. I., Freitag, G., Gold, V. J., & Kassorla, I. C. (1965). Experimental studies in childhood schizophrenia: Analysis of self-destructive behavior. *Journal of Experimental Child Psychology, 2*, 67–84.

Lovaas, O. I., & Simmons, J. Q. (1969). Manipulation of self-destruction in three retarded children. *Journal of Applied Behavior Analysis, 2*, 143–157.

Mace, F. C., Hock, M. L., Lalli, J. S., West, B. J., Belfiore, P., Pinter, E., & Brown, D. K. (1988). Behavioral momentum in the treatment of noncompliance. *Journal of Applied Behavior Analysis, 21*, 123–141.

Martin, P. L., & Foxx, R. M. (1973). Victim control of the aggression of an institutionalized retardate. *Journal of Behavior Therapy and Experimental Psychiatry, 4*, 161–165.

McGee, J., Menolascino, F. J., Hobbs, D. C., & Menousek, P. E. (1987). *Gentle teaching: A non-aversive approach to helping persons with mental retardation.* New York: Human Sciences Press.

Mirenda, P., Iacono, T., & Williams, R. (1990). Communication options for persons with severe and profound disabilities: State of the art and future directions. *Journal of the Association for Persons With Severe Handicaps, 15*, 3–21.

Musselwhite, C., & St. Louis, K. (1988). *Communication programming for persons with severe handicaps: Vocal and augmentative strategies* (2nd ed.). Boston: College Hill.

Neel, R. S., & Billingsley, F. F. (1989). *Impact: A functional curriculum handbook for students with moderate to severe disabilities.* Baltimore: Paul H. Brookes.

O'Neill, R. E., Horner, R. H., Albin, R. W., Storey, K., & Sprague, J. R. (1989). *Functional analysis: A practical assessment guide.* Sycamore, IL: Sycamore.

Plummer, S., Baer, D. M., & LeBlanc, J. M. (1977). Functional considerations in the use of procedural timeout and an effective alternative. *Journal of Applied Behavior Analysis, 10*, 689–706.

Reichle, J. E., & Yoder, D. E. (1979). Assessment and early stimulation of communication in the severely and profoundly mentally retarded. In R. L. York & E. Edgar (Eds.)., *Teaching the severely handicapped; vol. 4* (pp. 180–218). Seattle: American Association for the Education of the Severely/Profoundly Handicapped.

Repp, A. C., Felce, D., & Barton, L. E. (1988). Basing the treatment of stereotypic and self-injurious behaviors on hypotheses of their causes. *Journal of Applied Behavior Analysis, 21*, 281–289.

Rincover, A., Cook, R., Peoples, A., & Packard, D. (1979). Sensory extinction and sensory reinforcement principles for programming multiple adaptive behavior change. *Journal of Applied Behavior Analysis, 12*, 221–233.

Sailor, W., Guess, D., Rutherford, G., & Baer, D. M. (1968). Control of tantrum behavior by operant techniques during experimental verbal training. *Journal of Applied Behavior Analysis, 1*, 237–243.

Schroeder, S. R., Rojahn, J., Mulick, J. A., & Schroeder, C. S. (1990). Self-injurious behavior: An analysis of behavior management techniques. In J. L. Matson & J. R. McCartney (Eds.), *Handbook of behavior modification with the mentally retarded* (2nd ed., pp. 141–180). New York: Plenum.

Shevin, M., & Klein, N. K. (1984). The importance of choice-making skills for students with severe disabilities. *Journal of the Association for Persons With Severe Handicaps, 9*, 159–166.

Shodell, M. J., & Reiter, H. H. (1968). Self-mutilative behavior in verbal and nonverbal schizophrenic children. *Archives of General Psychiatry, 19*, 453–455.

Singer, G. H. S., Singer, J., & Horner, R. H. (1987). Using pretask requests to increase the probability of compliance for students with severe disabilities. *Journal of the Association for Persons With Severe Handicaps, 12*, 287–291.

Skinner, B. F. (1953). *Science and human behavior.* New York: Free Press.

Stokes, T. F., & Baer, D. M. (1977). An implicit technology of generalization. *Journal of Applied Behavior Analysis, 10*, 349–367.

Talkington, L. W., Hall, S., & Altman, R. (1971). Communication deficits and aggression in the mentally retarded. *American Journal of Mental Deficiency, 76*, 235–237.

Touchette, P. E., MacDonald, R. F., & Langer, S. N. (1985). A scatter plot for identifying stimulus control of problem behavior. *Journal of Applied Behavior Analysis, 18,* 343–351.

Wahler, R. G., & Fox, J. J. (1981). Setting events in applied behavior analysis: Toward a conceptual and methodological expansion. *Journal of Applied Behavior Analysis, 14,* 327–338.

Weeks, M., & Gaylord-Ross, R. (1981). Task difficulty and aberrant behavior in severely handicapped students. *Journal of Applied Behavior Analysis, 14,* 449–463.

White, R. (1959). Motivation reconsidered: The concept of competence. *Psychological Review, 66,* 297–323.

11

Promoting Generalization
Current Status and Functional Considerations

GLEN DUNLAP

INTRODUCTION

The overriding and fundamental goal of behavioral treatment has to do with personal welfare (Van Houten et al., 1988). The *effectiveness* of behavioral interventions must therefore be evaluated in terms of the extent to which such interventions solve significant problems and/or produce meaningful enhancements of a person's life-style (Horner, Dunlap, & Koegel, 1988). Demonstrations of behavior modification are not sufficient. The changes must represent meaningful outcomes and life-style adjustments for the person or persons being served (Baer, Wolf, & Risley, 1968).

When behavioral interventions fall short of this effectiveness criterion, they often do so because of insufficient generalization. Consider the following vignettes:

> John B is an adolescent with autism who is characterized by a pervasive lack of responsiveness to social stimuli. Since early childhood he has failed to acknowledge the presence of other people, to the extent that he typically does not even answer questions or requests that are presented to him in a very direct manner. During twice-weekly sessions with a private therapist, however, he has learned to respond to nearly every verbal initiative that his therapist has issued. In these

GLEN DUNLAP • Florida Mental Health Institute, University of South Florida, Tampa, Florida 33612.

Behavior Analysis and Treatment, edited by R. Van Houten & S. Axelrod. Plenum Press, New York, 1993.

sessions, John B. has looked like a new person. Unfortunately, his responsiveness has not changed at home, at school, or in any other context.

Mr. Scott is a skilled architect whose communication in public meetings is adversely affected by severe stuttering. Although he has become quite fluent when he reads aloud to his speech therapist, his public discourse has been unchanged. As a result of his stuttering problem, Mr. Scott still suffers distress, and he continues to avoid visible contracts where he might be expected to speak in public forums.

Beth B is a nonverbal 10-year-old girl who has severe intellectual disabilities. She frequently exhibits aggressive tantrum behaviors when she is asked to change activities or to participate in teaching interactions. Beth's teacher devised a communication system that provides Beth with the opportunity to express her frustrations, requests, and needs. With the communication system and carefully applied differential reinforcement, Beth's tantrums were eliminated during the school hours. Despite numerous attempts, however, Beth has not used the communication procedures outside of school, and her severe tantrums have persisted at home and in public community environments.

John, Scott, and Beth each received behavioral treatments that successfully changed behavior. New skills were acquired, and behavior problems were reduced. In addition, all of the targeted responses (responsivity, fluency, communication and violent tantrums) were important concerns. The ultimate effectiveness of the interventions, however, was minimal. John continues to display "autistic aloneness," Mr. Scott still speaks with anxiety and limited competence, and Beth's disruptions continue to exclude her from most extracurricular home and community-based opportunities. In other words, these behavioral interventions produced almost no benefit for the overall lifestyle functioning of these three individuals.

Fortunately, the problem of *generalization* has been explicitly recognized and has been a major focus of applied behavioral research over the past decade. Since the seminal work of Stokes and Baer (1977), generalization has been the subject of federally supported monographs (e.g., Albin, Horner, Koegel, & Dunlap, 1987; Haring, 1988; Haring et al., 1989), and several hundreds of research studies and literature reviews (e.g., Carr, 1980; Egel, 1982; Fox, 1989; Handleman, Gill, & Alessandri, 1988; Horner et al., 1988; Stokes & Osnes, 1986, 1989; Westling & Floyd, 1990). A substantial armamentarium has been developed for producing generalized results, and more importantly, principles of generalization have been articulated and refined.

This chapter is intended to review the current state of knowledge as it pertains to effective behavioral interventions and the production of generalized outcomes. The contributions and the limitations of the available technology will be discussed, and some conceptual refinements will be presented. A functional orientation to generalization, based on principles of stimulus control, will be advanced in order to suggest procedural recommendations for maximizing the probability of meaningful—and generalized—outcomes.

DEFINITION AND TECHNOLOGY OF GENERALIZATION

Issues of Definition and Description

Although generalization has been an applied concern for many years, the definition of the term, and of the outcomes that are to be labeled as generalization, remains unsettled (Baer, 1982; Johnston, 1979; Stokes & Osnes, 1988). Traditionally, generalization has not been indexed as a behavioral principle (see, e.g., Ferster, Culbertson, & Boren, 1975), and it was regarded earlier as primarily an accident of inadequate discrimination training (Stokes & Baer, 1977). As behavior analysts began to modify responding in real human environments, however, the common failure of the interventions to affect behavior in nontraining contexts became a visible and genuine problem (e.g., Lovaas, Koegel, Simmons, & Long, 1973; Redd & Birnbrauer, 1969). To consider generalization as an accident, as something that might or might not occur, was unacceptable. Stokes and Baer (1977) took the first formidable steps to define the problem, to organize the existing data base, and to establish a course for active technological development.

The definition of generalization that developed was acknowledged as applied and pragmatic. It focused on outcomes. It did not address functional relations or specific principles, but it did respond directly to the practical and prevailing exigencies of applied behavior analysis. Generalization was considered to be "the occurrence of relevant behavior under different, non-training conditions (i.e., across subjects, settings, people, behaviors, and/or time) without the scheduling of the same events in those conditions as had been scheduled in the training conditions" (Stokes & Baer, 1977, p. 350). The authors of this definition then indicated that generalization would certainly be said to occur when additional interventions were not required for extra-training effects and, further, that some generalization could be claimed when the additional interventions were less than those of the original program. Although this definition has some operational ambiguities, it served to focus the field's attention toward those procedures that succeed in producing behavior changes that transcend the immediate context of intervention.

Stokes and Baer's effort (1977) to integrate (and thus define) the topic of generalization has been met with acclaim and some controversy. On the plus side, the field has been galvanized and incited to generate substantial technological improvements. Without question, the focus on generalization has produced great benefits in terms of the effectiveness of behavioral interventions. The controversy has focused on the terminology (Cooper, Heron, & Heward, 1987; Johnston, 1979) and on the conceptual precision with which the phenomenon is addressed. Several authors, for example, have argued that greater productivity may result when generalization is defined and understood in terms of the principles of stimulus control and reinforcement (e.g., Horner, Bellamy, & Colvin, 1984; Kirby & Bickel, 1988).

Stimulus control refers to the influence that a discriminative stimulus exerts when it evokes a response. Reinforcement is responsible for the establishment and maintenance of a discriminative stimulus, because the stimulus becomes discriminative through a history of contingent reinforcement (Terrace, 1966). Generalization, then, is evident when an effective discriminative stimulus exerts control over a targeted response in a nontraining setting. From this perspective, the failure of a response to occur (or generalize) may be attributable to a number of factors, including (a) the discriminative stimulus not being present; (b) the discriminative stimulus being blocked or overshadowed by other stimuli in the environment; (c) another stimulus evoking a different response that is competitive with the targeted response; or (d) the same stimulus being discriminative for a different response in the nontraining setting because of a competing history of differential reinforcement in that setting. The concept of stimulus control offers advantages for an operational definition and description of generalization phenomena, and also for studying the phenomena in terms of specific behavioral principles.

Numerous authors have noted that the failure of desirable responses to occur in nontraining contexts can be manifested in various ways (Drabman, Hammer, & Rosenbaum, 1979; Stokes & Baer, 1977). Although it is likely that these manifestations are related to different principles, they merit description because they are commonly associated in discussions of generalization. *Stimulus generalization* refers to the occurrence of a response under nontraining stimulus conditions. That is, if a behavior change produced under one set of stimulus conditions is observed in different settings or in the presence of different people, then stimulus generalization may be said to have occurred. This is the type of generalization to which the bulk of the generalization technology is directed, and it is a phenomenon that is related directly to the principles of stimulus control. *Maintenance*, or generalization across time, is said to occur when a change in behavior persists after an intervention has ended. Maintenance usually refers to the durability of a response in a particular environment. Given a stability of prevailing antecedent stimuli, maintenance is interpreted best as a function of the contingencies of reinforcement (Koegel & Rincover, 1977; Whaley & Malott, 1971). *Response generalization* is a term that is applied when a change in a targeted response produces concomitant effects on other, nontargeted responses. Response generalization is tied to the notion of response classes and response covariation, and it is a function of reinforcer equivalence (e.g., Carr, 1988). Although maintenance and response generalization refer to fundamentally different phenomena, they are relevant to the broad concerns of promoting desirable performances in the absence of direct intervention, and they will be referred to in subsequent sections of this chapter.

Technology

The significant contribution of Stokes and Baer (1977) was the categorization of behavioral research in order to arrive at an implicit technology of generalization. This sorting served to highlight procedural commonalities and, thus, to suggest generic tactics that might facilitate the sought-after spread of effects. Stokes and Baer's categorization comprised nine general headings. Subsequently, with the aid of additional research, numerous articles have presented similar frameworks (e.g., Carr, 1980; Egel, 1982; Fox, 1989; Stokes & Osnes, 1988). A theme of each system is that it provides guidelines and strategies for promoting the generalization of treatment gains.

In the following paragraphs, a number of these useful strategies will be briefly summarized. There will be no attempt to develop the strategies in great detail, or to present numerous examples. Rather, the purpose is to give an overview of the state of the technology and to refer readers to illustrative publications. Later in the chapter, however, some of the strategies will be described more comprehensively. The summary begins by borrowing from Stokes and Osnes (1989), who organized tactics of generalization programming under three superordinate principles. The three principles are as follows: (a) exploit current functional contingencies; (b) train diversely, and (c) incorporate functional mediators.

Exploit Current Functional Contingencies

The strategies organized under this category pertain to decisions that can be made and actions that can be taken to ensure that learned behavior(s) will be supported by reinforcement contingencies in target nontraining contexts. It is often the case that generalization and maintenance of treatment gains are not realized because the conditions of training are not similar to the conditions of the generalization environments. Discrepancies may exist in the relevance of the behavior and/or in the prevailing contingencies of reinforcement and punishment. Therefore, when planning for generalization, it is important to create as close a fit as possible between the behavioral repertoires and the reinforcement schedules in the intervention and the generalization settings.

This fit may be accomplished in various ways. A first way is to focus on behaviors (i.e., to teach skills) that are likely to be performed and reinforced in the person's typical environments. Generalization and maintenance are much more likely to occur if the behaviors are useful, if they are expected, and if there are frequent opportunities for the response to be exhibited (Horner, Williams, & Knobbe, 1985). Similarly, behaviors will generalize and maintain more readily if they come into contact with extant contingencies of reinforcement. For example, the skill of walking, if performed with reasonable fluency and ease, is likely to generalize and maintain because it naturally facilitates access to a wide range of reinforcers.

A fit may also be accomplished by relying on the kinds of consequences (e.g., praise) that are ordinarily available in the generalization settings, and by avoiding the use of artificial reinforcers (e.g., candy, unusual tokens). This applies not only to the types of stimuli, but also to the schedules with which they are delivered (Koegel & Rincover, 1977). Sometimes, acquisition may be dependent upon the use of densely scheduled and uniquely salient reinforcers; if generalization and maintenance are to be anticipated, however, such schedules should be reduced substantially and brought into accord with naturally prevailing contingencies.

Although it is not truly a generalization strategy (because it actually represents direct intervention in multiple environments), a useful approach is to manipulate directly the consequences that occur in the target settings. Often, this can be accomplished with relatively little effort. For example, if tantrums have been eliminated in one setting but continue to occur in another because of the reactions of a classmate, it might be possible to change the seat location of one of the students. Or a teacher or aide might be provided with some brief behavioral training, which could represent much less effort than the initial direct intervention (e.g., Russo & Koegel, 1977). Similarly, it is often possible to program some simple reinforcement procedures to target especially desirable response patterns (e.g., Parsonson & Baer, 1978). Training significant others, including parents (Dangel & Polster, 1984), has been a popular method for extending the training environment (Lovaas et al., 1973; Nordquist & Wahler, 1973). By teaching caregivers and other people who have regular contact with a client to use successful interventions, a number of nontraining environments can be manipulated sufficiently to effect widespread life-style changes.

Train Diversely

The prescription to train diversely means that generalization and maintenance are more likely if the stimulus conditions of intervention incorporate breadth and variety, such that they are more liable to parallel or incorporate the conditions of generalization environments. One of the chief lessons of the generalization literature is that rigidly structured, unchanging, and artificial conditions of intervention result in very little generalization (G. Dunlap & Plienis, 1988). This appears to be related to the antecedent and consequent stimuli that are delivered in the process of establishing stimulus control. If a response in the process of acquisition comes under the control of a highly restricted range of stimulus arrangements, then future occurrences of the response are apt to be exhibited only when those few stimuli that come to control responding are present. In artificial training environments, the controlling stimuli might include a single therapist, a clearly discriminable training environment, or a distinctive reinforcer (e.g., Rincover & Koegel, 1975). The more unusual the controlling stimulus (or stimulus combination), the less likely it is that the stimulus would be present in a generalization setting, and thus, the less likely it is that generalized responding would occur. The recommendations that come from this observation are that the antecedent and consequent stimuli that are used in the intervention process be diversified and, in general, delivered in a manner that is less distinctive and discriminable. The literature has suggested a number of ways to diversify the training process.

Training in the presence of "sufficient exemplars" is a well-explored tactic for promoting generalization. This refers to the practice of intervening under multiple configurations of potentially relevant stimuli, including people, physical settings, and materials. If training is provided concurrently or sequentially in several settings (as opposed to only one setting), there is a higher probability that the response will be exhibited in subsequent generalization environments. The same rule applies to people (e.g., clinicians, teachers), requests and instructions (Schreibman & Carr, 1978), and objects (e.g., instructional materials). Thus, the recommendation has been to provide intervention in the context of a sufficient number of stimulus arrays. The call for sufficient exemplars also applies, in some circumstances, to various forms of response generalization (e.g., Baer, Peterson, & Sherman, 1967; Guess, Sailor, Rutherford, & Baer, 1968).

In addition to using sufficient stimulus exemplars, the call to train diversely also suggests that the conditions of training be made less discriminable. This recommendation applies to the distinctiveness of both antecedent stimuli and consequences. In general, much of this prescription is to make training arrangements as natural as possible, and to disguise as far as possible the specific interventions that are programmed to change responding. For example, incidental teaching procedures (Hart & Risley, 1982) take advantage of naturally occurring interactions, are embedded within ongoing activities, and exploit the moment-to-moment initiatives of targeted clients. In an excellent demonstration of this approach, McGee, Krantz, and McClannahan (1986) showed that incidental teaching procedures were successful in producing acquisition, retention, and generalization of sight reading by children with autism.

One process that might be especially functional in incidental and other naturalistic teaching approaches (Warren & Kaiser, 1988) could be the incorporation of a time delay between the presentation of a naturally occurring stimulus and an instructional prompt. In a study with autistic children, Charlop, Schreibman, and Thibodeau (1985) used a time-delay procedure (Halle, Baer, & Spradlin, 1981; Schuster, Gast, Wolery, & Guiltinan, 1988) to transfer stimulus control from a verbal prompt (e.g., "cookie") to a visual stimulus (e.g., the cookie). After the time-delay training, the children spontaneously verbalized requests for desired items, and these requests generalized across contexts that included different people, settings, and stimulus items. Charlop and Walsh (1986) used similar procedures to establish spontaneity in the verbal expression of affection. It is quite likely that the time-delay procedures that are incorporated in incidental teaching and similar teaching strategies contribute to the establishment of naturally occurring discriminative stimuli and, thus, enhanced generalization.

Reducing the discriminability of training has been achieved in many ways, most of which have to do with diminishing the salience or predictability of the stimulus presentations (e.g., Cuvo et al., 1980; G. Dunlap, Plienis, & Williams, 1987; Koegel & Rincover, 1977; Panyan & Hall, 1978; Schroeder & Baer, 1972). G. Dunlap and Johnson (1985) studied the productive responding of students with autism in unsupervised contexts and found that the students' productivity (and on-task responding) was enhanced when the presence of supervising teachers was scheduled in an unpredictable manner. In this vein, several studies have reported improved generalization when the contingencies of reinforcement are delayed or reduced in density to the point that their occurrence is not a frequent or salient part of the training context (e.g., G. Dunlap, Koegel, Johnson, & O'Neill, 1987; Fowler & Baer, 1981). These investigations point out the discriminative properties of reinforcers and illustrate how generalization can be promoted if not only the antecedents, but also the consequences are made less discriminable.

Incorporate Functional Mediators

A mediator has been defined as a "stimulus that occurs between the training and the occurrence of generalization in such a way that it facilitates or mediates that generalization, probably as a discriminative stimulus for the performance of the behavior" (Stokes & Osnes, 1989, p. 348). A functional mediator, then, is such a stimulus that is feasible and effective in serving the mediator role. Usually, a functional mediator is established during the course of training and is systematically introduced into generalization settings in order to produce desired responding. Functional mediators may be physical or social (e.g., verbal), and they may be produced by treatment agents or by the person being treated. It has also been suggested that audio (Rolider & Van Houten, 1985) and video recordings, as well as subsequent reenactments (e.g., Van Houten & Rolider, 1988), can be used to produce change in an environment when it is impossible or impractical for the provider of intervention to be present.

Common methods for incorporating functional mediators include picture prompt strategies for students with disabilities (e.g., Wacker, Berg, Berrie, & Swatta, 1985) and the use of self-management interventions, including self-recording or self-monitoring, for a variety of populations (e.g., Baer, Holman, Stokes, Fowler, & Rowbury, 1981; Bauman & Iwata, 1977; Gardner & Cole, 1984; Koegel & Koegel, 1988; Liberty, 1984; McCuller, Salzberg, &

Lignugaris/Kraft, 1987; Rhode, Morgan, & Young, 1983; Sowers, Verdi, Bourbeau, & Sheehan, 1985). In self-management training, it is typical that some kind of physical device (e.g., a checklist, a wrist counter) is used to prompt responding and/or to record occurrences of desirable or undesirable behaviors (L. K. Dunlap, Dunlap, Koegel, & Koegel, 1991). As the device is associated with training, it may acquire discriminative properties, so that when it is subsequently carried to nontraining contexts, it may function as a mediator, or facilitator, of generalization (e.g., Holman & Baer, 1979; Koegel, Koegel, & Ingham, 1986). Although physical stimuli, such as self-monitoring devices, are salient and serve well as functional mediators, it may also be possible to use more subtle stimuli, including self-verbalizations (e.g., Guevremont, Osnes, & Stokes, 1988; Osnes, Guevremont, & Stokes, 1987).

Another tactic that has received research attention is to use peers as functional mediators (Fowler, 1988). By including peers who will be present in generalization contexts in the course of training, it is hoped that the peers will become discriminative for continued rates of desirable responding. This approach is persuasive and is associated with a number of positive results (e.g., Dougherty, Fowler, & Paine, 1985), but its power remains somewhat tenuous in regard to the occasioning of behavior across settings (e.g., Odom, Hoyson, Jamieson, & Strain, 1985). It is, of course, likely that the strength of a mediator is dependent on multiple variables, ranging from the associations developed during the training process to the prevailing and historical contingencies that influence responding in the generalization settings. For social mediators such as peers, the complexity produced by multiple variables is multiplied, and consistently favorable outcomes are increasingly uncertain.

The three principles (exploit current functional contingencies, train diversely, and incorporate functional mediators) presented by Stokes and Osnes (1989) and briefly summarized above offer a parsimonious way to organize the prevailing technology of generalization. Included are numerous strategies that have been demonstrated to be effective to some degree with some individuals in some contexts. This technology, however, does not necessarily suggest ways to increase understanding of or functional control over the phenomenon of generalization. Therefore, the next section will focus on conceptual refinements and the additional power that they may contribute to the design and success of behavioral interventions.

CONCEPTUAL ADVANCES AND THEIR IMPLICATIONS

Although the literature now documents a variety of techniques that have been shown to promote or facilitate the occurrence of generalization, it is acknowledged, given the absolute importance of the endeavor, that facilitation is insufficient. What is needed is a technology with enough authority and precision that generalized behavior change can be assured. The development of such a technology will be dependent upon progress in the understanding and analysis of generalization (Baer, 1982). With improved analyses, the probabilities that are currently associated with our techniques should come closer to the certainties to which we aspire.

There have been a number of contributions that have brought behavioral scientists to a more knowledgeable position. Koegel and Rincover (1977), for example, presented data that distinguished parameters of extratherapy responding. In two experiments, these authors illustrated a difference between stimulus generalization and maintenance by continuously evaluating responses in therapy and extratherapy environments. Their results showed that (a) children's responses sometimes generalized to the extratherapy setting, and sometimes did not generalize; (b) the responses that did generalize did not maintain in the extratherapy setting; (c) the speed of extinction in the extratherapy setting was related to the schedule of reinforcement that had been used in the therapy; and (d) extratherapy responding could be maintained by thinning the reinforcement schedule in therapy, or by presenting the reinforcer intermittently (and noncontingently) in the extratherapy context. These results helped to distinguish functionally the operations underlying stimulus generalization and maintenance, and they suggested different considerations for practitioners (e.g., Egel, 1982): The schedules of reinforcement operating within and outside of the therapy environment should be carefully examined in relation to maintenance of behavior change, and the manipulation of antecedent stimuli should be of principal concern in regard to generalization (Albin & Horner, 1988; Sidman & Willson-Morris, 1974).

These same authors, in an earlier report (Rincover & Koegel, 1975), shed light on the functions of stimulus control by assessing the generalization failures exhibited by children with autism. They discovered that generalization across settings had not occurred in some cases because, in the course of training, irrelevant cues had been established (inadvertently) as discriminative stimuli for compliant responding. For example, one child's responding did not generalize until the table and chairs (the "irrelevant" cues) that were present during training were brought into the extratherapy setting. When they were, the child's correct responding increased dramatically. This study showed that generalization failures may be related to unanticipated (and sometimes very peculiar) patterns of stimulus control. The study also demonstrated how a careful analysis of failures can uncover the functional stimuli and produce the sought-after generalization.

Horner et al., (1984) took the subject of error analysis and developed a framework for defining error types and for relating particular error configurations to aspects of the training procedures. Based on the principles of stimulus control, this model provided a conceptual refinement of generalization that has contributed another level of exactness to the design of instructional interventions (Albin & Horner, 1988). As these few examples suggest, the advances that have occurred in the applied interpretation of generalization are based on long-standing principles of behavior analysis. Increased emphasis has been placed on the precise study of environmental variables that govern responding in a particular setting and at a particular time. From such detailed examinations, it has been possible to operationalize processes and stimulus-response relationships that can be transposed into recommendations for generalization programming. In the following discussion, three broad areas of notable importance will be presented: stimulus generalization and general case programming, contextual factors and competing events, and response generalization and functional equivalence.

Stimulus Generalization and General Case Programming

As has been indicated throughout this chapter, the notion of stimulus control is fundamental to current conceptualizations of stimulus generalization (Kirby & Bickel, 1988). *Stimulus control* refers to the influence that specific stimuli or stimulus arrangements exert over individual responses or response classes; it is observed when responding occurs at different rates in the presence of different stimuli. It is a pervasive phenomenon that explains why organisms behave differently in the presence of different environmental contexts.

Stimulus control can be developed through a variety of differential reinforcement procedures (Terrace, 1966). In training circumstances, for example, reinforcement typically follows instances of desired performances. These reinforced behaviors occur in the presence of planned stimulus presentations (e.g., verbal requests, instructional materials) as well as a large variety of contextual and ambient stimuli (e.g., the particular service provider, the furniture, the color of the carpeting). As reinforcement is provided and the response is exhibited, some of the stimuli (or combinations of stimuli) come to acquire control over the response. Thus, in future circumstances, if the same stimuli or combinations are presented, the response will be repeated. In this manner, instructions often become reliable antecedents to specific responses. And further, one would expect, if the stimuli or stimulus combinations are replicated in a new context (e.g., a new setting, or a new set of materials), one would see evidence of stimulus generalization.

Although this interpretation seems straightforward and simple to engineer, it has become increasingly clear that stimulus control can be an extremely complex phenomenon. This is the case for several reasons: first, it is often very difficult to predict which of a very large number of stimuli (or stimulus combinations) will actually come to control responding (e.g., G. Dunlap, Koegel, & Burke, 1981; Lovaas, Koegel, & Schreibman, 1979; Rincover & Koegel, 1975). Second, although a stimulus may come to control responding in one context in which it is associated with other (conditional) stimuli, the stimulus may *not* exert control in another context if the conditional stimuli are absent. Related to the above, an individual's prior history with other stimuli that are associated with the same or different responses may interfere with (i.e., block or mask) the stimulus-response relationships observed in training (Horner & Billingsley, 1988).

It may be argued that these and other sources of complexity have contributed to a lack of precision in the prevailing technology of generalization. Consider, for example, the well-researched tactic of training sufficient exemplars. This strategy suggests that if training is conducted across enough stimulus conditions, then the response will be displayed in other stimulus conditions that have not been associated directly with the intervention. The deficiencies in this tactic have been that there is no a priori means of determining sufficiency, and there have been no guidelines for specifying the optimal training exemplars. An increased focus on stimulus control has helped to overcome these weaknesses (Horner et al., 1984).

General case programming is an approach that has extended considerably the precision with which generalized outcomes are achieved (Horner, McDonnell, & Bellamy, 1986; Horner, Sprague, & Wilcox, 1982). Derived from principles of direct instruction (Englemann & Carnine, 1982), the general case approach places great emphasis on (a) pretraining analyses of the generalization contexts, (b) the selection and sequencing of training examples, and (c) a careful specification of the desirable ranges of stimulus control and response variation (Albin & Horner, 1988). The first step in general case programming is to define the set of stimulus conditions (the "instructional universe") under which the trained response is to occur. For example, in teaching a particular student to tie his or her shoes, the instructional universe might consist of only two types of shoes (e.g., sneakers and dress shoes), but it also might include long laces, short laces, and a variety of settings and postures (e.g., sitting on a chair, sitting on the floor, standing). In this shoe-tying example, the initial assessment of stimulus conditions would reveal requirements both for the establishment of stimulus control and for the response topographies in need of training; the specific motor responses involved in tying short laces in a standing position are apt to be more exacting than those required for tying long laces while seated.

The definition of the instructional universe is followed by the selection and sequencing of teaching examples. Multiple examples are always required, and they should be designed to sample the range of stimulus variation and response requirements. Negative examples are also included. In tying shoes, for instance, a teacher might include as negative examples tasseled loafers or even high-top basketball shoes, depending upon the prevailing style of popular dress. Such examples of footwear would be presented as situations where shoe tying would not be appropriate. The minimum number of examples are selected that adequately sample the range of stimulus and response variation. When examples are selected, the next steps are to teach and to test for generalization with untrained stimulus configurations.

Using the general case approach, Horner and his colleagues have demonstrated powerful outcomes in teaching generalized skills to individuals with disabilities in such areas as street crossing (Horner, Jones, & Williams, 1985), grocery shopping (Horner, Albin, & Ralph, 1986; McDonnell & Horner, 1985), telephone use (Horner, Williams, & Steveley, 1987), table busing (Horner, Eberhard, & Sheehan, 1986), vending machine use (Sprague & Horner, 1984), and several other important areas of adaptive living. These studies have demonstrated that a technology of generalization can become much more precise if care is taken to analyze the stimulus functions in training and in generalization environments.

Thomas Haring and his associates (Haring et al., 1989) have also employed analyses of controlling stimuli to advance the technology of generalization. These investigators extended the principles associated with sufficient exemplar training to produce generalization across different *sets* of stimuli, a phenomenon they refer to as "between-class generalization." This paradigm, first reported by Haring (1985), involves the identification of distinct sets of stimuli and associated response classes that are functionally related to the stimulus sets. Some of the sets are then selected for training. The initial training involves teaching an appropriate response to one of the stimuli within each of the selected sets. Subsequently, additional stimuli are trained within each of the initial sets until within-set generalization occurs. (This, of course, is an instance of sufficient-exemplar training.) Generalization to the untrained sets is then probed, and if necessary, additional sets are trained until generalization is observed across different, untrained stimulus sets. When combined with the principles of general case programming, this strategy can produce very widespread gains.

One demonstration (Haring, 1985) of between-class generalization involved the toy play of four children with moderate and severe mental retardation. In this study, each child was exposed to eight different sets of toys that involved distinctive movements for appropriate play (e.g., "airplanes" were to be moved in a flying posture, "snakes" were to be manipulated on the floor in a wriggling motion). Each set had five examples that shared defining features of the stimulus class (e.g., all airplanes included a fuselage and wings) but that varied along a number of nondefining variables (e.g., the five airplanes differed in color, size, and/or amount of detail). When the author used the between-class training procedures described above, extensive generalization occurred to untrained items within the generalization sets of these movement toys. Interestingly, however, generalization did not occur to sets of "reactive" toys (i.e., toys that produced an observable reaction, such as wind-up figures and musical instruments). This generalization failure may have been predicted by the fact that the idiosyncratic response topographies and/or functional effects of the reactive toys were not accounted for in the identification and selection of the training examples. Thus, the study not only provided an important illustration of between-class generalization, it also offered another demonstration that generalization cannot be anticipated if the range of stimulus and response variations is not adequately considered in the design of training (Albin & Horner, 1988).

Contextual Factors and Competing Events

The work on error analyses and general case programming has highlighted the importance of adequate assessment of the stimulus events that are to be associated with responding in generalization settings. Such specific stimuli as a toy or a shoe, however, are not the only factors that are relevant to stimulus control and generalized responding. Stimulus generalization also depends upon many other characteristics of the environment in which responding is desired. These include a disparate collection of variables that may affect established stimulus-response relationships in a manner that competes with anticipated generalization. Such factors have been subsumed under many different headings, including "setting events" (e.g., Bailey & Pyles, 1989; Wahler & Fox, 1981) and "context" (e.g., Dumas, 1989). For the purposes of this discussion, *contextual events* will refer in a broad sense to any unplanned stimuli or circumstances that influence responding in ways other than what has been developed in the course of training.

Contextual events that interfere with desired generalization can be viewed as instances of antagonistic stimulus control, which are usually related to learning histories and/or competing reinforcers. The stimuli that control unwanted response patterns can be virtually anything, ranging from the presence of specific individuals (who may have been associated with reinforcement for problem behaviors) to conditions of overcrowding (which may evoke escape responding) or a distracting ambience (which may mask or block the intended stimulus control). Though focused research in this area is limited, the effects of contextual events are increasingly recognized as powerful determinants of generalization. The message that this recognition has put forth is a clear one: Simply because appropriate stimulus control is developed in one context does not mean that it will hold in another context.

Although the effects of contextual events are pervasive, they are notably clear in two areas that pertain to intervention in developmental disabilities: parent training, and reduction of serious behaviors. These areas will be discussed as examples of contextual influences. In *parent training*, professionals typically attempt to teach parents to use effective behavioral procedures with their children. The techniques that are taught include reinforcement and various strategies of instruction and behavior management. The hope and expectation is that the skills that parents acquire in the course of training will generalize to the many and diverse situations in which parent-child interactions occur. Indeed, generalization of the effects of parent training has been the subject of many investigations (e.g., Sanders & Glynn, 1981). It is also evident, however, that there are considerable differences in the extent to which generalization occurs across parent participants and circumstances (Robbins & Dunlap, 1990; Wahler, 1980). These differences can be attributed increasingly to contextual variables, including specific setting characteristics and other environmental factors that affect functioning.

In a recent report, Strain, Cordisco, and Laus (1989) analyzed differences in the observed generalization of skills that families had acquired in the authors' parent training program. They categorized families as demonstrating three different degrees of generalization (from full generalization to none) and then compared these data with dimensions of the contexts in which the generalization was assessed. The contextual dimensions were defined in terms of complexity; that is, the settings were rated in terms of the extent to which they permitted an undistracted parental focus on the child's responding, the extent to which the parent-child interactions were visible to strangers, and the apparent complexity of the child's behavior. The data suggested that the extent to which generalization occurred was highly related to these contextual dimensions. Further, when the authors provided interventions that were designed to remove or mitigate the effects of the contextual distractors, the parents quickly demonstrated their previously learned skills (i.e., generalization occurred).

Other studies have suggested that even more indirect contextual events may also affect the generalization and maintenance of learned parent-child interactions. For example, data provided by Robbins, Dunlap, and Plienis (1991) suggest that parents' ability to instruct and interact productively with their young autistic children may be related to the life-style pressures that they experience from sources not directly related to child rearing. Earlier, Wahler (1980) reported data from a parent training study with low-income mothers and their children who had been referred for oppositional behavior. Wahler's data showed that, over time, aversive interactions between the mothers and their children were associated significantly with days in which the mothers experienced few social contacts with friends. In other words, social contacts appeared to be a setting event that affected the probability that parenting skills would be exhibited in the generalization (home) context. These data suggest that, in some instances, the generalized performance of skills learned in parent training curricula may be a function of life-style events that are not typically regarded as integral to generalized outcomes.

Contextual factors may also be considered in efforts to produce generalized reductions of behavior problems (G. Dunlap, Johnson, Winterling, & Morelli, 1987). In treating behavior problems, a behavior analyst will usually conduct a functional assessment (Lennox & Miltenberger, 1989) and then manipulate stimuli and arrange contingencies to decrease the problem and increase desirable alternative responses. This general strategy works well within the treatment setting, but it often fails to produce generalization. One reason is that the stimulus arrangements and contingencies that were altered in treatment may still persist and, thus, reinforce the problem behavior in the additional settings. For example, self-injury is still apt to function to obtain attention or to terminate an activity, unless the maintaining contingencies are directly modified. In addition, however, there is the problem of those stimuli that have a history of controlling the undesirable responding. Even when training develops a preferable pattern of stimulus control, the introduction of the trained stimulus into a generalization environment does not guarantee that it will evoke the desired behavior. Instead, those other stimuli that have a history of controlling the problem behavior may compete with the influence of the newly trained repertoire (Horner, Albin, & Mank, 1989). Therefore, in efforts to reduce previously established behavior problems, it is unlikely that generalization will be achieved unless contingencies are managed *and* competing stimuli are identified, removed, and/or reconditioned (Horner & Billingsley, 1988).

Other contextual factors may also affect the generalized reduction of behavior problems. Certain environments, for example, may contain setting events that increase the probability of problem behaviors. Some classrooms have poor temperature regulation, are overcrowded, include teachers who complain a great deal, or include classmates whose incessant teasing produces high levels of stress and anxiety. Any of these conditions might increase the likelihood that a previously established stimulus would occasion aggression, self-injury, or other undesirable responses (Bailey & Pyles, 1989). In such circumstances, efforts to produce generalization might first require that such setting factors be identified and ameliorated.

Though it is possible to produce generalized reductions of behavior problems through procedures such as self-management (Gardner & Cole, 1984) and delayed contingencies (G. Dunlap & Plienis, 1988), a complete understanding and precise management of generalized response reduction will be dependent upon further analyses of the stimulus factors and contextual events that control problem behaviors in multiple settings. At the present time, it is clear that confidence in managing behavior problems must be associated with an adequate assessment of the controlling variables.

Response Generalization and Functional Equivalence

Stimulus generalization, including the influence of contextual factors, refers to a dispersion of intervention effects across locales, individuals, and other stimulus dimensions. Response generalization refers to phenomena in which a change in one response produces concomitant changes in other responses. The changes can be in any direction. An increase in a response might produce an increase or a decrease in a different response; alternatively, suppression of a response might produce an accompanying suppression of additional behaviors, or it might generate acceleration of some behaviors. Those behaviors that are affected indirectly are manifestations of response generalization. They are often referred to as collateral or side effects.

Response generalization is viewed as a necessary ingredient in education because it is impossible to teach directly all of the individual behaviors that must be acquired for a successful life. Thus, the expectation is that instruction in some responses will lead to additional gains that cannot be attributed to direct instruction. Imitation is a clear and common example (Baer et al., 1967). Imitation training usually begins with a student being prompted to mimic a motor movement that has been demonstrated by a teacher. When that behavior is established, a second motor movement is modeled, and its mimicry is similarly prompted and reinforced. Eventually, generalized imitation is established. This is evident when novel movements are presented and the learner copies the movements without the need for any assistance. This type of generative performance is essential not only for imitation, but also for the development of language and all other forms of complex responding.

Response generalization is also observed in other interventions, especially with persons who have developmental disabilities. Researchers have long sought more efficient methods for developing repertoires of competence in persons with severe disabilities. Thus, investigations have focused on the effects of skills that might lead to patterns of widespread acquisition and adaptive performance. Robert Koegel and his colleagues (e.g., Koegel & Koegel, 1988) have explored several strategies for increasing the responsiveness of children who are described as autistic. The assumption of these investigators has been that by heightening the extent to which such children respond to relevant environmental stimuli, their learning rate and desirable behavior will increase and become more widespread. In other words, by directly manipulating the frequency and persistence of the children's responding, indirect (collateral) benefits will be realized in a manner that is apt to be more efficient and extensive than would be possible through teaching each new behavior in an individual, step-by-step progression. This research emphasis has led to numerous studies in the areas of stimulus overselectivity (e.g., Koegel & Schreibman, 1977), self-monitoring (e.g., Koegel & Koegel, 1990), and motivation (e.g., G. Dunlap & Koegel, 1980). As an example in the area of motivation, Koegel, O'Dell, and Dunlap (1988) targeted responsivity by reinforcing the observable attempts of very severely handicapped learners with severe autism as they participated in speech therapy. Over time, the strategy of increasing the children's attempts resulted in improved (i.e., more consistent and more accurate) speech production and more positive affect than a comparative condition in which vocal topographies were addressed with a traditional shaping program. Although surprising, these results may be related to improved attentiveness and task engagement that were reinforced more directly under the attempts as opposed to the shaping contingency.

Other research in the area of autism and related disabilities has even more direct pertinence to the concept of response generalization. For example, numerous investigations have demonstrated that the suppression of certain stereotypic behaviors can lead to collateral improvements in various forms of adaptive responding, such as toy play (Koegel, Firestone, Kramme, & Dunlap, 1974) and discrimination learning (Koegel & Covert, 1972). Other studies have shown the reverse; that is, that increasing rates of desirable responding can lead to reductions in stereotypies and other problem behaviors (e.g., G. Dunlap, Dyer, & Koegel, 1983; Eason, White, & Newsom, 1982; Santarcangelo, Dyer, & Luce, 1987). This latter observation, in fact, serves as the basis for efforts to reduce behavior problems through positive educational programming. By establishing repertoires of desirable performance, collateral reductions in problem behaviors are apt to occur.

Perhaps the clearest manifestation of response generalization is evident in the notion of *functional equivalence*. Functional equivalence is a phenomenon in which two or more topographically different responses are maintained by the same class of reinforcing stimuli (Carr, 1988). For example, a student may obtain a teacher's attention through various means—a tantrum, raising her hand, or throwing a pencil at a classmate. In this example, each of these different responses is maintained by the attention of the teacher. The responses thus are said to be functionally equivalent.

Functional equivalence relates to response generalization because a change in the rate of one topography will affect the rates of other, functionally equivalent topographies. In the case described above, suppose that a teacher alters the schedule with which he provides attention following the student's hand raising. Instead of occasionally recognizing the student when her hand is raised, he now delivers attention immediately following every instance of the response. For the student, the act of raising her hand has become a highly consistent (and thus efficient) method for obtaining teacher attention. Given that tantrums and pencil throwing are less efficient, it is likely that these topographies will decline. This concomitant reduction in the rate of the problem behaviors is an example of response generalization. Demonstrations of this phenomenon have been articulated in extensive reports of functional communication training (e.g., Bird, Dores, Moniz, & Robinson, 1989; Carr & Durand, 1985; Durand, in press; Durand & Carr, 1987), as well as in other analyses of functional equivalence (e.g., Carr & Kemp, 1989).

Response generalization refers to a broad category of events that has not been adequately explored in the applied literature. The recent experimental work on skill development, pivotal responses, and functional equivalence (and its pertinence to problem behaviors) is changing this status. Increasingly, practitioners are developing effective ways to affect multiple responses in a durable manner by invoking the concepts of response generalization. This trend holds great promise for current intervention and for the further development of even more powerful applications (Carr, 1988; G. Dunlap, Johnson, & Robbins, 1990).

IMPLICATIONS AND GUIDELINES: A FUNCTIONAL PERSPECTIVE

Few efforts to modify behavior can have significance if their results do not include generalization. Only when behavior is changed sufficiently to be clinically significant, and only when the change is evident in authentic settings and contexts, can the criterion of effectiveness be fully proclaimed.

Over recent years, the categorization and analysis of generalization strategies has led to improved practice and to a foundation upon which further developments are sure to occur. From Stokes and Baer's implicit technology (1977), a rich core of information and principles has been elaborated. These principles have tended to be applied refinements and elaborations of an existing science of human behavior. The data continue to show that responding, whether in treatment or generalization contexts, is a direct function of learning histories and environmental events. Programming for generalization involves no special tricks, and no magical formulas are apt to be discovered. Rather, further advances in applied interventions will continue to require more precise analyses and subsequent translation of those analyses into an increasingly robust technology. This empirically based process does not occur overnight, but it does produce gains that are evident in the improving effectiveness of behavioral interventions.

The knowledge that has accumulated over the past decade suggests a number of guidelines for intervening in a manner that is likely to result in functional outcomes. These guidelines account for the "problem" of generalization either through circumvention or through careful programming of stimuli and reinforcement contingencies.

1. *Plan for generalization from the beginning.* Included in any plan (e.g., Individualized Education, Habilitation, or Behavior Plans) for behavior change should be a clear statement about the contexts in which the change is expected to occur. This statement should contain specific descriptions of the targeted behaviors (including any expected response generalization), as well as a delineation of the physical settings and social contexts. The point is that it is important to know from the outset the desired outcomes of the behavioral intervention, including the "wheres," "with whoms," "whens," and other questions that relate to under what circumstances the behavior change is expected to be seen. This applies to efforts both to teach new behavior and to reduce problem behaviors. Specification of these parameters is necessary for adequate goal setting, as well as for planning the intervention and evaluation procedures.

It is important to note that designations of "everywhere" and "all the time" are inadequate. These terms imply no discrimination and do not facilitate programming or assessment. Even when a teacher or clinician expects a behavior change to be pervasive, it is important to specify conditions.

2. *Assess the relevant stimulus and reinforcement conditions in the identified contexts.* When the scope of the anticipated behavior change is described operationally, assessment should be conducted in the targeted contexts. It is essential to have information about the stimulus conditions and reinforcement contingencies that exist in each of the pertinent situations. In the development of instructional programs, for example, a crucial step includes the identification of the stimulus parameters that must eventually come to control the target response (Horner, McDonnell, & Bellamy, 1986). It would be of minimal value to teach an adolescent male with severe disabilities to discriminate bathrooms on the basis of the word *men* if, in fact, the bathrooms in his typical habitats are designated by symbols rather than words. If generalization is to occur, some assessment of the actual contexts must precede instruction. Recent work in the area of general case instruction provides an excellent format for such assessment.

Similarly, assessment should account for contextual factors and setting events. Frequently, generalization does not occur because the generalization environment includes conditions that are not present in training. The presence of different people, sounds, lighting, or other stimuli may represent distractors that can interfere with the performance of established repertoires (or with stimulus control). The example with parent training (provided by Strain et al., 1989) that was described earlier offers one illustration. Observing these events during a preintervention assessment alerts the trainer to factors that must be accounted for in the process of instruction.

Assessment should also include an evaluation of the reinforcement contingencies that are present in the different contexts. Some classrooms, homes, and other environments are characterized by schedules of reinforcement that may be antagonistic to generalization. If so, it may be very difficult to produce generalized change until some modifications are made in those settings directly. Direct assessment of such possibilities might suggest a more profitable and efficient emphasis of intervention.

There is no single instrument that is capable of describing all of these dimensions and their potential effects on desired behavior change. A knowledge of the generalization literature, however, indicates that direct observation of controlling antecedent stimuli, contextual factors, and reinforcement contingencies is extremely useful for designing effective interventions.

3. *Provide intervention in relevant settings under naturally occurring conditions.* Obviously, the best way to ensure that behavior change will occur in a particular context is to provide the intervention in that context. The more different the contexts, the less likely it is that the controlling stimuli (or stimulus combinations) will be present and exert their expected influence. Often, however, it is neither feasible nor practical to conduct a specialized intervention in each and every setting. In such circumstances, the context(s) in which the need or the problem is the greatest should be selected, and all efforts to facilitate transfer should be undertaken.

4. *Make use of the existing technology of generalization.* The literature is currently replete with discussions and reviews of strategies for promoting generalization. This chapter has summarized some of that literature in accordance with Stokes and Osnes's three superordinate principles (1989): exploit current functional contingencies, train diversely, and incorporate functional mediators. These principles, and the techniques that they encompass, have been demonstrated to be useful in many situations and with many populations.

5. *For questions about stimulus generalization, attend to the functions of stimulus control.* If there is one dominant message that has been conveyed by the last decade's research in generalization, it has been to strengthen our appreciation of the fact that antecedent stimulus conditions govern the presence or absence of particular responses. Therefore, intervention must include a precise identification and manipulation of the specific stimuli that are to evoke desired behaviors. The more explicit and exact that this process is, the greater the probability will be of generalized performance.

6. *For questions of maintenance, attend to the functions of reinforcement schedules.* Stimulus control will not maintain without a suitable schedule of reinforcement. The durable performance of desired repertoires is dependent upon the effectiveness and efficiency of the response in obtaining reinforcing outcomes. Therefore, maintenance can be assured only when the response fits into a naturally prevailing context of reinforcement, or when relevant environments are designed to provide specifically programmed support.

7. *For generalized response suppression, attend to the generalization of functional alternatives.* The research showing generalized response suppression is remarkable for its limitations (G. Dunlap et al., 1987). Efforts to reduce behavior problems through direct contingency management do not tend to generate a spread of effect, and thus they require systematic replication across multiple environments. The alternative is to focus attention on a desirable response (or responses) that can be established as a replacement (Evans & Meyer, 1985). The work by Carr and his colleagues on functional equivalence provides perhaps the best example of how the mechanism of response generalization can provide durable reductions in behavior problems through positive programming (e.g., Carr, 1988; Durand & Carr, 1990).

Problem behaviors are not different from other responses. Behavioral repertoires of any sort are established, generalize, and maintain as a result of their efficiency in operating upon the environment. A basic difference in the modification of existing problem behaviors is that these behaviors have already demonstrated their functionality and have usually persisted despite considerable efforts to discourage them. Therefore, as voluminous data attest, the simple manipulation of reinforcing and punishing events is apt to be successful only insofar as the contingencies can be consistently enforced. Because this strategy can be extremely difficult (especially with long-standing behavior problems in typical environments), a common response has been to limit participation in typical settings and to rely on increasing restriction to artificial settings in which contingencies can be more carefully engineered. The problem of generalization is thereby ameliorated.

A much preferable option is the one that has been suggested implicitly throughout this chapter. That option is to focus attention on the functional properties of the response as it pertains to the various contexts in which it is performed. This requires a delineation of the stimulus and reinforcement parameters (i.e., the environmental conditions) that govern the identified behavior. When such an assessment has been conducted, the existing principles of behavior analysis should serve to identify those conditions under which a preferred repertoire will be developed. In the case of problem behaviors, the behavior analyst's responsibility is to establish a functionally alternative response and to use the knowledge of generalization principles to create transfer across relevant locales.

Generalization is a phenomenon that is indistinct from the focus and purview of behavior analysis. Its study relies on the same methodology and principles that govern all behavior. Like all questions that impinge upon behavior analysis, the questions of generalization are vulnerable to empirical investigation and progressive intervention. Continued progress will continue to be dependent upon an appreciation and exploitation of the rich legacy of behavior analytic research.

ACKNOWLEDGMENTS.   Preparation of this manuscript was supported in part by U.S. Department of Education, National Institute on Disability and Rehabilitation Research Cooperative Agreement No. G0087C0234.

References

Albin, R. W., & Horner, R. H. (1988). Generalization with precision. In R. H. Horner, G. Dunlap, & R. L. Koegel (Eds.), *Generalization and maintenance: Lifestyle changes in applied settings* (pp. 99–120). Baltimore: Paul H. Brookes.

Albin, R. W., Horner, R. H., Koegel, R. L., & Dunlap, G. (Eds.). (1987). *Extending competent performance: Applied research on generalization and maintenance.* Eugene: University of Oregon.

Baer, D. M. (1982). The role of current pragmatics in the future analysis of generalization technology. In R. B. Stuart (Ed.), *Adherence, compliance, and generalization in behavioral medicine* (pp. 192–212). New York: Brunner/Mazel.

Baer, D. M., Holman, J., Stokes, T. F., Fowler, S. A., & Rowbury, T. (1982). In S. Bijou & R. Ruiz (Eds.), *Behavior modification: Contributions to education* (pp. 39–61). Hillsdale, NJ: Lawrence Erlbaum.

Baer, D. M., Peterson, R. F., & Sherman, J. A. (1967). The development of imitation by reinforcing behavioral similarity to a model. *Journal of the Experimental Analysis of Behavior, 10,* 405–416.

Baer, D. M., Wolf, M. M., & Risley, T. R. (1968). Some current dimensions of applied behavior analysis. *Journal of Applied Behavior Analysis, 1,* 91–97.

Bailey, J. S., & Pyles, D. A. M. (1989). Behavioral diagnostics. In E. Cipani (Ed.), *The treatment of severe behavior disorders: Behavior analysis approaches* (pp. 85–107). Washington, DC: American Association on Mental Retardation.

Bauman, K. E., & Iwata, B. A. (1977). Maintenance of independent housekeeping skills using scheduling plus self-recording procedures. *Behavior Therapy, 8,* 554–560.

Bird, F., Dores, P. A., Moniz, D., & Robinson, J. (1989). Reducing severe aggressive and self-injurious behaviors with functional communication training. *American Journal on Mental Retardation, 94,* 37–48.

Carr, E. G. (1980). Generalization of treatment effects following educational intervention with autistic children and youth. In B. Wilcox & A. Thompson (Eds.), *Critical issues in educating autistic children and youth* (pp. 118–134). Washington, DC: Department of Education, Office of Special Education.

Carr, E. G. (1988). Functional equivalence as a mechanism of response generalization. In R. H. Horner, G. Dunlap, & R. L. Koegel (Eds.), *Generalization and maintenance: Lifestyle changes in applied settings* (pp. 221–241). Baltimore: Paul H. Brookes.

Carr, E. G., & Durand, V. M. (1985). Reducing behavior problems through functional communication training. *Journal of Applied Behavior Analysis, 18,* 111–126.

Carr, E. G., & Kemp, D. C. (1987). Functional equivalence of autistic leading and communicative pointing: Analysis and treatment. *Journal of Autism and Developmental Disorders, 19,* 561–578.

Charlop, M. H., Schreibman, L., & Thibodeau, M. G. (1985). Increasing spontaneous verbal responding in autistic children using a time delay procedure. *Journal of Applied Behavior Analysis, 18,* 155–166.

Charlop, M. H., & Walsh, M. E. (1986). Increasing autistic children's spontaneous verbalizations of affection: An assessment of time delay and peer modeling procedures. *Journal of Applied Behavior Analysis, 19,* 307–314.

Cooper, J. O., Heron, T. E., & Heward, W. L. (1987). *Applied behavior analysis.* Columbus, OH: Charles E. Merrill.

Cuvo, A. J., Klevans, L., Borakove, S., Borakove, L. S., Van Landuyt, J., & Lutzker, J. R. (1980). A comparison of three strategies for teaching object names. *Journal of Applied Behavior Analysis, 13,* 249–258.

Dangel, R. F., & Polster, R. A. (Eds.). (1984). *Parent training: Foundations of research and practice.* New York: Guilford.

Dougherty, B. S., Fowler, S. A., & Paine, S. (1985). The use of peer monitors to reduce negative interactions during recess. *Journal of Applied Behavior Analysis, 18,* 141–153.

Drabman, R. S., Hammer, D., & Rosenbaum, M. S. (1979). Assessing generalization in behavior modification with children: The generalization map. *Behavioral Assessment, 1,* 203–219.

Dumas, J. E. (1989). Let's not forget the context in behavioral assessment. *Behavioral Assessment, 11,* 231–247.

Dunlap, G., Dyer, K., & Koegel, R. L. (1983). Autistic self-stimulation and intertrial interval duration. *American Journal of Mental Deficiency, 88,* 194–202.

Dunlap, G., & Johnson, J. (1985). Increasing the independent responding of autistic children with unpredictable supervision. *Journal of Applied Behavior Analysis, 18,* 227–236.

Dunlap, G., Johnson, J., Winterling, V., & Morelli, M. A. (1987). The management of disruptive behavior in unsupervised settings: Issues and directions for a behavioral technology. *Education and Treatment of Children, 10,* 367–382.

Dunlap, G., Johnson, L. F., & Robbins, F. R. (1990). Preventing serious behavior problems through skill development and early intervention. In A. C. Repp & N. N. Singh (Eds.), *Current perspectives in the use of non-aversive and aversive interventions with developmentally disabled persons* (pp. 273–286). Sycamore, IL: Sycamore Press.

Dunlap, G., & Koegel, R. L. (1980). Motivating autistic children through stimulus variation. *Journal of Applied Behavior Analysis, 13,* 619–627.

Dunlap, G., Koegel, R. L., & Burke, J. C. (1981). Educational implications of stimulus overselectivity in autistic children. *Exceptional Education Quarterly, 2,* 37–49.

Dunlap, G., Koegel, R. L., Johnson, J., & O'Neill, R. E. (1987). Maintaining performance of autistic clients in community settings with delayed contingencies. *Journal of Applied Behavior Analysis, 20,* 185–191.

Dunlap, G., & Plienis, A. J. (1988). Generalization and maintenance of unsupervised responding via remote contingencies. In R. H. Horner, G. Dunlap, & R. L. Koegel (Eds.), *Generalization and maintenance: Lifestyle changes in applied settings* (pp. 121–142). Baltimore: Paul H. Brookes.

Dunlap, G., Plienis, A. J., & Williams, L. (1987). Acquisition and generalization of unsupervised responding: A descriptive analysis. *Journal of the Association for Persons With Severe Handicaps, 12,* 274–279.

Dunlap, L. K., Dunlap, G., Koegel, L. K., & Koegel, R. L. (1991). Using self-monitoring to increase students' success and independence. *Teaching Exceptional Children, 23*(3), 17–22..

Durand, V. M. (in press). *Functional communication training.* New York: Guilford.

Durand, V. M., & Carr, E. G. (1987). Social influences on "self-stimulatory" behavior: Analysis and treatment application. *Journal of Applied Behavior Analysis, 20,* 119–132.

Durand, V. M., & Carr, E. G. (1990). *Functional communication training to reduce challenging behavior: Maintenance and application across settings.* Manuscript submitted for publication.

Eason, L. J., White, M. J., & Newsom, C. (1982). Generalized reduction of self-stimulatory behavior: An effect of teaching appropriate play to children. *Analysis and Intervention in Developmental Disabilities, 2,* 157–169.

Egel, A. L. (1982). Programming the generalization and maintenance of treatment gains. In R. L. Koegel, A. Rincover, & A. L. Egel (Eds.), *Educating and understanding autistic children* (pp. 281–299). San Diego, CA: College-Hill Press.

Englemann, S., & Carnine, D. W. (1982). *Theory of instruction: Principles and applications.* New York: Irvington.

Evans, I. M., & Meyer, L. H. (1985). *An educative approach to behavior problems.* Baltimore: Paul H. Brookes.

Favell, J. E., & Reid, D. H. (1988). Generalizing and maintaining improvement in problem behavior. In R. H. Horner, G. Dunlap, & R. L. Koegel (Eds.), *Generalization and maintenance: Lifestyle changes in applied settings* (pp. 171–196). Baltimore: Paul H. Brookes.

Ferster, C. B., Culbertson, S., & Boren, M. C. P. (1975). *Behavioral principles* (2nd ed.). Englewood Cliffs, NJ: Prentice-Hall.

Fowler, S. A. (1988). The effects of peer-mediated interventions on establishing, maintaining, and generalizing children's behavior changes. In R. H. Horner, G. Dunlap, & R. L. Koegel (Eds.), *Generalization and maintenance: Life-style changes in applied settings* (pp. 143–170). Baltimore: Paul H. Brookes.

Fowler, S. A., & Baer, D. M. (1981). "Do I have to work all day?" The timing of delayed reinforcement as a factor in generalization. *Journal of Applied Behavior Analysis, 14,* 13–24.

Fox, L. (1989). Stimulus generalization of skills and persons with profound handicaps. *Education and Training in Mental Retardation, 24,* 219–229.

Gardner, W. I., & Cole, C. L. (1984). Aggression and related conduct difficulties in the mentally retarded: A multi-component behavior model. In S. E. Breuning, J. L. Matson, & R. P. Barrett (Eds.), *Advances in mental retardation and developmental disabilities,* vol. 2 (pp. 41–84). Greenwich, CT: JAI Press.

Guess, D., Sailor, W., Rutherford, G., & Baer, D. M. (1968). An experimental analysis of linguistic development: The productive use of the plural morpheme. *Journal of Applied Behavior Analysis, 1,* 297–306.

Guevremont, D. C., Osnes, P. G., & Stokes, T. F. (1988). The functional role of preschoolers' verbalizations in the generalization of self-instructional training. *Journal of Applied Behavior Analysis, 21,* 45–55.

Halle, J. W., Baer, D. M., & Spradlin, J. E. (1981). Teacher's generalized use of delay as a stimulus control procedure to increase language use in handicapped children. *Journal of Applied Behavior Analysis, 14,* 389–409.

Handleman, J. S., Gill, M. J., & Alessandri, M. (1988). Generalization by severely developmentally disabled children: Issues, advances, and future directions. *Behavior Therapist, 11,* 221–223.

Haring, N. G. (Ed.). (1988). *Generalization for students with severe handicaps: Strategies and solutions.* Seattle: University of Washington Press.

Haring, T. G. (1985). Teaching between-class generalization of toy play behavior to handicapped children. *Journal of Applied Behavior Analysis, 18,* 127–139.

Haring, T. G., Breen, C., Laitinen, R., Weiner, J., Bednersh, F., Bernstein, D., & Kennedy, C. (Eds.). (1989). *Complex models of generalization: Extending repertoires of critical skills.* Santa Barbara: University of California.

Hart, B. M., & Risley, T. R. (1982). *How to use incidental teaching for elaborating language.* Lawrence, KS: H & H Enterprises.

Holman, J., & Baer, D. M. (1979). Facilitating generalization of on-task behavior through self-monitoring of academic tasks. *Journal of Autism and Developmental Disorders, 9,* 429–446.

Horner, R. H., Albin, R. W., & Mank, D. M. (1989). Effects of undesirable, competing behaviors on the generalization of adaptive skills. *Behavior Modification, 13,* 74–90.

Horner, R. H., Albin, R. W., & Ralph, G. (1986). Generalization with precision: The role of negative teaching examples in the instruction of generalized grocery item selection. *Journal of the Association for Persons With Severe Handicaps, 11,* 300–308.

Horner, R. H., Bellamy, G. T., & Colvin, G. T. (1984). Responding in the presence of nontrained stimuli: Implications of generalization error patterns. *Journal of the Association for Persons With Severe Handicaps, 9,* 287–296.

Horner, R. H., & Billingsley, F. F. (1988). The effect of competing behavior on the generalization and maintenance of adaptive behavior in applied settings. In R. H. Horner, G. Dunlap, & R. L. Koegel (Eds.), *Generalization and maintenance: Lifestyle changes in applied settings* (pp. 197–220). Baltimore: Paul H. Brookes.

Horner, R. H., Dunlap, G., & Koegel, R. L. (Eds.) (1988). *Generalization and maintenance: Lifestyle changes in applied settings.* Baltimore: Paul H. Brookes.

Horner, R. H., Eberhard, J., & Sheehan, M. (1986). Teaching generalized table bussing: The importance of negative teaching examples. *Behavior Modification, 10,* 457–471.

Horner, R. H., Jones, D. N., & Williams, J. A. (1985). A functional approach to teaching generalized street crossing. *Journal of the Association for Persons With Severe Handicaps, 10,* 71–78.

Horner, R. H., McDonnell, & Bellamy, G. T. (1986). Teaching generalized skills: General case instruction in simulation and community settings. In R. H. Horner, L. H. Meyer, & H. D. B. Fredericks (Eds.), *Education of learners with severe handicaps: Exemplary service strategies* (pp. 289–314). Baltimore: Paul H. Brookes.

Horner, R. H., Sprague, J., & Wilcox, B. (1982). Constructing general case programs for community settings. In B. Wilcox & G. T. Bellamy (Eds.), *Design of high school programs for severely handicapped students* (pp. 61–98). Baltimore: Paul H. Brookes.

Horner, R. H., Williams, J. A., & Knobbe, C. (1985). The effect of "Opportunity to perform" on the maintenance of skills learned by high school students with severe handicaps. *Journal of the Association for Persons With Severe Handicaps, 10,* 172–175.

Horner, R. H., Williams, J. A., & Steveley, J. D. (1985). Acquisition of generalized telephone use by students with severe mental retardation. *Research in Developmental Disabilities, 8,* 229–247.

Johnston, J. M. (1979). On the relation between generalization and generality. *Behavior Analyst, 2,* 1–6.

Kirby, K. C., & Bickel, W. K. (1988). Toward an explicit analysis of generalization: A stimulus control interpretation. *Behavior Analyst, 11,* 115–129.

Koegel, R. L., & Covert, A. (1972). The relationship of self-stimulation to learning in autistic children. *Journal of Applied Behavior Analysis, 5,* 381–388.

Koegel, R. L., Firestone, P. B., Kramme, K. W., & Dunlap, G. (1974). Increasing spontaneous play by suppressing self-stimulation in autistic children. *Journal of Applied Behavior Analysis, 7,* 521–528.

Koegel, R. L., & Koegel, L. K. (1988). Generalized responsivity and pivotal behaviors. In R. H. Horner, G. Dunlap, & R. L. Koegel (Eds.), *Generalization and maintenance: Lifestyle changes in applied settings* (pp. 41–66). Baltimore: Paul H. Brookes.

Koegel, R. L., & Koegel, L. K. (1990). Extended reductions in stereotypic behavior of students with autism through a self-management treatment package. *Journal of Applied Behavior Analysis, 23,* 119–127.

Koegel, R. L., Koegel, L. K., & Ingham, J. C. (1986). Programming rapid generalization of correct articulation through self-monitoring procedures. *Journal of Speech and Hearing Disorders, 51,* 24–32.

Koegel, R. L., O'Dell, M. C., & Dunlap, G. (1988). Producing speech use in nonverbal autistic children by reinforcing attempts. *Journal of Autism and Developmental Disorders, 18* 525–538.

Koegel, R. L., & Rincover, A. (1977). Research on the differences between generalization and maintenance in extra-therapy responding. *Journal of Applied Behavior Analysis, 10,* 1–12.

Koegel, R. L., & Schreibman, L. (1977). Teaching autistic children to respond to simultaneous multiple cues. *Journal of Experimental Child Psychology, 24,* 299–311.

Lennox, D. B., & Miltenberger, R. G. (1989). Conducting a functional assessment of problem behavior in applied settings. *Journal of the Association for Persons With Severe Handicaps, 14,* 304–311.

Liberty, K. A. (1984). Self-monitoring and skill generalization: A review of current research. In M. Boer (Ed.), *Investigating the problem of skill generalization: Literature review I* (pp. 37–53). Seattle: University of Washington Research Organization.

Lovaas, O. I., Koegel, R. L., & Schreibman, L. (1979). Stimulus overselectivity and autism: A review of research. *Psychological Bulletin, 86,* 1236–1254.

Lovaas, O. I., Koegel, R. L., Simmons, J. Q., & Long, J. S. (1973) Some generalization and follow-up measures on autistic children in behavior therapy. *Journal of Applied Behavior Analysis, 6,* 131–166.

McCuller, G. L., Salzberg, C. L., & Lignugaris/Kraft, B. (1987). Producing generalized job initiative in severely retarded sheltered workers. *Journal of Applied Behavior Analysis, 20,* 413–420.

McDonnell, J. J., & Horner, R. H. (1985). Effects of in vivo and simulation-plus-in-vivo training on the acquisition and generalization of grocery item selection by high school students with severe handicaps. *Analysis and Intervention in Developmental Disabilities, 5,* 323–344.

McGee, G. G., Krantz, P. J., & McClannahan, L. E. (1986). An extension of incidental teaching procedures to reading instruction for autistic children. *Journal of Applied Behavior Analysis, 19,* 147–157.

Nordquist, V. M., & Wahler, R. G. (1973). Naturalistic treatment of an autistic child. *Journal of Applied Behavior Analysis, 6,* 79–87.

Odom, S. L, Hoyson, M., Jamieson, B., & Strain, P. S. (1985). Increasing handicapped preschoolers' peer social interactions: Cross-setting and component analysis. *Journal of Applied Behavior Analysis, 18,* 3–16.

Osnes, P. G., Guevremont, D. C., & Stokes, T. F. (1987). Increasing a child's prosocial behaviors: Positive and negative consequences in correspondence training. *Journal of Behavior Therapy and Experimental Psychiatry, 18,* 71–76.

Panyan, M. C., & Hall, R. V. (1978). Effects of serial versus concurrent task sequencing on acquisition, maintenance, and generalization. *Journal of Applied Behavior Analysis, 11,* 67–74.

Parsonson, B. S., & Baer, D. M. (1978). Training generalized improvisation of tools by preschool children. *Journal of Applied Behavior Analysis, 11,* 363–380.

Redd, W. H., & Birnbrauer, J. S. (1969). Adults as discriminative stimuli for different reinforcement contingencies with retarded children. *Journal of Experimental Child Psychology, 7,* 440–447.

Rhode, G., Morgan, D. P., & Young, K. R. (1983). Generalization and maintenance of treatment gains of behaviorally handicapped students from resource rooms to regular classrooms using self-evaluation procedures. *Journal of Applied Behavior Analysis, 16,* 171–188.

Rincover, A., & Koegel, R. L. (1975). Setting generality and stimulus control in autistic children. *Journal of Applied Behavior Analysis, 8*, 235–246.

Robbins, F. R., & Dunlap, G. (1990). *Some relationships between task difficulty, parent teaching skills, and child behavior problems in young children with autism*. Manuscript submitted for publication.

Robbins, F. R., Dunlap, G., & Plienis, A. J. (1991). Family characteristics, family training, and the progress of young children with autism. *Journal of Early Intervention, 15*, 173–184.

Rolider, A., & Van Houten, R. (1985). Suppressing tantrum behavior in public places through the use of delayed punishment mediated by audio recording. *Behavior Therapy, 16*, 181–194.

Russo, D. C., & Koegel, R. L. (1977). A method for integrating an autistic child into a normal public school classroom. *Journal of Applied Behavior Analysis, 10*, 579–590.

Sanders, M. R., & Glynn, T. (1981). Training parents in behavioral self-management: An analysis of generalization and maintenance. *Journal of Applied Behavior Analysis, 14*, 223–237.

Santarcangelo, S., Dyer, K., & Luce, S. C. (1987). Generalized reduction of disruptive behavior in unsupervised settings through specific toy training. *Journal of the Association for Persons With Severe Handicaps, 12*, 38–44.

Schreibman, L., & Carr, E. G. (1978). Elimination of echolalic responding to questions through the training of a generalized verbal response. *Journal of Applied Behavior Analysis, 11*, 453–463.

Schroeder, G. L., & Baer, D. M. (1972). Effects of concurrent and serial learning on generalized vocal imitation in retarded children. *Developmental Psychology, 6*, 293–301.

Schuster, J. W., Gast, D. L., Wolery, M., & Guiltinan, S. (1988). The effectiveness of a constant time-delay procedure to teach chained responses to adolescents with mental retardation. *Journal of Applied Behavior Analysis, 21*, 169–178.

Sidman, M., & Wilson-Morris, M. (1974). Testing for reading comprehension: A brief report on stimulus control. *Journal of Applied Behavior Analysis, 7*, 327–332.

Sowers, J., Verdi, M., Bourbeau, P., & Sheehan, M. (1985). Teaching job independence and flexibility to mentally retarded students through the use of a self-control package. *Journal of Applied Behavior Analysis, 18*, 81–85.

Sprague, J. R., & Horner, R. H. (1984). The effects of single instance, multiple instance, and general case training on generalized vending machine use by moderately and severely handicapped students. *Journal of Applied Behavior Analysis, 17*, 273–278.

Stokes, T. F., & Baer, D. M. (1977). An implicit technology of generalization. *Journal of Applied Behavior Analysis, 10*, 349–367.

Stokes, T. F., & Osnes, P. G. (1986). Programming the generalization of children's social behavior. In P. S. Strain, M. J. Guralnick, & H. Walker (Eds.), *Children's social behavior: Development, assessment and modification* (pp. 407–443). Orlando, FL: Academic Press.

Stokes, T. F., & Osnes, P. G. (1988). The developing applied technology of generalization and maintenance. In R. H. Horner, G. Dunlap, & R. L. Koegel (Eds.), *Generalization and maintenance: Lifestyle changes in applied settings* (pp. 5–19). Baltimore: Paul H. Brookes.

Stokes, T. F., & Osnes, P. G. (1989). An operant pursuit of generalization. *Behavior Therapy, 20*, 337–355.

Strain, P. S., Cordisco, L., & Laus, M. (1989, May). *Parent training generalization: Problems in technology or problems in living?* Paper presented at the 15th annual convention of the Association for Behavior Analysis, Milwaukee, WI.

Terrace, H. S. (1966). Stimulus control. In W. K. Honig (Ed.), *Operant behavior: Areas of research and application* (pp. 271–344). Englewood Cliffs, NJ: Prentice-Hall.

Van Houten, R., Axelrod, S., Bailey, J. S., Favell, J. E., Foxx, R. M., Iwata, B. A., & Lovaas, O. I. (1988). The right to effective treatment. *Behavior Analyst, 11*, 111–114.

Van Houten, R. & Rolider, A. (1988). Recreating the scene: An effective way to provide delayed punishment for inappropriate motor behavior. *Journal of Applied Behavior Analysis, 21*, 187–192.

Wacker, D. P., Berg, W. K., Berrie, P., & Swatta, P. (1985). Generalization and maintenance of complex skills by severely handicapped adolescents following picture prompt training. *Journal of Applied Behavior Analysis, 18*, 329–336.

Wahler, R. G. (1980). The insular mother: Her problems in parent-child treatment. *Journal of Applied Behavior Analysis, 13*, 207–219.

Wahler, R. G., & Fox J. J. (1981). Setting events in applied behavior analysis: Toward a conceptual and methodological expansion. *Journal of Applied Behavior Analysis, 14*, 327–338.

Warren, S. F., & Kaiser, A. P. (1988). Research in early language intervention. In S. L. Odom & M. B. Karnes (Eds.), *Early intervention for infants and children with handicaps* (pp. 89–108). Baltimore: Paul H. Brookes.

Westling, D. L., & Floyd, J. (1990). Generalization of community skills: How much training is necessary? *Journal of Special Education, 23*, 386–406.

Whaley, D., & Malott, R. W. (1971). *Elementary principles of behavior.* Englewood Cliffs, NJ: Prentice-Hall.

12

Providing Outclinic Services
Evaluating Treatment and Social Validity

David P. Wacker and Mark W. Steege

Overview

The implementation and evaluation of effective behavioral treatments is most commonly conducted in controlled settings, such as inpatient units, residential facilities, or classrooms. This occurs because those settings provide opportunities for direct observation over extended time periods. Direct observation of trends in behavior, when coupled with measures of treatment integrity, provides the information needed to evaluate functional control (i.e., the relation between the independent and dependent variables can be directly assessed within subjects over time and across treatment conditions). Functional control over behavior is a necessary condition for defining an effective treatment, and thus the majority of behavioral research is completed within controlled settings.

This situation poses a dilemma for behavioral psychologists who work within less controlled settings, such as community-based or outclinic settings or in hospitals or mental health centers. Most of us who provide services in outclinics subscribe to the necessity of functional control; yet the establishment of functional control within an outclinic is a difficult process. A quick review of research published in the *Journal of Applied Behavior Analysis*, for example, suggests that few studies have been published that specifically involved outclinic evaluations (Steege, 1989). When one reviews other behavioral journals, it becomes clear that very few published reports are available of

David P. Wacker • Department of Pediatrics, University Hospital School, University of Iowa, Iowa City, Iowa 52242.   Mark W. Steege • School Psychology Program, University of Southern Maine, Gorham, Maine 04038.

Behavior Analysis and Treatment, edited by R. Van Houten & S. Axelrod. Plenum Press, New York, 1993.

attempts to establish functional control within outclinic settings (Charlop, Parrish, Fenton, & Cataldo, 1987).

This is a disturbing situation because many psychological services are provided through outclinics, yet the technology needed for establishing the effectiveness (or functional control) of those services may be questionable. What is most common is for the therapist to use indirect measures of treatment effectiveness (e.g., child behavior checklists, interview data, or survey reports) that follow a descriptive assessment. During assessment, indirect measures also are used to identify target behavior; through interviews or informal observation, possible maintaining conditions are hypothesized. In other words, evaluation is conducted within a case study design with limited control.

Our initial approach to this situation was to put in our time in the outclinics for which we were required to provide service, and to conduct our research in other settings where better control was possible. This is, we believe, common for applied behavior analysts. Whenever the opportunity occurred, many of us chose to discontinue our involvement in outclinics so that we could be more "productive." Therefore, even though a substantial amount of our service time was devoted to outclinic work, very little of what we accomplished in those settings was evaluated sufficiently to establish functional control. This is problematic given (a) our belief in the necessity of establishing functional control to define effective treatments, and (b) that many (in our case, the majority of) treatments were being recommended through outclinics.

Approximately 4 years ago, we decided to attempt to establish functional control directly within the two outclinics for which we (applied behavior analysts) had primary responsibility: the Behavior Management Clinic, and the Self-Injurious and Aggressive Behavior Service. Both clinics are conducted within the department of pediatrics at the University of Iowa and are intended to provide tertiary-level services; clients frequently travel more than 100 miles to receive diagnostic evaluations and treatment recommendations. In most cases, even weekly services to a particular individual are not possible, given pragmatic constraints within either our hospital or locally. Consumers are typically scheduled every 90 to 120 minutes, with up to seven consumers evaluated per day; both clinics are in operation 1 day per week. The Behavior Management Clinic is intended to serve children of average intelligence who display conduct problems at school or home. The Self-Injurious and Aggressive Behavior Service provides evaluations for children and young adults who are developmentally disabled and who display self-injurious, aggressive, destructive, or stereotypic behavior.

The goal for both clinics was clear: We wanted to change our assessment approach from one that was primarily descriptive to one that was functional, and we wanted to base our treatments directly on our results of assessment (i.e., we wanted the clinics to provide prescriptive assessments; Wacker,

Steege, & Berg, 1990). By using a combination of direct assessment and functional analysis as our primary method of assessment and by basing our treatment recommendations directly on assessment, we believed that our recommendations would be more valid and that we would recommend more effective treatments.

Four questions or concerns are immediately apparent when one attempts to conduct functional analyses within an outclinic setting. First, can functional analyses be conducted with any degree of confidence within the pragmatic constraints of an outclinic setting? In other words, can we establish functional control over a target behavior with sufficient experimental rigor? In addressing this question, the answer seemed to be related to replication. If replication of initial assessment results could be built into the assessment process, then we would have greater confidence in the results of our assessment.

The second question involves the treatment selected based on assessment. Quite simply, are different treatments recommended as a result of differences in our assessment results? If not, then there is little need to conduct modified functional analyses, regardless of the "success" achieved in conducting those analyses.

Third, are the treatments we recommend actually implemented in local settings, and if so, are they effective? This third question, although certainly important, is to a large extent out of our control because of the maintaining conditions available in local settings. We may recommend an effective treatment but if it is not or cannot be carried out, then we are unable to evaluate the efficacy of the recommended treatment (Elliott, Witt, Galvin, & Peterson, 1984; Reimers, Wacker, & Koeppl, 1987). This question ultimately involves what Wolf (1978) referred to as *social validity*. In making recommendations to consumers in a clinic setting, two distinct aspects of this situation influence the probability of treatment success (Reimers, 1986): (a) the effectiveness of the recommended treatment, and (b) the acceptability of the recommended procedures. As discussed by several authors (Reimers et al., 1987), acceptability is most likely based on a unique interaction between the target behavior (e.g., severity), the recommended procedure (e.g., positive or reductive), and the consumer (e.g., history with similar treatments and available time).

Although a number of methods are available for evaluating social validity, the use of acceptability measures appears most reasonable in the context of an outclinic. Acceptability was originally referred to as "judgements by lay persons, clients, and others of whether treatment procedures are appropriate, fair, and reasonable for the problem or client" (Kazdin, 1981, p. 493). It is, in short, an evaluation of the social validity of procedures recommended to a consumer.

Acceptability becomes an issue when several effective procedures are available for treatment. In the case of self-injury maintained by social attention, a number of equally effective treatments may be available, including various differential reinforcement procedures, extinction, time out, and functional communication training. To make matters even more complex, we usually recommend treatments that are made up of several components (e.g., differential reinforcement of appropriate behavior, plus time out). The consumer's view of different treatments, or of different components within a treatment package, may vary substantially from the therapist's and may be idiosyncratic across consumers. Measuring the acceptability of recommended treatments may facilitate treatment implementation and thus influence treatment success (Kazdin, 1981). Put another way, if the treatment is not attempted, there is virtually no chance that the problem will be resolved (Witt & Elliott, 1985).

It is for the above reasons that we attempt to assess acceptability either formally (through developed checklists; Reimers & Wacker, 1988) or informally (through interviews or follow-up site visits or phone calls). We are still left, however, with a descriptive analysis; we can often establish the acceptability of a recommended treatment to a consumer, but we are just as often unable to influence more acceptable judgments.

Several authors (see Reimers et al., 1987, for a review) have discussed acceptability as being composed of a number of interrelated factors, the most common being the severity of the problem, the time needed to implement the treatment, and the type of treatment recommended. Group analyses have shown that, in general, the more severe the problem, the more options for treatment will be judged acceptable (e.g., time-consuming treatments become possible). For any individual case, however, the acceptability of a given treatment is unknown.

Given both the idiosyncratic nature of acceptability and our continued belief that social validity (based on acceptability) is important, we have attempted to identify if recommended treatments are acceptable, but we have only recently begun to measure them systematically. What appears clear is that for long-term use of treatment in applied settings, acceptability must be high. If acceptability is low, there appears to be a very reduced probability of the treatment even being attempted 3 months after the evaluation (Reimers & Wacker, 1988). Given this finding, we need to devote much more future effort to establishing and promoting the acceptability of our recommended treatments.

A related fourth question involves the *need* to conduct a functional analysis to identify effective treatment: Does knowing the function of a behavior provide for more effective treatments? We believe that it does, to the extent that functional analysis permits identification of the class (positive or negative reinforcement) of maintaining contingencies. As Iwata, Pace, Kalsher, Cowdery, and Cataldo (1990) have discussed, identifying the class of maintaining contingencies permits the therapist to fit the treatment to the maintaining contingency. For example, time out would not be recommended for behavior maintained by negative reinforcement (escape), and graduated guidance might be questionable if behavior is maintained by positive reinforcement (social contact). Completion of a functional analysis rules out certain classes of treatments because those treatments are not a good match for the variables maintaining the behavior.

The primary purpose of this chapter is to present our outclinic assessment model that is based on direct assessment and functional analysis procedures. For the purposes of this chapter, we illustrate the approach with case examples from the Self-Injurious and Aggressive Behavior Service (also see Northup et al., 1991), but the same model is used in both clinics. In describing and evaluating the clinics, we attempt to provide preliminary answers to the first two questions raised previously: Do we demonstrate functional control, and are different treatments selected? Through our outreach components, however, we also attempt to provide tentative answers to the third question on social validity.

COMPONENTS OF THE CLINICS

Within both clinics, we use a combination of direct and indirect measures to define the target behavior. As discussed recently by Mace and Lalli (1991), we believe that descriptive measures are useful for defining target behavior, but they must be followed by an experimental analysis to identify maintaining conditions. A schematic of the services provided in the Self-Injurious and Aggressive Behavior Service was previously provided by Wacker, Steege, Northup, et al. (1990), and so we present here a similar schematic of the Behavior Management Clinic (see Figure 1).

As shown in the figure, historical and descriptive information is collected prior to the clinic day and primarily involves parent and teacher reports. Information on estimated frequency and intensity of behavior across home and school situations, duration of problem behavior, previous attempts at treatment, and so forth are compiled. At least two examiners independently read the descriptive information and present the information at a morning staffing session on the clinic day. The purposes of the session are to identify the primary target behavior and to generate hypotheses of maintaining conditions from the available descriptive information. To partially verify or reject those hypotheses, the evaluation is then conducted in two parts: (a) a functional analysis, usually with one parent or a therapist interacting with the child under controlled conditions, and (b) a behavioral interview to verify information obtained from the surveys and checklists. Given that we normally have only 90 to 120 minutes to complete the assessment, the functional analysis and behavioral interview are usually conducted during the same session.

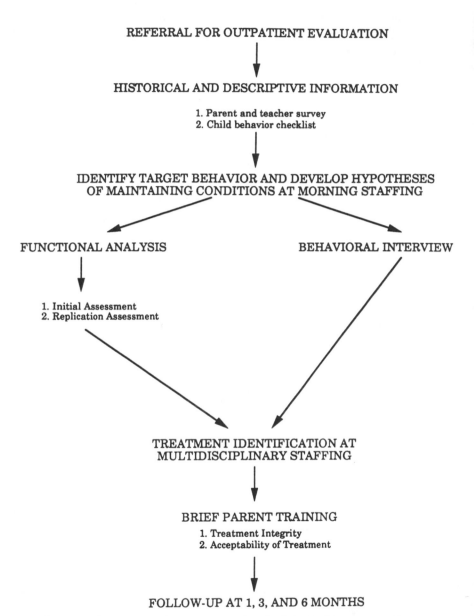

FIGURE 1. Components of assessment within the Behavior Management Clinic.

Both clinics involve multidisciplinary teams including a physician, nurse, social worker, and speech therapist, and the evaluations are completed at alternative times. When all evaluations are completed, a multidisciplinary staffing session occurs, and treatment recommendations are generated. Following the staffing session, the recommendations are provided to parents, and brief training occurs. The purposes of training are to facilitate both the integrity and acceptability of the treatment. Following training, parents complete an acceptability survey (Reimers & Wacker, 1988), which they also complete at 1-, 3-, and 6-month intervals following the evaluation. Phone contact, outreach, and videotaping are also frequently conducted, with the primary purpose being to assess and (if needed) to improve treatment integrity or to make modifications in the treatment.

Thus, the model comprises three primary components: a descriptive analysis of target behavior, a functional analysis of maintaining conditions, and a follow-up of treatment integrity. These same components are used in both clinics.

FUNCTIONAL ANALYSIS COMPONENT

Given that the efficacy of the model ultimately can be reduced to the utility of the functional analysis, it is important to consider this component separately from the other components. The functional analysis is based directly on the research reported by Iwata, Dorsey, Slifer, Bauman, and Richman (1982) and Carr and Durand (1985). Descriptions of our use of functional analysis procedures in outclinic settings were provided by Cooper (1989) and Cooper, Wacker, Sasso, Reimers, and Donn (1990) for the Behavior Management Clinic, and by Steege (1989) and Northup et al. (1989) for the Self-Injurious and Aggressive Behavior Service.

When considering the application of functional analysis procedures as conducted in tightly controlled settings over extended periods of time to outclinic settings, the primary issue becomes one of the generalizability of the independent variable. Put succinctly, is it possible to modify the procedures in such a way as to meet the pragmatic limitations of the clinic and yet still demonstrate experimental control? This issue involves immediate replication of the effects during our evaluation with sufficient internal validity. After a year of testing various methods, we have settled on the basic method provided in Figure 2.

As shown in the top panel of Figure 2, the generic method for conducting functional analyses occurs within two phases; an initial assessment phase, where various maintaining conditions are evaluated, and a replication phase, where the results of the initial assessment are replicated within a reversal design. Each condition continues for approximately 10 minutes, permitting the entire evaluation to be completed within 90 minutes. Control over

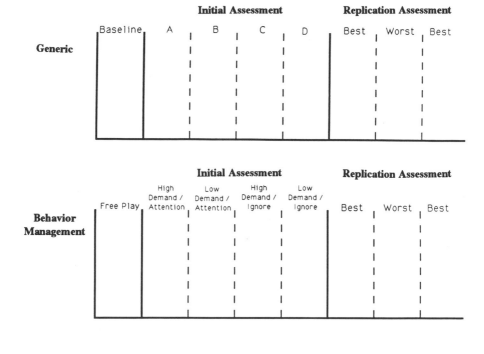

FIGURE 2. Methods of conducting functional analyses in outclinic settings. Portions adapted from Cooper et al. (1990) and Northup et al. (1989).

behavior is assessed primarily within the replication phase, with the overall design constituting a rapidly changing reversal or multielement design.

Various versions of this analysis are used in both clinics, with the "ideal" versions used in the Behavior Management Clinic and the Self-Injurious and Aggressive Behavior Service shown in the middle and bottom panels, respectively. In the Behavior Management Clinic, we typically evaluate the effects of parental attention (high or low) and task demands (high or low) on child behavior. The target behavior has most frequently involved completing academic tasks (representing homework) or picking up toys, depending on the age of the child. When a maintaining condition is identified in the initial assessment, it is repeated twice during replication, with a contrast condition separating the two presentations of the maintaining condition. A similar approach is used in the Self-Injurious and Aggressive Behavior Service, with the initial assessment evaluating the maintaining conditions discussed by Carr and Durand (1985).

Depending on the target behavior, numerous variations of this approach to assessment are possible. If, for example, the descriptive evaluation identifies the target behavior as being stereotypic, then high and low levels of social and sensory consequences might be provided contingently for stereotypic behavior. As a second example, the assessment might involve only an analysis of appropriate manding (e.g., signing). We use this approach when the client is not displaying aberrant behavior during the outclinic evaluation (this occurs fairly frequently for clients who have low frequencies but high intensities of aberrant behavior) and one objective of treatment is to teach appropriate communicative responding. During the initial assessment, the client can request attention, escape from a demanding task, or a tangible item by displaying an appropriate mand, such as signing "Please."

The use of multielement designs for evaluating our assessment results provides us with answers to the first two questions posed in the overview to this chapter: (a) Can functional analyses be conducted, and (b) are different treatments recommended? Relative to the first question, the replication phase of assessment permits an analysis of the control established by an independent variable over the target behavior. If the replication assessment results in the expected changes in behavior (based on the results of the initial assessment), then we believe that we have identified a maintaining variable. We view these results with caution because we have not, of course, evaluated the stability of functional control over time or ruled out a wide range of stimulus conditions that may be either present or absent in the outclinic environment. What we have done, at the very least, is identify a maintaining variable that may prove to be important to subsequent treatment.

When the results of this direct assessment are considered in conjunction with historical information, even greater confidence is possible relative to the maintaining variable. For example, assume that the target behavior is hand biting, and that hand biting has been stable in terms of frequency of occurrence over time. The local intervention involves redirection ("Hands down") to a task. At least two explanations are possible: Hand biting occurs to gain staff attention, or it occurs to avoid the task. Interviewing staff can certainly be useful for further clarifying the respective roles of attention and escape, but our direct assessment with replication can offer more definitive information. This is especially true if the task used during assessment is very similar to the local task, and if local staff serves as the "therapists" by actually conducting the assessment conditions.

Relative to the second question, the results of assessment, if replication occurs, definitively lead to different treatments. In the above example, a differential reinforcement of appropriate behavior (DRA) approach using staff attention might be used if attention is identified as the maintaining condition, whereas escape extinction might be used if negative reinforcement is identified.

During the first 2 years we conducted these assessments at the Self-Injurious and Aggressive Behavior Service, replication of initial assessment results have occurred more than 80% of the time, and predicted changes in behavior have occurred during the replication phase. During follow-up phone contacts, substantial reductions in target behavior were reported 3 to 6 months following the evaluation about 50% of the time.

Is it fair to conclude that our outclinic assessment actually constitutes a functional analysis? We believe that it does, in that a direct relationship is identified between an independent and a dependent variable. Given the brief duration of the assessment and the fact that we have *not* directly established treatment effects based on the assessment, however, it may be more prudent to label the procedure simply as direct assessment.

FOLLOW-UP/OUTREACH

When the evaluation is completed and the parents, teachers, or care providers have been shown the procedures, a measure of acceptability (Kazdin, 1981) is completed using the survey developed by Reimers and Wacker (1988). The survey, which is composed of 16 items, asks the consumers to rate their understanding of the procedures, the anticipated effectiveness of the procedures, problems (side effects, time needed to implement the procedures, etc.), and overall acceptability. These factors, based on the work of Elliott et al. (1984), are related to consumer use of treatment; we send similar surveys to the consumers at 1, 3, and 6 months. The primary purpose of obtaining acceptability ratings is to assist us in conducting more thorough evaluations of maintenance. Our preliminary results (Reimers & Wacker, 1988) obtained in the Behavior Management Clinic indicate that if the consumers do not rate the procedures as being effective in the clinic, there is a substantially decreased probability that they will be using the procedures 3 months later. As discussed previously, the social validity of our approach, although important, has not been established. Instead, we have thus far completed only a descriptive analysis of follow-up results and must now begin to more systematically evaluate social validity.

Most treatments involve multiple components and thus are best considered as treatment packages. Any given component in the package may cause a treatment to be rated as acceptable or as unacceptable by parents or local staff. At least three levels of analysis appear needed: (a) the general acceptability of the proposed treatment package ("Is this recommended approach, in general, acceptable?"), (b) the acceptability of the individual components (e.g., use of time out or extinction in conjunction with DRA), and (c) the delivery of the treatment package (e.g., by whom, when, for how long). In addition, reasons for acceptability ratings need to be identified.

We have found, for example, that if local staff believe (as measured by rating forms and surveys) that the behavior is maintained by an underlying physiological variable (e.g., a reaction to some unspecified pain, a chemical imbalance, or an allergy), then our approach is frequently unacceptable and not attempted. This is a tricky situation in that an underlying (and often immeasurable) cause of behavior is assumed, and we are not eliminating that cause. From the consumer's standpoint, therefore, our recommendation is *not* socially valid. We have not been successful in many cases in resolving this difficulty.

During follow-up phone contacts and outreach visits, our primary intent is to assess treatment integrity. Given pragmatic concerns, most follow-up is conducted by phone, and after obtaining descriptive information, we ask the consumer to provide two examples of when and how they have used the procedures. A simple checklist is then used to determine if the treatment is being implemented as intended. If it is, and the results are poor after 1 month, then adjustments in treatment are made. When direct observation is possible, we observe the consumer actually providing the treatment and then rate integrity. If improvement in integrity is needed, we again model the procedures.

CONDUCTING EVALUATIONS IN THE SELF-INJURIOUS AND AGGRESSIVE BEHAVIOR SERVICE

Evaluations of self-injury, stereotypy, destruction, and aggression involve two components: behavioral interviews, and functional analysis (direct assessment) of specific maintaining conditions. Behavioral interviews are conducted with parents, classroom teachers, group home staff, and/or interdisciplinary team members (e.g., psychologist, speech/language therapist, physical therapist, social worker) who are familiar with and who accompany the referred individual to the outclinic evaluation. The behavioral interview adheres to a hypothesis-testing model, with the interviewer directing questions to interviewees in an attempt to confirm or disconfirm hypotheses about the maintaining conditions of the target behavior. The primary goals of the behavioral interview are to (a) obtain a complete description of each target behavior, (b) identify specific activities and times when the target behavior occurs, (c) identify specific consequences that immediately follow the occurrence of the target behavior, (d) specify previous treatment interventions, and (e) determine the effectiveness of previous treatments.

Given that consumers' adherence in implementing recommended interventions is enhanced by explaining the possible interventions (Reimers & Wacker, 1988), time is spent discussing different treatment options (e.g., differential reinforcement procedures, functional communication training). Therefore, secondary goals of the behavior interview involve determining (a) the degree to which consumers understand and consider acceptable the possible treatments, and (b) the applicability of treatments to home, school, or community settings.

The functional analysis, as discussed, is used to identify maintaining conditions. Specific behaviors can be described in terms of their form (i.e., topography) or their function (i.e., variables maintaining the occurrence of the target behavior). A behavior analysis that focuses on describing target behaviors in terms of topography does not provide information about the variables maintaining the target behaviors. For example, a detailed operationalization of the form of a child's self-injury, although necessary for recording and measuring the behavior, does not provide much information about the variables (e.g., social attention, or escape from demanding tasks/ activities) that currently maintain the behavior. Thus, the primary goal of the functional analysis is to identify maintaining conditions for the purpose of developing specific treatments based on those conditions. By identifying variables controlling occurrences of maladaptive behavior, individually tailored treatments that address the function rather than the form of the behavior can be designed (Iwata et al., 1990).

The functional analysis procedure used in the clinic, as described by Steege, Wacker, Berg, Cigrand, and Cooper (1989), involves recording the individual's behavior within a variety of analogue conditions using a 6-second partial interval recording system. Rather than using an evaluation system with preestablished analogue conditions, we base the design of each assessment on the contextual variables (activities included in the IEP, specific caregivers, etc.) associated with each person. For example, assessment of demand conditions for a school-aged child usually involves prompting the child to participate in a functional instructional activity that was included in his or her special education IEP, such as a domestic living activity (e.g., grooming) or a vocational activity (e.g., janitorial work). The functional analysis of behavior is conducted by trained therapists or local staff and parents, who in turn are responsible for completing the conditions of assessment.

When local staff or parents serve as therapists, a trained staff member is present and serves as a coach. The coach prompts therapist behavior, explains the assessment conditions, and in general functions to facilitate the integrity of the conditions. Regardless of who serves as therapist, data are recorded on the presentation of the independent variables as well as the target behavior. Table 1 depicts the various assessment conditions, the presence or absence of the primary therapist, and the specific activity of each condition.

TABLE 1. Assessment Conditions Used in the Self-Injurious
and Aggressive Behavior Service

Condition	Therapist/Parent	Task	Activity
Alone	Absent	None	None
Alone with tasks	Absent	Play items	None
DRO (free play)	Present	Play task	Therapist provides continuous attention except when target behavior occurs
Social attention	Present	None	Therapist attends to patient contingent upon occurrence of target behavior
Escape	Present	High demand	Therapist provides brief breaks from task contingent upon occurrence of target behavior
Tangible	Present	None (preferred stimulus present)	Therapist provides patient with preferred stimulus contingent upon occurrence of target behavior

During each of the assessment conditions, an observer records occurrences and nonoccurrences of prespecified target behaviors (both appropriate and inappropriate behaviors), with each assessment condition lasting approximately 10 minutes. During approximately 33% of the observation sessions, a second trained observer simultaneously but independently records occurrences of target behavior using the same 6-second partial interval observation system. By comparing the observation results of the two observers on an interval-by-interval basis, interobserver agreement can be determined.

In summary, each evaluation involves a behavioral interview and a direct assessment of behavior. The goals of both methods are similar; assessment data are used to prescribe individually tailored treatment interventions with the emphasis of the interview being descriptive (target behavior and acceptability), and the functional analysis comprising an investigation of hypotheses of maintaining conditions.

In the following case examples, we discuss the application of the behavioral assessment procedures, the design of treatment interventions, methods of determining consumers' acceptability of treatments, and the applicability of treatments to local settings. These case examples illustrate the outclinic–outreach service continuum available in the Self-Injurious and Aggressive Behavior Service.

Case Example 1

Sally was a 22-year-old woman who resided in a residential facility in a community approximately 100 miles from the clinic. Referral to the outpatient clinic for behavioral assessment of Sally's stereotypic, self-injurious, and aggressive behaviors was made by the social worker and case manager from the residential facility where Sally lived. Sally was ambulatory, nonverbal, and diagnosed as severely mentally retarded. By parent report, Sally had engaged in stereotypic and self-injurious behavior for approximately 15 years. Her stereotypy was defined as repetitively rubbing her hands and hand mouthing. Self-injury was defined as self-scratching (hands, legs, and torso) that led to tissue damage (open and bleeding wounds). One year prior to the evaluation, Sally began to display aggressive behavior, including striking, kicking, and biting others. Sally's day programming was provided in a work activity center where she was expected to perform a variety of prevocational activities (e.g., sorting items by color).

During the behavioral interview with Sally's parents and the local social worker, it was determined that Sally's stereotypic and self-injurious behaviors occurred primarily during situations in which she was not actively engaged in structured activities (break times, between activities, etc.). Aggressive behaviors occurred primarily when staff attempted to restrain her physically from engaging in stereotypic or self-injurious behaviors. Previous intervention strategies addressing stereotypy and self-injury included verbal reprimands and physical restraint, with staff restraining Sally's hands to prevent problem behaviors. Treatment for aggressive behaviors included a time-out procedure where Sally was placed in her bedroom with no contact with staff or peers for 30 minutes.

The functional analysis involved measuring occurrences and nonoccurrences of stereotypic, self-injurious, and aggressive behaviors during the following analogue conditions: (a) alone, (b) alone/structured task, (c) social attention, and (d) escape. The results of the functional analysis are depicted in Figure 3.

Throughout the evaluation, occurrences of stereotypic and self-injurious behavior occurred most consistently during conditions in which Sally was not actively engaged in structured activities (alone and social attention conditions). Aggressive behavior occurred only when the therapist attempted physically to prevent Sally from exhibiting stereotypic or self-injurious behaviors. Equally important, there were no occurrences of target behaviors when Sally was either engaged in or prompted to participate in functional activities (alone/task and escape conditions). These data suggested that Sally's stereotypic and self-injurious behaviors were maintained by positive reinforcement (i.e., staff attention) when she had nothing else to do, and that aggressive behavior appeared to be maintained by negative reinforcement (i.e., escape from staff's physical restraint). These results were then replicated.

Following the completion of the functional analysis, the therapists reviewed the assessment results with Sally's interdisciplinary team members by phone. Based on the assessment data, a treatment package that included

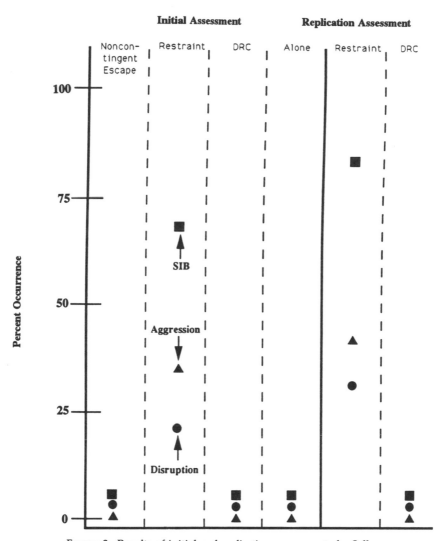

FIGURE 3. Results of initial and replication assessments for Sally.

the following components was recommended: (a) increased opportunities for participation in functional activities and decreased "downtime," and (b) redirection (i.e., prompting Sally to engage in age-appropriate recreation-leisure activities). The acceptability of the treatment intervention to the vocational setting was rated as high, with administrative staff from the vocational setting agreeing to identify a set of staff persons who would be responsible for implementation. Outreach by the therapists to Sally was conducted 2 weeks later. Consistent with the clinic evaluation, self-injury and stereotypy occurred during times when Sally was not engaged in structured activities, and aggression occurred when staff attempted physically to restrain occurrences of stereotypy or self-injury.

The results of the functional analysis and of observations of Sally's and staff's behavior within the vocational setting were presented to the local staff. The treatment package of environmental restructuring and redirection was also presented. Following the presentation, discussions of the application of the treatment intervention within the vocational setting ensued, with participation from direct care, interdisciplinary, and administrative staff. Phone consultation follow-up also was scheduled. All occurrences of aggressive behavior were eliminated immediately, with occurrences of self-injury and stereotypy reduced to near-zero levels.

Case Example 2

Don was 21 years old and lived in a residential facility in the community where the Self-Injurious and Aggressive Behavior Service is located. A referral for an outclinic evaluation of Don's self-injurious, disruptive, and aggressive behavior was made by interdisciplinary team members from the residential setting. Don was ambulatory, nonverbal, and visually impaired, and he was diagnosed as being severely mentally retarded. Don had engaged in self-injurious, disruptive, and aggressive behavior for several years. Self-injury was identified as self-scratching (face, hands, ankles), whereas disruptive behavior was described as throwing objects and screaming; aggression involved striking others.

During the behavioral interview, it was determined that all aberrant behaviors occurred exclusively during mealtimes. Specifically, these behaviors occurred when Don had completed his meal and was attempting to leave the dining area. When staff prevented him from leaving the dining area by physically prompting him to remain in his chair or by restraining him, he first engaged in self-injury; if staff then continued to restrict him, he became disruptive (i.e., throwing plates, glasses, silverware) and aggressive (striking staff). Staff responded to disruptive and aggressive behavior with a time-out strategy by removing Don from the dining table and placing him in a chair in the hallway of the group home for 15 minutes. During a phone conversation between the therapist and staff from the vocational day program that Don attended, it was determined that self-injurious, disruptive, and aggressive behaviors did not occur at lunchtime at the day program, where Don was permitted to leave the dining area when he completed his meal.

The functional analysis involved measuring occurrences and nonoccurrences of self-injurious, disruptive, and aggressive behaviors during a series of mealtime analogue conditions in which Don was provided with brief snacks. These conditions were (a) noncontingent escape from dining area, (b) restraint (staff restricting Don to the dining area), (c) differential reinforcement of communication (staff physically prompting Don to sign "Please" manually, then allowing him to leave the dining area), and (d) alone (Don alone in the dining area). The results of the functional analysis are shown in Figure 4.

The results showed that self-injurious, disruptive, and aggressive behavior occurred only during the assessment condition in which the primary therapist physically prevented Don from leaving the dining area after he had completed his snack (restraint condition). Of equal interest was the finding that when Don was alone at the dining table, he did not attempt to leave the area following completion of his snack. These data suggested that Don's self-

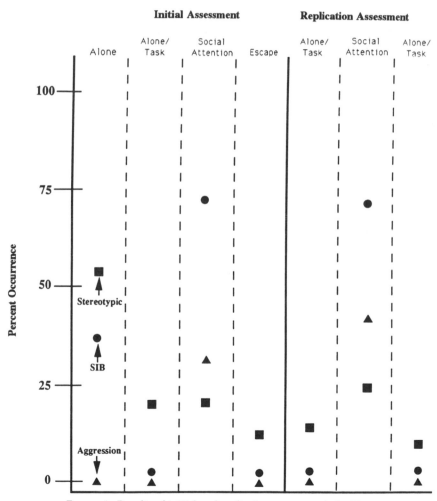

FIGURE 4. Results of initial and replication assessments for Don.

injurious, disruptive, and aggressive behaviors were maintained by negative reinforcement (escape from the physical restraints that staff were using to restrict him). It was further hypothesized that his behavior of standing and walking away from the dining table was maintained by escape from the group activity. To further evaluate this hypothesis, we conducted an assessment of Don's "exiting behavior" within small groups and when alone. The results of this evaluation suggested that Don demonstrated avoidance of small group situations.

Based on the results of these evaluations, the treatment intervention consisted of a functional communication training procedure whereby Don was prompted by staff to sign "Please" following completion of meals and snacks and was then permitted to spend up to 30 minutes alone in his bedroom. The treatment intervention was discussed with interdisciplinary team members from the residential program, and the treatment procedure with Don was demonstrated; the team members rated the procedure as being acceptable. An outreach was provided to the group home 1 week after the outclinic evaluation by the two therapists who conducted the evaluation. Following an observation of Don during mealtime, an in-service session was conducted that provided a demonstration of the treatment procedure with Don. Monthly phone consultations were conducted over a 6-month period. It was reported that Don was routinely signing "Please" after the completion of meals at both his residential and vocational settings, occurrences of self-injurious and aggressive behaviors had been eliminated within the first month, and disruptive behavior occurred less than once per month.

Case Example 3

Rick was an 8-year-old with severe multiple disabilities who lived with his parents in a metropolitan area within 30 miles of the outclinic. Rick's mother reported that Rick had engaged in self-injury (i.e., hand mouthing and hand biting, leading to wounds and contusions on his right hand) since he was approximately 2 years old. Rick was nonambulatory and had no functional communication skills. A referral for an outclinic evaluation of Rick's self-injurious behavior was made by his parents.

Behavioral interviews indicated that self-injury occurred primarily during situations when Rick was not engaged in activities with either his mother or his father. They responded to occurrences of self-injury with mild verbal reprimands (e.g., "Stop, Rick, you're hurting yourself") and by engaging him in activities. They reported an increase in both the intensity and frequency of occurrence of hand-mouthing and hand-biting behaviors within the past year.

A functional analysis was conducted using Rick's mother as the primary therapist during alone, demand, social attention, and differential reinforcement of other behavior (DRO) conditions (the other behavior comprised playing together with toys). The results of this assessment showed that self-injury occurred at the highest frequencies during the social attention condition, suggesting that Rick's self-injury was maintained by positive reinforcement (i.e., social attention contingent upon occurrences of self-injury). After the initial assessment, an additional assessment using a differential reinforcement of communication (DRC) condition was conducted. The DRC strategy involved physically prompting Rick to activate a pressure-sensitive microswitch that played a prerecorded message ("Mom, come here. Mom, come here."). When Rick pressed the switch, his mother was directed to approach and engage him in an age-appropriate leisure activity and to provide positive social interactions. Self-injury was ignored.

The results of the assessment are provided in Figure 5. They demonstrated that Rick's self-injury was maintained by social attention. Moreover,

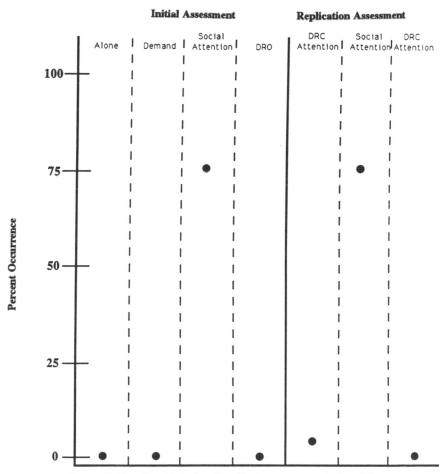

FIGURE 5. Results of initial and replication assessments for Rick.

when social attention was provided contingent upon occurrences of an alternative behavior, a marked decrease in self-injury occurred.

At the conclusion of the outclinic evaluation, Rick's mother was provided with a pressure-sensitive microswitch, a tape recorder, and a prerecorded tape. A follow-up schedule of telephone calls was established. An outreach to Rick's school 2 weeks following the outclinic evaluation was conducted, and an in-service session with Rick's classroom teacher and interdisciplinary team members demonstrating the application of the DRC procedure to the school setting was provided. The DRC procedure was modified to include pretaped messages for Rick's classroom teacher, teacher associate, and non-handicapped peers (e.g., "Susan, come here," "Steve, come here"). Follow-up phone calls indicated that the treatment was effective in reducing occurrences of self-injury both at home and at school.

CONSIDERATIONS AND LIMITATIONS

There are several advantages of conducting functional analyses of behavior in outclinic settings and not relying solely on descriptive information obtained during interviews or surveys. Regardless of the expertise of the interviewer, interviewees often do not have sufficient information to allow for a thorough analysis of the behaviors of concern. The functional analysis of behavior provides an empirical analysis of maintaining conditions, thus confirming or disconfirming hypotheses about controlling variables generated from the descriptive information. During the functional analysis, treatment interventions also can be implemented briefly to evaluate their efficacy. By asking consumers to observe and participate in the evaluation, their acceptance of the treatment can be ascertained.

The use of brief functional analysis procedures is new (Steege, 1989), however, and a number of questions or concerns need to be addressed. One obvious potential limitation of conducting behavioral assessments of aberrant behavior in outclinic settings is the limited amount of assessment data that can be collected during the evaluation. Behavioral assessment procedures conducted in more controlled settings (e.g., Iwata et al., 1982; Steege et al., 1989) generally involve multiple observations of the client's behavior within each assessment condition. Assessment continues until a stable pattern of behavior emerges, which can often take several weeks. Stability of responding cannot be assessed in an outclinic, and thus caution is warranted in interpreting the results.

The validity of an evaluation, however, should not be based on the amount of data collected. Rather, the degree to which an evaluation provides information that is useful in prescribing effective and efficient treatment interventions determines its validity. If the results of the outpatient evaluation are ambiguous, then additional assessments conducted in the community or on an inpatient basis are warranted. Outpatient evaluations appear to be most useful when single maintaining conditions control behavior; multiple maintaining conditions involve more complicated analyses that most often require further assessment.

A second limitation involves the evaluation of the efficacy of the treatment based on the assessment. Again, in more controlled settings, we can evaluate treatments directly and make subtle changes. To measure the efficacy of a treatment intervention adequately, both the dependent and the independent variables need to be evaluated, a process that we are seldom able to complete in the outclinic. Phone contacts simply provide information about the overall effectiveness of treatment, requiring that we make inferences based on indirect data about the reasons for effectiveness.

Finally, the degree of control possible in an outclinic setting is often a function of the behavior observed. We frequently find that the patient responds differently, by report, in our setting than in the natural setting. If we were able to observe the patient over time, more accurate patterns of behavior might be possible. As is also obvious in the case examples provided, we often fail to complete our "ideal" assessment of initial and replication phases. In these situations, even more caution is needed in interpreting the results.

SUMMARY

There are, of course, a number of reasons for not attempting to conduct functional analyses in outclinic settings. From a practical standpoint, they can be difficult to implement, are time-consuming relative to staff time, and can be frustrating if the patient refuses to cooperate. From a conceptual standpoint, it is questionable if the analyses conducted are comparable to what would be obtained through a more thorough analysis. It is, frankly, easy to state that such an approach is impossible and instead conduct descriptive evaluations that rely heavily on indirect data.

For a number of other practical and conceptual reasons, we have decided to attempt to conduct functional analyses in our outclinics and to invest our time and resources in the development of direct assessment approaches. Although still in a preliminary phase, we believe that our results have been sufficiently successful to warrant continued development and evaluation. In both clinics, our "success" rate (as defined by the elimination or substantial reduction of target behavior 6 months following assessment) is approximately 50%. We do not interpret this success rate as being either particularly good or bad, because there is very little with which to compare it. When we compare this success rate to that of our own descriptive (interview data or less systematic observation) evaluations, we are convinced that it is easily the higher of the two, but a number of potentially confounding variables make comparisons in assessment approaches impossible.

What is possible for us to begin to assess directly are the answers to the questions posed previously. First, can functional analyses be conducted in outclinics? Our initial results indicate that they can be conducted and that the information obtained, if not overinterpreted, is very useful for identifying treatments. Second, are different treatments selected based on the results of assessment? We are most confident of an affirmative response to this question. The functional analysis, by directly evaluating maintaining conditions, provides direction for treatment selection by identifying classes of treatment (positive or negative reinforcement).

Third, are the treatments effective? We are not sure. A number of uncontrolled conditions occur in natural settings that almost certainly moderate our results. Further assessments involving direct observation of treatment integrity are needed to answer this question more fully. Fourth, is a functional analysis needed to prescribe effective treatment? This is not necessarily the case. As recently reported by Repp, Felce, and Barton (1988), effective treatments can be based on descriptive data and on hypotheses generated from those data. If functional analyses are conducted, however, we believe that there is a much improved probability that the *class* of treatments recommended will match the maintaining variables, leading to more successful interventions.

REFERENCES

Carr, E., & Durand, V. M. (1985). Reducing behavior problems through functional communication training. *Journal of Applied Behavior Analysis, 18,* 111–126.

Charlop, M., Parrish, J., Fenton, L., & Cataldo, M. (1987). Evaluation of hospital-based outpatient pediatric psychology services. *Journal of Pediatric Psychology, 12,* 485–503.

Cooper, L. (1989, May). Functional analysis of conduct disorders in an outclinic setting. In D. Wacker (Chair), *Functional analysis of severe behavior problems: Recent applications and novel approaches.* Symposium conducted at the annual meeting of the Association for Behavior Analysis, Milwaukee, WI.

Cooper, L., Wacker, D., Sasso, G., Reimers, T., & Donn, L. (1990). Using parents as therapists to assess the appropriate behavior of their children through a functional analysis: Application to a tertiary diagnostic clinic. *Journal of Applied Behavior Analysis, 23,* 285–296.

Elliott, S., Witt, J., Galvin, G., & Peterson, R. (1984). Acceptability of positive and reductive behavioral interventions: Factors that influence teachers' decisions. *Journal of School Psychology, 22,* 353–360.

Iwata, B., Dorsey, M., Slifer, K., Bauman, K., & Richman, G. (1982). Toward a functional analysis of self-injury. *Analysis and Intervention in Developmental Disabilities, 2,* 3–20.

Iwata, B., Pace, G., Kalsher, M., Cowdery, G., & Cataldo, M. (1990). Experimental analysis and extinction of self-injurious escape behavior. *Journal of Applied Behavior Analysis, 23,* 11–27.

Kazdin, A. (1981). Acceptability of child treatment techniques: The influence of treatment efficacy and adverse side effects. *Behavior Therapy, 12,* 493–506.

Mace, F. C., & Lalli, J. (1991). Linking descriptive and experimental analysis in the treatment of bizarre speech. *Journal of Applied Behavior Analysis, 24,* 553–562.

Northup, J., Wacker, D., Sasso, G., Steege, M., Cigrand, K., Cook, J., & DeRaad, A. (1991). A brief functional analysis of aggressive and alternative behavior in an outclinic setting. *Journal of Applied Behavior Analysis*, *24*, 509–522.

Northup, J., Wacker, D., Steege, M., Cigrand, K., Sasso, G., & Cook, J. (1989, May). *Outpatient evaluation of self-injurious and aggressive behavior using functional analysis.* Paper presented at the annual meeting of the Association for Behavior Analysis, Milwaukee, WI.

Reimers, T. (1986). *Acceptability of behavioral treatment recommendations: Social validation in an outclinic.* Unpublished doctoral dissertation, University of Iowa, Iowa City.

Reimers, T., & Wacker, D. (1988). Parents' ratings of acceptability of behavioral treatment recommendations made in an outpatient clinic: A preliminary analysis of the influence of treatment effectiveness. *Behavioral Disorders*, *14*, 7–15.

Reimers, T., Wacker, D., & Koeppl, G. (1987). Acceptability of behavioral interventions: A review of the literature. *School Psychology Review*, *16*, 212–227.

Repp, A., Felce, D., & Barton, L. (1988). Basing the treatment of stereotypic and self-injurious behavior on hypotheses of their causes. *Journal of Applied Behavior Analysis*, *21*, 281–289.

Steege, M. (1989, May). Functional analysis of self-injurious behavior in an outclinic setting. In D. Wacker (Chair), *Functional analysis of severe behavior problems: Recent applications and novel approaches.* Symposium conducted at the annual meeting of the Association for Behavior Analysis, Milwaukee, WI.

Steege, M., Wacker, D., Berg, W., Cigrand, K., & Cooper, L. (1989). The use of behavioral assessment to prescribe and evaluate treatments for severely handicapped children. *Journal of Applied Behavior Analysis*, *22*, 23–33.

Wacker, D., Steege, M., & Berg, W. (1990). Best practices in assessment and intervention with persons who are severely handicapped. In A. Thomas & J. Grimes (Eds.), *Best practices in school psychology*, Vol. 2 (pp. 81–92). Washington, DC: National Association of School Psychologists.

Wacker, D., Steege, M., Northup, J., Reimers, T., Berg, W., & Sasso, G. (1990). Use of functional analysis and acceptability measures to assess and treat severe behavior problems: An outpatient clinic model. In N. Singh & A. Repp (Eds.), *Aversive and non-aversive treatment: The great debate in developmental disabilities* (pp. 349–359). Sycamore, IL: Sycamore.

Witt, J. C., & Elliott, S. N. (1985). Acceptability of classroom management strategies. In T. R. Kratochwill (Ed.), *Advances in school psychology, vol. 4* (pp. 251–288). Hillsdale, NJ: Lawrence Erlbaum.

Wolf, M. M. (1978). Social validity: The case for subjective measurement or how applied behavior analysis is finding its heart. *Journal of Applied Behavior Analysis*, *11*, 203–214.

V

Advancing the State of the Art

13

A Model for Developing and Evaluating Behavioral Technology

J. M. JOHNSTON

THE FIRST 30 YEARS

What has come to be recognized as a technology of behavior has been developing over the past 30 years or so. As is probably typical of the early years of a new technology's development, there has been no plan or set of standards guiding this evolution; each contributor has simply brought along his or her history and motivating circumstances. Thus, a handful of basic animal laboratory researchers, a core of academics, a lot of practitioners, and miscellaneous entrepreneurs and interested parties have had assorted impacts on how this technology has progressed.

The resulting capability for solving behavioral problems may be characterized in as many ways as there are points of view. Basic researchers might worry that the relationship between the techniques routinely used in the field and the basic principles of behavior is too tenuous for comfort. Applied researchers, who constitute an influential segment of the field, are likely to be proud of the technological accomplishments while worrying about how to overcome obvious shortcomings. Depending on their needs, some practi-

ACKNOWLEDGMENT. I would like to thank Dr. Bill Hopkins for his comments on an earlier version of this chapter.

J. M. JOHNSTON • Department of Psychology, Auburn University, Auburn, Alabama 36849.

Behavior Analysis and Treatment, edited by R. Van Houten & S. Axelrod. Plenum Press, New York, 1993.

tioners might describe the technology as powerful and exciting, whereas others might complain that it is too undeveloped and inconsistent in its effectiveness to depend upon. Many other users or recipients of behavioral technology may be largely untrained in the field, and probably know so little about it that they do not even have evaluative opinions.

There has for some years now been a modest literature describing various concerns about behavioral technology (e.g., Baer, 1981; Baer, Wolf, & Risley, 1987; Deitz, 1982; Fawcett, 1985; Hayes, 1978; Hayes, Rincover, & Solnick, 1980; Hopkins, 1970; Michael, 1980; Pierce & Epling, 1980). Although these worries are invariably offered in the constructive style of a family member, perhaps the most common theme is a sense of dissatisfaction with various facets of the technology and how it is developed and delivered. There seems to be an increasing realization that the future development of behavioral technology will require a degree of planning and management that exceeds its relatively informal traditions.

TECHNOLOGY VERSUS CRAFT

What does it mean to refer to a behavioral technology? What distinguishes technology from common sense, folklore, skilled experience, or craft? The following conception has emerged from practices in the natural sciences: *Behavioral technology* refers to behavior change procedures the nature of whose influence has been established by experimental analysis in the terms of the natural science of behavior and for which applied empirical evaluation has established reliable and general effects.

This definition is rich with implications that may not be obvious. For example, it makes a distinction between behavior change procedures that may be effective—even consistently so—for reasons that are unknown or merely suspected, and those that work because of variables whose role has been certified by experiment. The definition says that it is the mechanism of a procedure's action, rather than its source or the consistency of its effectiveness, that should determine its status as technology. In other words, what is central to the meaning of technology is that how it works has been fairly well established by experimentation.

Were it not for this experimental requirement, the practitioner's repertoire might consist largely of procedures that worked at least once for their originator but about which little else is known. Without this criterion, the technology's growth might come from premature proselytizing of procedures by their creators. Eventually, what would appear to be a legitimate, wide-ranging, and capable technology could be only a Hollywood back-lot facade, hiding a miscellany of uncertain procedural details, untested convictions about their rationales, and naively optimistic promises of effectiveness.

Understanding the nature of a procedure's effects involves a number of requirements. For example, it means that the component elements of a procedure must be identified and separately analyzed to determine the contribution of each to the aggregate effect. This process will almost certainly modify the original procedure by more effective arrangements of useful elements and elimination of impotent features. It will also identify those components and parameters that are critical to the procedure's effects and that must not be modified in field applications. Component analysis is thus the first step in learning what makes a procedure effective or prevents it from being ineffective.

A research program concerning rumination in retarded individuals exemplified this analytical style. An initial study showed that feeding satiation quantities of food to clients would greatly reduce their rates of ruminating (Rast, Johnston, Drum, & Conrin, 1981). This was followed by a series of studies attempting to identify the components of the feeding procedure that might contribute to this effect. Eventually, the caloric density of the diet, oral and esophageal stimulation, stomach distention, and other variables were each shown to play a role (Rast, Johnston, & Drum, 1984; Rast, Johnston, Ellinger-Allen, & Drum, 1985; Rast, Johnston, Ellinger-Allen, & Lubin, 1988).

Understanding the nature of a procedure's influence, however, means more than just component analysis. It also requires understanding the means by which the components separately or collectively accomplish their effects. Understanding mechanisms of action is really part of the component analysis process, which requires a series of thematic studies that eventually generate an entire literature from the contributions of different investigators. This requirement for experimental analysis also means that verbal "analysis" cannot suffice. The details of a procedure's influence on behavior cannot be established by careful extrapolation, reasoned speculation, or personal conviction. This kind of interpretation is tempting because of the convenience and apparent fit of our guesses; however, if everyone engaging in such speculations leaves the subsequent experimental responsibilities to someone else, the latter may accumulate like garbage waiting to be taken out—and eventually may be worth as much.

The definition's insistence that candidate technologies be understood "in the terms of the natural science of behavior" provides a critical qualification for the manner in which a procedure's influence is understood. Not only must a procedure be described in the technical language of the science, the understanding of how and why it works must be at the level of the basic principles of behavior as established by the science. This is quite different from the nominal process of verbally describing a procedure and its workings in technical terms in the absence of experimental verification and on the sole basis of superficial similarities between procedural elements and behavioral principles. For example, the popular applied procedure usually referred to as "time out" is seminally derived from early laboratory research. The variety of procedures now used in applied settings that are described as time out, however, go well beyond our experimentally based understanding of that label. As a result, there is much that practitioners do not know about the important variables that influence the effectiveness of this procedure, and it often does not work as expected.

Aside from the obvious benefit of improving a procedure's effectiveness, the importance of this definitional requirement lies in the continuity that this practice encourages between science and technology. It encourages technologists to keep abreast of scientific advances, and scientists to be sensitive to the needs of practitioners. When both groups look at behavior in the same fundamental terms, the definition also maintains consistency in the approach to understanding behavior and the methods developed to manage it. The requirement of developing an experimental understanding of procedures in terms of the basic principles of behavior thus prevents the technology from drifting away from the science and devolving into quasi technology (i.e., something that looks like technology but really is not).

After a procedure has been experimentally developed, explained, and refined, its relevance, usefulness, and requirements under practical conditions must be assessed. This second empirical process can only be accomplished by using members of the target population behaving in the setting of interest, although a procedure's development will already have involved target subjects and settings, at this stage it must be evaluated under conditions that closely approximate everyday reality. Examining a procedure under fairly routine conditions (i.e., without benefits such as extra staff or disruptions such as those imposed by experimental design that are often necessary for good experimentation) may prevent sound experimental analyses, but there should be no important experimental questions remaining at this point. Most analysis has presumably been completed, and the goal is now evaluation.

Although this goal may often be satisfied by quantitative description rather than experimental analysis, it also calls for more than a demonstration or two. Establishing the effects of a procedure under routine field conditions means that any variation in the effects already established that depends on the everyday details of population, setting conditions, or administration must be identified and described. The focus here is to learn how the circumstances of routine use might modulate the effects of a procedure that have already been thoroughly determined during its experimental development. At the same time, it is important to examine the administrative requirements for proper application of a procedure (i.e., staffing, scheduling, physical resources, and financial costs). Although the findings of such tests may lead to the need for further experiments, there may be no experimental question driving this phase of research. For example, a program of research concerning techniques of breast self-examination (BSE) for detection of lumps followed an experimental phase that developed BSE training procedures with a series of evaluation studies focusing on just these issues (Pennypacker & Iwata, 1990).

STRATEGIES OF TECHNOLOGICAL RESEARCH

Developing New Procedures

Ideas about possible technological solutions to behavioral problems may emerge from the complete range of the field's interests, including behavioral theory, the literature on basic processes, the study of human behavior, informal observation in field settings, or the experiences of those who are responsible for managing behavior. Whatever the genesis of a technological idea, it should spawn an array of sometimes overlapping questions that will guide the experimental agenda for developing, analyzing, refining, and evaluating a technological product. Answering the following questions will help guide practitioners and applied researchers in the development of new procedures.

What Is the Nature of the Problem?

This first question should be pursued with thoroughness and breadth. It is important to identify all of the roles that behavior plays in the definition of the problem. (References here to behavioral problems broadly include any undesirable situations in which behavior plays a role, whether involving behavioral excesses or deficits.) Different interested parties will probably have different ways of defining a problem involving behavior, and the researcher should be careful to examine all points of view. For instance, the challenge of managing the behavior of elementary school children conveniently defines disruptive child behavior as the problem. A more penetrating interpretation, however, may reveal that the actions of parents, teachers, administrators, and other children all are part of the problem and may need to be a part of the solution (Winett & Winkler, 1972).

The challenge at this early point is not to target specific behaviors but to consider the dimensions of the problem from different perspectives. Winett and Winkler's concern (1972) about early studies in elementary classrooms was that only the teacher's or principal's point of view was acknowledged, and that it was not often reinterpreted by behavior analysts as possibly representing a problem involving weak teaching methods that failed to reinforce academic behaviors. Furthermore, the exercise may sometimes require not just looking at the problem from the perspective of various interested parties but considering the different environments that are or may in the future be involved. The problem may be defined one way in the presenting settings, but somewhat differently when considering other settings that may create different behavioral demands. This is the familiar issue of generality that behavior analysts face when planning intervention programs that require training settings that may differ substantially from those in which the behavior needs to occur routinely (Johnston, 1979).

Another way to phrase this issue is as follows: In what ways does behavior contribute to the problem, and what changes in behavior may be relevant to its solution? It may not be possible to answer these questions by simple observation; formal measurement or even experimentation may be required to uncover facts and to identify contingencies. Because the convictions about the nature and causes of the problem that are established at this early stage will guide the remainder of the effort to develop a solution, it is important that the analysis of the problem is accurate and complete.

A project in a large salvage plant showed how easy it is to misdiagnose the nature of a problem. Productivity in one division of the plant had greatly improved when a performance-feedback contingency was implemented. After a few months, however, performance deteriorated to pretreatment levels, and it was immediately assumed that the feedback system has lost its effectiveness. This assumption was reassessed when the effects of the hotter summer weather on the temperatures inside the plant were shown to match the decrement in productivity. Instead of attempting to solve the productivity problem with revisions of the feedback contingencies, it seemed that efforts should instead focus on reducing the temperatures in the work area (Johnston, Duncan, Monroe, Stephenson, & Stoerzinger, 1978).

What Are the Goals for the Procedure?

Establishing the nature of the problem should lead directly to deciding on the goals that the procedure must accomplish. This, however, is not a trivial or bureaucratic task. These goals will constitute the standards by which the procedure's effectiveness is judged. Such goals should reflect the multifaceted features of the presenting behavioral problems, and so they must be detailed. They must describe not only a state of affairs in which the central problems no longer exist, but also specific changes in particular behaviors and environments.

In doing so, the goals must recognize vested interests by assessing the concerns of all parties and deciding how they should be taken into account (Wolf, 1978). This does not necessarily mean that the priorities of each party must be accommodated; sometimes, these interests may need to be modified. For instance, the earlier reference to the interest that school officials and teachers often have in schoolchildren being still, quiet, and docile must be balanced with the primary interest of parents and the society in having well-educated children, which is not necessarily compatible with students being quietly in their seats all of the time.

Goals must also address not just the immediate and central functions of a procedure or technology, but also its long-term and peripheral effects. Goals must look beyond the initial application of a procedure to the realities of routine application in the absence of any special resources. Maintaining the proper application of a procedure over a long period may require designing contingencies into the procedure that will maintain necessary behaviors on the part of certain individuals, and this must be the focus of additional goals. For instance, ensuring that special education teachers continue to use certain procedures in the classroom throughout the year may require that certain supporting behaviors of the principal, resource teachers, and others be maintained throughout the year as well.

What Are the Behaviors of Interest?

The discussion thus far should suggest that procedures will usually have to focus on not just one or two target behaviors, but many. Although the colloquial definition of the problem may highlight only a few behaviors in a few individuals, it is the technologist's responsibility to approach the situation with sufficient thoroughness to identify all of the behaviors in different individuals whose management will be necessary to attain the goals of the technology or procedure.

The importance of fully identifying all of the individuals and behaviors of interest lies in facilitating an understanding of the web of interlocking social contingencies that may exist in the presenting situation or that might evolve as a result of an intervention. Such contingencies may aid in explaining the behaviors of interest, require modification in order to accomplish desired behavioral changes, or be fruitfully managed to support procedural goals. Whatever their treatment, ignoring the consequences that the behavior of some individuals contingencies arranged by procedural design. For instance, an organizational behavior management program in a company may focus on how supervisory personnel interact with subordinates, but if the development of a program does not consider how the behavior of subordinates may in turn influence the behavior of managers, the intervention may lose its effectiveness over time. If the recommended interactions do not lead to reinforcement for the efforts of managers, they will probably stop complying with the management program.

What Are the Controlling Variables?

As behaviors are identified that must be taken into account, interest naturally extends to the variables that have influenced them in the past, are doing so currently, or might exert influence in the future. Historical influences may be difficult to trace, and understanding them may not always be necessary to designing effective procedures. Sometimes, however, understanding the etiology of a pattern of behavior may lead to new treatment directions, if not techniques aimed at prevention. For example, if it can be determined that a pattern of self-injurious behavior in a retarded individual is probably the result of a history of social reinforcement from staff, a treatment program that includes extinction may be attempted instead of one using punishment procedures (e.g., Lovaas & Simmons, 1969).

Contemporary controlling variables will usually require some management, whether to ensure that they do not interfere with the effects of procedural variables or so that they can be usefully incorporated into the technology. Sometimes it can even be easier to manipulate current controlling variables than to develop procedures that can override their effects. For instance, if a retarded individual who spends a lot of time screaming cannot talk or otherwise communicate his or her needs, a program that focuses on teaching appropriate communication skills might be more appropriate, if not more effective, than one that merely tries to punish screaming.

Anticipating the importance of controlling variables that might eventually develop as the procedure is routinely used may be difficult, but this interest may need to be thoroughly pursued if the procedure is to meet long-term goals reliably. The potential problem is that as a procedure continues to be applied, some of its contingencies may change in ways that have not been anticipated, with the result that it can lose the initial level of effectiveness or even be abandoned. This is not an uncommon finding for consultants in different areas, who may set up an elaborate intervention program and monitor its successful operation for a time, only to find later that the program is in shambles because of complicating factors that had not been considered when it was developed. This might be the case, for example, if a performance improvement program for line workers in a manufacturing facility did not consider that the union would eventually get involved.

What Are the Relevant Principles and Procedures?

It is only after answering the above questions that principles and procedures can be knowledgeably pursued. The challenge is to design the bits and pieces of a procedure into an integrated and often complex whole. There should be no necessary expectation here that the first combination of elements will remain intact throughout the experimental processes of analysis, refinement, and evaluation. In some cases, this might still be a fairly early stage of the larger task of developing and evaluating a multifaceted procedure. (For example, a technology for treating certain types of alcoholism might include a controlled-drinking training component, a social skills component, a family-relations component, and so forth.) In those cases in which the definition of the problem and its controlling variables have been given considerable attention, the designation of treatment procedures might be the culmination of an extensive experimental program. At some point, however, everything that has been learned should suggest a reasonable combination of procedural elements as a focus for further analytical attention.

Finally, this last point should suggest that the above questions concerning the steps in developing a new procedure are not meant to be interpreted as a rigid sequence. The questions necessarily overlap somewhat to provide a thorough and seamless guide for the researcher; each problem and research agenda will proceed as circumstances and data dictate. All of these questions, however, must be clearly answered before a proposed procedure is likely to qualify as a completed technology.

Analyzing and Refining New Procedures

What Are the Procedure's Effects?

It is all too common in contemporary practice to proceed rather quickly from the idea for a procedural solution to its evaluation in the field. From the perspective proposed here, this would almost certainly assure unnecessary limitations on the effectiveness and efficiency of the resulting procedure. The seriousness and permanence of these limitations would depend on whether a proper analytical literature evolved as the procedure grew more familiar to applied researchers and practitioners. The conception of natural science technology proposed here, however, clearly requires the analytical steps discussed in this section in order to understand fully and to refine a procedure's workings so as to augment its effectiveness in the field.

Perhaps the most useful focus at this early analytical stage is to be thorough in searching out all of the effects of the procedure that may occur in the different individuals involved. This includes not just looking for the initial effects expected on target behaviors but examining the durability of these effects and the emergence of unplanned changes in behavior, all in the context of intervention goals. Examples of the failure to look carefully at the diverse effects of an intervention are widely evident in governmental regulations and statues designed to control specific behaviors in particular groups of individuals. Economic contingencies are often at the root of such management programs, and the result is all too often the discovery of loopholes that enable targeted individuals to obtain funds (or avoid paying fees or taxes) in ways not anticipated by those who designed the programs.

Of course, trying out a new procedure requires decisions about subjects and setting conditions. Although it may seem reasonable, if not necessary, to conduct analytical research under conditions as close as possible to typical field conditions, this may sometimes only prevent sound experimentation. Even if it is otherwise desirable, the selection of target subject and setting must not impose serious methodological compromises on technological research. There should be no confusion between the present analytical goals and the later challenge of evaluation. Analyzing how a procedure works and improving its effectiveness do not necessarily require fully realistic field conditions for every study, and if methodological conflicts arise, they must not weaken the experimental effort. For instance, not all experiments aimed at developing improved techniques for teaching reading skills have to be conducted in a regular elementary classroom. More controlled settings may be required by some experimental questions; the generality of the answers obtained can be pursued in subsequent experiments.

What Are the Components and Their Effects?

The term *procedures* is used in this chapter as a generic reference to a set of operations that can always be broken into smaller components. The focus of this stage of analysis is to identify the different functional components and their individual or interactive contributions to the overall effects of the whole procedure. This knowledge is important to the effectiveness and efficiency of the procedure because it helps to identify those components that are critical to the procedure's effectiveness, and because it permits weak components to be strengthened or omitted. This kind of analysis also begins providing some information about the procedure's reliability and generality.

This process of breaking a procedure into its constituent parts always raises the issue of how far the analysis should proceed. Because each component can usually be broken down into further subcomponents, it is reasonable to ask how *reductio ad infinitum* is prevented from becoming *reductio ad absurdum*. At every point, the investigator's concern is with the effects of each bit of procedure on responding. The analytical partitioning therefore should continue until the effects on responding can no longer be traced to separable components.

It may be interesting to break down components until the effects on responding disappear. For instance, if a procedural element with clear effects is divided into two parts, and one produces the same effects and the other yields no effects, then the analysis has accomplished its purpose, and the ineffective element may be safely dropped in the interest of efficiency. The process, however, can get far more complicated. If each element separately produces an effect that is less than that obtained by their combination, it may suggest either a simple combination of effects or an interaction effect, perhaps revealing that the component should be left intact. Such information is not available without carrying the analysis to this point; the rumination research referred to earlier followed this experimental strategy. Although the field is not now accustomed to such thoroughness in applied research, we unwittingly pay the inevitable price for a cruder level of analysis in procedures that are too often weak and inconsistent in their effects.

How Do Components Produce Their Effects?

This question urges even further analysis of the procedure's components in the interest of explaining their basic mechanisms, which will often be close to the fundamental processes of conditioning. This analytical focus thus may sometimes blur the artificial distinction between studying a procedure versus studying behavior. Although the organization and language of this chapter may suggest that procedures are the primary target of experimentation, it is unwise to argue for this general priority. A procedure's effectiveness is inevitably limited by the extent of ignorance about the behaviors at which it is aimed and the environmental conditions under which it must work. The earlier questions concerning the behaviors of interest and their controlling variables represent a balancing focus.

Such analyses will often lead to discoveries that allow the procedure to be made more effective or more efficient. Greater effectiveness can come in the form of improvements that augment the degree or rapidity of the procedure's effects, but it can also come from identifying the conditions under which the procedure will not work. Identifying the limits of the procedure's generality will permit practitioners to avoid applying it inappropriately, which will in turn avoid the failures that would otherwise lead to a reputation of inconsistent effectiveness. The research cited earlier concerning rumination in retarded individuals provides a good example of this point. The original satiation-feeding procedure was powerfully effective, although it had serious practical limitations because of excess weight gain (Rast et al., 1981). Analyses of the procedure led to an understanding of the variables that made it work, which led to variations of the procedure that avoided the side effect of weight gain (Rast et al., 1984; Rast et al., 1985; Rast et al., 1988).

How Can the Procedure Be Improved?

The data accumulated from analyzing the procedure will naturally lead to its evolution into a more effective technology. This process of refinement is ongoing, as emerging evidence suggests revisions to either the procedure itself or to the circumstances of its application; these changes may themselves need to be the subject of analysis. The result of this entire effort to analyze and refine the procedure is the evolution of an increasingly effective set of operations in the context of an experimental style of decision making in which procedural refinements result from a growing understanding of the target behaviors, their environmental influences, and the workings of the procedure. The project concerning breast self-examination reported by Pennypacker and Iwata (1990) is an all-too-rare example of this style of procedural improvement.

Evaluating and Refining Procedures

What Are the Effects Under Applied Conditions?

As revisions to the procedure become minor and its effects usefully consistent, interest will shift to assessing its effectiveness under conditions that fairly closely approximate those of routine practice. Although this should still be considered a research activity, the goal now becomes description rather than explanation. The answers to this question may be available from simple measurement under field conditions. Although the procedure will have to be controlled and monitored as would be required with an experiment's independent variable, a comparison condition is not needed in order to describe or evaluate the procedure's effects (Johnston, 1988).

In fact, excessively careful management of the procedure may violate the conditions that might customarily be expected in the field, thus providing an optimistic picture of its operation and effectiveness that may rarely be attained in practice. The question guiding this stage of research does not ask primarily about the effects of the procedure; those have already been well established. This emphasis is now on the effects that can be expected under routine field conditions. Thus, attention may focus on how the procedure's effects are modulated by target subjects, environmental variables, administrative complications, and so forth. This stage is particularly important when the technology depends on the behavior of many other people, especially if they are paraprofessionals or nonprofessionals. This is often the case in applications in the business world, for example.

What Refinements Are Necessary, and What Are Their Effects?

Initial trials of the procedure will probably suggest further refinements, which may then raise the question of new effects. It may even be the case that new questions are raised about behaviors or controlling variables that require additional explanation. Thus, although procedural evaluation may not start with an experimental agenda, one may emerge when the procedure does not work as expected.

This was the experience of Wolf and his colleagues, as reported in a chapter by Braukmann et al. (1975). In training "teaching parents" to staff home-style residential facilities for predelinquent and delinquent boys, an initial attempt was very academically oriented. The early applications of this program, however, showed the researchers that this training was not achieving the effects that they wanted, and they then had to modify the teaching-parent training program substantially.

Do the Conditions of Application Maintain the Procedure?

This question can only be answered by monitoring the procedure's operations and effects under routine field conditions for an extended period of time. Regardless of initial success, a procedure cannot be considered effective if all of its components do not continue to operate as designed for as long as its effects are necessary. This is why a procedure's development must focus as much on understanding the variables that may influence its operation and maintenance in the field as on how to change the target behaviors that may define the problem to nonprofessionals. The need to ensure that a procedure can be sustained under routine conditions may sometimes be a more difficult challenge than resolving the presenting problem.

Does the Procedure Meet Its Original Goals?

The concluding challenge for a new procedure is raised by comparing its effects with its original goals. This does not require an experimental effort, although the derivation of its goals may suggest empirical techniques for this final stage of evaluation. For instance, if one goal is that certain client groups must feel that the technology has satisfactorily resolved a problem, then those groups should be asked for their evaluation in some manner (Wolf, 1978). Although questionnaires may be a familiar mechanism, other tactics that measure more functional behavior may provide more revealing data (Barrett, Johnston, & Pennypacker, 1986).

Before the reader leaves this section on the development, analysis, and evaluation of procedures, it is once again important to point out that its organization should not suggest that these guiding questions should be or are normally pursued in a rigidly sequential manner. Such a research program is naturally made up of the work of different investigators over an extended period, and the organization suggested here may be clear only in retrospect. This informality, however, should not depreciate the priorities that characterize good technological research. Despite the slow pace of interactions through professional meetings and journal publications, there should still be a collective sense of the current status and needs of an area of technology, much as basic science topics reveal a relatively organized development in the literature.

RESEARCH VERSUS PRACTICE

A Division of Labor

The discussion of this model of developing and evaluating behavioral technology implies an important division of labor between technological research and technological application. This distinction is not common in contemporary behavior analysis, although it is rather easily made in established natural science technologies such as medicine and engineering. The differences between the responsibilities for developing versus delivering technology have pervasive implications for how new technology is developed and evaluated.

A description of technological or applied research must first distinguish it from basic research. The primary dimension for this distinction is the nature of the experimental question. The wide range of questions that the natural science of behavior pursues have in common a search for the most fundamental facts of behavior, a detailed identification of those variables that generally influence the interactions between organisms and environments. Basic science questions ask about the fundamental relations between general variables and behavior and usually follow the answers with further basic questions.

In contrast, the questions directing technological research are typically questions whose answers will fairly directly improve ways of controlling behavior for practical purposes. Although the process of developing, analyzing, and improving applied procedures is an experimental venture with the same methodological standards as basic research, its focus is usually quite practical. Analysis, for example, is most often at the level of understanding the contributions of components of a complex procedure. Only a minority of studies would pursue a more detailed analysis of the mechanisms of critical components, which might then reach the level of basic principles. Of course, a sizable portion of technological research is addressed to the evaluation of procedures, and many of these studies are descriptive rather than analytical.

Although this distinction can usually be made easily, it becomes more difficult near the boundary separating these related experimental endeavors. For instance, technological research may sometimes lead to discoveries about general characteristics of behavior (e.g., the research by Lovaas and his students concerning stimulus overselectivity; see Lovaas, Keogel, & Schreibman, 1979), and basic research can lead an enhanced ability to control behavior (e.g., see basic research literatures concerning time-out contingencies). The occasional difficulty of this discrimination, however, is exciting. Research in a natural science and the more analytical portions of its technology should come together at some points in a symbiotic and synergistic miscegenation. Whether a particular study should be considered basic or applied is unimportant; the distinction has only strategic value in guiding the development of the field.

In addition to applied research, the other major facet of technological activity is application of the results of this research for the practical control of behavior. The questions here are not usually experimental in nature (or at least they would only infrequently be so in the case of a mature technology). Instead, application involves an assessment of the goals of the application, the selection of the proper procedures, the details of their administration in a particular situation, and the tracking of their results. In the shadows of these obvious concerns is a further array of interests that cannot be ignored: logistical realities, social and political constraints, measurement requirements, transfer of effects to other circumstances, and ethical considerations.

Although the interests of those delivering technology are practical rather than experimental in nature, this does not mean that there are no empirical concerns. Even when applying thoroughly researched and reliable technologies, it may often be necessary to measure behavior. Furthermore, empirical responsibilities may become unavoidably experimental when a procedure does not have the effects that were expected. Then, efforts to modify the established procedure substantially or to use a different procedure may take on the style, if not the substance, of an experiment. In this sense, routine technological practice is never very far from the style of its research history. The more successful that history, however, the less often experimentation will be required in the context of service delivery.

Priorities and Contingencies

The primary importance of this distinction between technological research and practice lies in the different requirements for doing each well. Technological research is motivated by the need to develop maximally and consistently effective behavior change procedures, which can be achieved only through the scientific process. It is an effort to discover and understand that is guided by practical problems, and experimentation is the required method.

Technological application, in contrast, is motivated by the need to change behavior to solve practical problems, and the availability of established technology permits this to be done without the inefficiencies of scientific method. The only real questions are about how to adapt well-researched procedures to the unique features of each case. If the technology were developed in accordance with the model described in this chapter, actual experimentation in the context of service delivery should not often be necessary. In general, then, pure practice is not primarily a challenge of discovery, understanding, and explanation (at least in the scientific sense) any more than is the practice of medicine or engineering. Its focus is on efficiently ameliorating practical problems with behavior.

These different goals frequently conflict, and the means by which they are attained are often incompatible. Discovery requires control, but the price of control is unrepresentative artificiality. Practical behavior management requires accepting many of the givens of field circumstances, but its price is a lack of control. Each has many features that make it an inferior occasion for accomplishing the other, and attempting to combine them may often only limit achievements in both directions.

Separating the two technological activities allows each to pursue its mission with minimum compromises. The methodological requirements for sound research need not always be jeopardized by all of the practical considerations that service delivery must respect. Similarly, applications of established technology need not be burdened by the methodological necessities of science when there is no experimental question to be answered, although there may be circumstances in which some aspects of scientific method (most often measurement) are desirable. Practical application can therefore accept the full range of its responsibilities, including some that are often abandoned in efforts to secure publication in research journals (e.g., maintaining the effectiveness of a procedure over long periods).

As an example of the conflict, consider the matter of selecting subjects and settings for research. Ideally, these decisions are guided solely by the experimental question. But when studies are conducted by individuals more oriented by training, interests, and employment toward practice than research, these decisions are often influenced by practical factors in ways that may weaken the value of the study as an experiment. For instance, a study may require only a few subjects to answer its question, but an entire class, ward, or other grouping of individuals may be selected, perhaps because the study's analytical function is misinterpreted in the context of service delivery or because of political contingencies in the applied setting. As a result of this decision, inferior measurement practices may be designed to accommodate the large number of subjects, thus limiting the conclusions that can be defended. In another case, although a study might not require subjects from the target population to behave under target conditions, a decision to use them may burden the study with constraints inherent in field conditions that prevent the question from being clearly answered.

Researchers Versus Practitioners

These distinctions suggest that it may be important to reflect the different needs of applied research versus application in how individuals are accepted into graduate programs, how they are trained, and how they are employed. The repertoires and interests required to be maximally effective in each career direction may have less in common than is traditionally assumed. Those interested in technological research need to be good scientists above all, and the applied aspects of their training must not interfere with this priority. Of course, they also need to know the applied literature, as well as to be fully familiar with the populations and service delivery settings in their areas of interest. Technological researchers also must develop a sound command of the basic literature, because they are the bridge between the science and its application.

Although there will certainly be considerable overlap in core areas, students planning a service delivery career require other skills. They must not only know the applied literature, but also acquire both clinical skills and the skills necessary to work in service delivery bureaucracies. Because these skills are difficult to teach entirely in the classroom, the students will need considerable field experience. And although it borders on heresy to note this, there are good arguments that those trained for service delivery careers need not be thoroughly trained as researchers and should not generally be encouraged to conduct research. (Most practitioners in medicine and engineering are neither trained nor tempted to do research, and for good reasons.)

The implications for professional training of this approach to developing versus delivering technology clearly conflict with the scientist-practitioner model that has, in spite of increasing attacks, dominated applied psychology for 40 years (see Barlow, Hayes, & Nelson, 1984, for a brief review of this history). Although this topic cannot be explored here, it is easy to observe that this model is exemplified in the careers of relatively few individuals. It is simply the case that those who attempt to be well trained and effective as both scientist and practitioner often run afoul of conflicting contingencies. It is especially clear that the contingencies of service settings and goals tend to encourage compromises in the nature of research questions and methods, and the result is often a weak applied research literature.

These observations should not suggest that there are not important benefits to those scientists and practitioners whose specific circumstances permit them to pursue intersecting interests together. Furthermore, it is in no way undesirable for a small cadre of students to aim for scientist-practitioner careers. Those who are able to achieve in such a capacity are often especially valuable to the field. These special circumstances and few shining examples, however, do not provide a strong argument that the scientist-practitioner model is therefore appropriate as a *general* approach to training either applied researchers or practitioners.

Practitioners and Technological Development

What is the role of practitioners in this model of developing, analyzing, and evaluating new technology? The role that emerges from these arguments is more limited than traditions might suggest. Although a handful of true scientist-practitioners may competently contribute as researchers to the process of technological development, most practitioners are neither trained nor interested in doing so. Their contributions to the development of technology as "pure" practitioners should generally be limited to communicating the demand for particular technologies, reporting serendipitous discoveries that emerge from field experience, and uncovering and reporting problems with new technologies that were not identified during their development and evaluation.

Although these functions do not involve research obligations, such services are an invaluable adjunct to technological development. Even though the need for technology is often obvious in the culture at large, practitioners are the ones who are usually most sensitive to these needs and capable of seeing technological needs and possibilities. As a result of their frontline status, the ideas for technology may often originate with practitioners, although their development must be turned over to researchers.

The value of practitioners in making serendipitous observations that may eventually lead to important advances is well established in fields such as medicine. Practitioners' vast experience makes their accidental discovery of interesting facts about behavior more common than rare. Describing such observations to researchers assures that the discovery will receive the proper scientific attention.

Although this model assumes that practitioners will only be applying technology that has completed its full course of development, analysis, and evaluation, new procedures will still present practitioners with some problems and shortcomings. Identifying such difficulties to researchers is another important role for practitioners. For the reasons discussed above, however, it is not appropriate to impose the responsibility of formal evaluation on practitioners. Evaluation is a research task, and it can be most effectively conducted by those who are trained and motivated to do good research.

A discussion of this approach to developing new technologies must acknowledge that contemporary applied behavioral research does not generally have this analytical focus, and existing behavior change procedures have not usually emerged from such histories. As a result, few applications today yield the consistently effective results that would permit practitioners to play purely a service delivery role. They often find themselves in situations in which procedures do not generate desired results, thus forcing an effort in a service delivery context to revise the procedure or to try new procedures for which there is no research history describing their application or predicting their effectiveness. It is at this point that service delivery becomes research, and the client's role becomes that of experimental subject.

In the abstract, this situation could be avoided by declining to offer services for which an adequate science-based technology has not been fully developed. More realistically, psychology and behavior analysis long ago established service delivery domains in the culture that cannot now be abandoned, even when there is insufficient technological capability to guarantee an effective service. Furthermore, behavior analysts may sometimes rightfully argue that at least they can often offer a better approximation than can other helping professions. Whatever the rationale, given that behavioral services are going to be offered, perhaps it should be considered an ethical obligation to disclose the limitations of the technology upon which the services will depend.

Once the practitioner has undertaken the obligation of providing a behavior change service, there is no recourse but to use the traditional experimental style of contemporary applied behavior analysis, which involves adjusting existing procedures or creating new procedures that will attain intervention goals. The real issue, however, is not how to use a weak technology well, but how to improve the technology so that this situation will not be necessary. Although some may personally enjoy the challenge of creating a novel solution to a behavioral problem in the field, the goal for the professional must be to develop the technology so thoroughly that it can be easily applied with consistently effective results, often by persons without formal and extensive advanced training in behavior analysis. Achieving this goal will require accepting a new model of technological research and service.

CONFRONTING A NEW MODEL

How behavioral technology is developed and delivered may be one of the most important issues facing the field of behavior analysis. This chapter has very briefly outlined a new model of technological development and service based on traditions that have evolved in the natural sciences over many years. The common rejoinders to these arguments are that (a) behavior is fundamentally different from other natural phenomena, and we will never be able to learn enough to create a technology as effective as those created by the physical sciences (and, therefore, we need not try); (b) our ability to control relevant variables in the environment is inevitably so limited that we can never develop a technology of comparable effectiveness to those of medicine and engineering (and again, therefore, we need not try); or (c) we really do not need to change the way we do applied research and professional training, because we are doing pretty well (better than everyone else, anyway) and making reasonable progress in our capabilities.

The tragedy implicit in these rebuttals is that we may have lost the vision and hope that stems from the deterministic assumption guiding all science. Without the conviction that we can eventually learn everything about behavior, however long it may take, we may accommodate the more comfortable alternative assumption that we have no choice but to make do with little more than we know at present. Perhaps the remarkable advances in the natural sciences are discouraging, rather than encouraging, to us. After all, how can we hope ever to learn enough about behavior or to have enough control over the environment to perform feats as fantastic as gene therapy or planetary exploration? Perhaps our social science heritage has so dominated our development that we never even had the dream that natural scientists are increasingly realizing. Have we succumbed to the belief, implied by the above rejoinders, that a behavioral technology can never be so effective that it does not routinely require experimentation in the context of service delivery? Perhaps we have been seduced by short-term contingencies and are satisfied merely by being able to outperform others in the human services arena.

Confronting a new model of behavioral technology is likely to be a difficult experience. The history of science, however, suggests that the acceptance of novel and often threatening ideas or discoveries about the nature of our world and the support of the scientific endeavors that such ideas or discoveries prompt ultimately depends on the development of effective technologies and their application to practical problems in ways that improve the daily lives of ordinary citizens. If this is so, then the acceptance of Skinner's arguments about the nature of human behavior and how we should study it, as well as the cultural support of the science that has resulted from these positions, will depend on the effectiveness of the behavioral technology that we can deliver.

This is a considerable burden for behavioral technology. When we further consider the exacerbating constraints of our relatively paltry supply of research personnel and our financial resources, it should be easy to appreciate how important it is for our technological efforts to be maximally effective and efficient. We simply cannot allow ourselves the luxury of unproductive literatures and weak procedures. It is time to apply our behavioral skills to managing our own behavior and to redefine our conception of behavioral technology and how it is developed and applied.

REFERENCES

Baer, D. M. (1981). A flight of behavior analysis. *Behavior Analyst, 4*(2), 85–91.

Baer, D. M., Wolf, M. M., & Risley, T. R. (1987). Some still-current dimensions of applied behavior analysis. *Journal of Applied Behavior Analysis, 20*(4), 313–327.

Barlow, D. H., Hayes, S. C., & Nelson, R. O. (1984). *The scientist practitioner: Research and accountability in clinical and educational settings.* New York: Pergamon.

Barrett, B., Johnson, J. M., & Pennypacker, H. S. (1986). Behavior: Its units, dimensions, and measurement. In R. O. Nelson & S. C. Hayes (Eds.), *Conceptual foundations of behavioral assessment* (pp. 156–200). New York: Guilford.

Braukmann, C. J., Fixsen, D. L., Kirigin, K. A., Phillips, E. A., Phillips, E. L., & Wolf, M. M. (1975). Achievement Place: The training and certification of teaching parents. In W. S. Wood (Ed.), *Issues in evaluating behavior modification* (pp. 131–152). Champaign, IL: Research Press.

Deitz, S. M. (1982). Defining applied behavior analysis: An historical analogy. *Behavior Analyst, 5*(1), 53–64.

Fawcett, S. B. (1985). On differentiation in applied behavior analysis. *Behavior Analyst, 8*(2), 143–150.

Hayes, S. C. (1978). Theory and technology in behavior analysis. *Behavior Analyst, 1*(1), 25–33.

Hayes, S. C., Rincover, A., & Solnick, J. V. (1980). The technical drift of applied behavior analysis. *Journal of Applied Behavior Analysis, 13*, 275–285.

Hopkins, B. L. (1970). The first twenty years are the hardest. In R. Ulrich, T. Stacknick, & J. Mabry (Eds.), *Control of human behavior, vol. 2.* Glenview, IL: Scott, Foresman.

Johnston, J. M. (1979). On the relation between generality and generalization. *Behavior Analyst, 2*(2), 1–7.

Johnston, J. M. (1988). Comparing behavior change procedures: Some strategic and tactical limits. *Behavior Analyst, 11,* 1–9.

Johnston, J. M., Duncan, P. M., Monroe, C., Stephenson, H., & Stoerzinger, A. (1978). Tactics and benefits of behavioral measurement in small businesses. *Journal of Organizational Behavior Management, 1,* 164–178.

Johnston, J. M., & Pennypacker, H. S. (1980). *Strategies and tactics of human behavioral research.* HIllsdale, NJ: Lawrence Erlbaum.

Lovaas, O. I., Koegel, R. L., & Schreibman, L. (1979). Stimulus overselectivity and autism: A review of research. *Psychological Bulletin, 86,* 1236–1254.

Lovaas, O. I., & Simmons, J. Q. (1969). Manipulation of self-destruction in three retarded children. *Journal of Applied Behavior Analysis, 2*(3), 143–157.

Michael, J. (1980). Flight from behavior analysis. *Behavior Analyst, 3*(2), 1–21.

Pennypacker, H. S., & Iwata, M. M. (1990). Mammacare: A case history in behavioral medicine. In P. Blackman & H. LeJeune (Eds.), *Behavior analysis in theory and practice: Contributions and controversies* (pp. 259–288). Hillsdale, NJ: Lawrence Erlbaum.

Pierce, W. D., & Epling, W. F. (1980). What happened to analysis in applied behavior analysis? *Behavior Analyst, 3*(1), 1–9.

Rast, J., Johnston, J. M., & Drum, C. (1984). A parametric analysis of the relation between food quantity and rumination behavior. *Journal of the Experimental Analysis of Behavior, 41,* 125–135.

Rast, J., Johnston, J. M., Drum, C., and Conrin, J. (1981). The relation of food quantity to rumination behavior. *Journal of Applied Behavior Analysis, 14*(2).

Rast, J., Johnston, J. M., Ellinger-Allen, J., & Drum, C. (1985). Effects of nutritional and mechanical properties of food on ruminative behavior. *Journal of the Experimental Analysis of Behavior, 42,* 195–206.

Rast, J., Johnston, J. M., Ellinger-Allen, J., & Lubin, D. (1988). Effects of pre-meal chewing on ruminative behavior. *American Journal of Mental Retardation, 93*(1), 67–74.

Winett, R. A., & Winkler, R. C. (1972). Current behavior modification in the classroom: Be still, be quiet, be docile. *Journal of Applied Behavior Analysis, 5,* 499–504.

Wolf, M. M. (1978). Social validity: The case for subjective measurement or how applied behavior analysis is finding its heart. *Journal of Applied Behavior Analysis, 11*(2), 203–214.

14

The Development and Evaluation of the Self-Injurious Behavior Inhibiting System

A Personal Perspective

Thomas R. Linscheid

I was asked to write this chapter to describe my experiences during the development and initial evaluation of a new technology. Specifically, the new technology is called the Self-Injurious Behavior Inhibiting System, or SIBIS. As anyone who has been working in the field of behavior disorders in individuals with mental retardation or developmental disabilities over the last few years knows, SIBIS has become a focal point in the controversy regarding the use of aversive procedures. The reason for focusing upon SIBIS is, no doubt, attributable to its utilization of contingent electrical stimulation (or "electric shock") as a punishing stimulus. It should be stated at the outset that SIBIS was never conceptualized as the sole treatment or the sole method of intervention for individuals who have self-injurious behavior. Unfortunately, at times during the controversy, individuals and opposing advocacy groups have attempted to paint this issue as one between treatment with this method and treatment with exclusively positive educational methods.

What I will do in this chapter is to provide a brief overview of the history and development of the device and my experiences during the initial introduction and clinical evaluation of the device. I will also address some of the concerns I have regarding the opposition that the introduction of this device

Thomas R. Linscheid • Ohio State University and Columbus Children's Hospital, Columbus, Ohio 43205.

Behavior Analysis and Treatment, edited by R. Van Houten & S. Axelrod. Plenum Press, New York, 1993.

has engendered and discuss my concerns regarding the need for scientific integrity, the open exchange of information, and the open-mindedness required in the evaluation of any new treatment procedure or device. In the historical descriptions I will be reporting from the best of my recollections. This chapter should not be considered to be a definitive history, as I will not concern myself with the exact dates of meetings, names of people who were involved, and so forth. Rather, I will be giving the reader a feel for the general course of events and thinking that went into the development of SIBIS.

Just mentioning the words *electric shock* generally conjures up negative concepts and feelings in most people (Matson & DiLorenzo, 1984). For this reason, I feel it important to relate how I came to be involved with the use of contingent electrical stimulation in the treatment of behavior problems. Because there are few people in this country who have experience in using contingent electric shock in treatment, most people have formed their opinion of contingent electric-shock treatment based on secondary information (through reading, word of mouth, or the media). Unfortunately, these sources are often inaccurate or biased, leading to conclusions based on misinformation, emotional reactions, or confusion with other applications of electric shock (e.g., electroconvulsive therapy).

As an example, I recently attended a presentation by an acknowledged opponent of SIBIS who stated that the device gave six jolts of electricity. The speaker appeared deliberately to leave the impression that a client is hit with six distinct shocks, separated by some unreported time interval, for each self-inflicted blow to the head. In reality, SIBIS delivers an electrical current that cycles on and off 16 times within two-tenths of a second. Subjectively, the shock is perceived as only one occurrence and is described by all who have felt it as being of a very short duration. The cycling on and off of the current was specifically programmed into the device to reduce the total amount of time electric current was in contact with the skin while providing the same subjective experience. The speaker was first of all incorrect, and secondly presented the information in a way to make the device seem more intense and painful than it is. Specifications about the duration, intensity, and nature of the electrical current are readily available in a published article (Linscheid, Iwata, Ricketts, Williams, & Griffin, 1990). A minimal effort by this speaker to obtain the article and thereby present accurate information seems not to have occurred.

My first experience with electric shock came in the mid-1970s while I was working at the Georgetown University Child Development Center, a university-affiliated facility. This interdisciplinary-based training program was located administratively within the medical school's department of pediatrics, and from time to time, as a behavioral psychologist, I would receive consultation requests from pediatric specialists regarding their inpatients. Once such consultation was in regard to a 9-month-old infant who had been in the hospital more than 6 weeks with a diagnosis of rumination.

Rumination is a condition in which food is voluntarily regurgitated from the stomach into the mouth and either rechewed or allowed to run from the mouth; in the process, a significant amount of food is lost.

Rumination in infants is somewhat rare in pediatric practice but, when it does occur, can have very serious medical problems. Indeed, an early study that followed 44 of these cases found that 11 of them eventually died from the weight loss and malnutrition resulting from the frequent vomiting and food loss (Kanner, 1957). Often these infants come from nonstimulating or deprived environments, and merely placing them into the hospital with "mothering" provided by nurses and volunteers can quickly reduce the rate of rumination. Some cases, however, do not respond to this approach or to other traditional treatments (e.g., thickened foods, positioning boards).

The patient in question had been losing weight steadily since approximately 6 months of age. During his hospital stay a multitude of medical tests had been performed, and all other reasons for his vomiting had been ruled out. More traditional forms of treatment had proven ineffective. On the initial consultation, the recommendation was made to provide contingent attention to this infant whenever he was not ruminating, particularly after meals, and to withdraw attention at the onset of rumination. Withdrawal of attention was accomplished by placing the infant into his crib and picking him up again only when the rumination had ceased. This suggestion was based on the assumption that rumination was reinforced by self-stimulation or social attention, and therefore providing positive social attention for periods of nonruminating would serve to decrease the frequency of rumination.

Although the suggestion was implemented for a period of a week or so, no change in rate of rumination or increases in weight gain were noted. At this point I was approached by the frantic pediatrician, who was very distressed about the deteriorating medical condition of his patient and practically demanded that we do something to produce a significant and rapid change in the rate of rumination. I remember clearly his specific statement: "Don't you psychologists do electric shock when someone's life is in danger?" During my graduate and advanced training I had some limited experience with the use of contingent electric shock in animal research, but I had absolutely no experience with nor had ever even considered the use of electric shock as a treatment with humans. To be honest, the pediatrician's suggestion frightened me.

A search of the literature at that time did reveal one case study reporting the successful treatment of an infant with rumination using contingent electrical stimulation (Lang & Melamed, 1969). Despite knowing that the treatment had been successful with another patient, I was still in the dilemma of having no experience with the treatment and no equipment in order to effect it. Two or three days later I encountered the same pediatrician, who again asked us to conduct the treatment and emphasized its importance for the child's survival. After discussing the possible treatment carefully with the child's parents and obtaining their consent, it was decided to try to locate some equipment that could be used for this purpose. I was assisted at this time by a graduate student from another university, who was able to obtain the loan of a device usually used to produce electric stimulation for use in animal operant conditioning studies. After the equipment was obtained, the next major decision had to do with the intensity of the stimulation that we would use. We used the Lang and Melamed (1969) study as a guide, but we decided to start with the lowest setting possible and increase the intensity to a point at which we saw what we hoped would be a very mild but definitely observable response in the child.

On the first day of treatment, electrode leads from the electric-shock device were connected to the infant's leg, and a hand-held activation button made it possible for the observer to administer the electric stimulation. The plan was to observe the infant constantly while he was awake and to provide the electrical stimulation for each instance of rumination. A timing device made it possible to deliver a half-second electrical stimulation that would cycle on and off in half-second intervals as long as the button was depressed. We initiated the electric shock on the first sign of rumination and terminated it when the rumination ceased.

Baseline data revealed 36 to 40 episodes of rumination per day. On the first day of treatment the frequency fell to 6 episodes, and by the third day of treatment no rumination was noted. The infant begin to gain weight after the first day of reduced ruminating and gained more than 2 pounds within the first week. When the shock was actually administered the infant displayed a mild startle reaction, as if he had heard an unusual sound. On only one occasion did any whimpering or crying occur, and this was brief. An effort was made to treat the child in several different locations and to create a homelike setting in order to prepare him for the transition to his home. After 10 days, treatment was discontinued, and the child returned home with his parents. No further episodes of rumination occurred, and at a 3-month follow-up the child had gained so much weight that it was necessary to place him on a diet (Cunningham & Linscheid, 1976).

For me, the most striking aspect of this case was the distinction between what my perceptions of an electric-shock treatment entailed and the realities of the treatment process. I had assumed that the shock would result in great emotional distress with crying and observable pain, that the program would involve severe limitation in this child's mobility, and all sorts of other dire results that could only be tolerated because the alternative was death for the child. None of this happened. The child's response to the shock was minimal; he remained happy and interactive. He was free to crawl about his room because we had used a long cord for the electrodes, and his mother was able to maintain a fairly normal mother-infant interaction pattern with him. If anything, I was "shocked" by how simple, nonintrusive, and effective the program proved to be.

Over the next 3 years, two more infant ruminators were referred for treatment. Both of these cases were treated as successfully and rapidly as the first case had been. Because of our success, I was invited to present a grand-rounds lecture to the department of pediatrics of the medical school. Prior to this lecture, an article was published describing the successful treatment of rumination in a child by using the contingent administration of lemon juice squirted into the child's mouth (Sajwaj, Libet, & Agras, 1974). Near the end of the lecture, I made the suggestion that on the next case I would try lemon juice instead of electric shock, as it seemed to be more acceptable to the general public. In the question-and-answer period that followed the lecture, one of the prominent physicians from the department of pediatrics stood up to make a comment. He had been very much bothered that I would try something different in the future (i.e., lemon juice). He stated strongly that he believed the treatment using the contingent electric shock that we had employed had saved the life of the three infants, that it had worked rapidly and with only the most minor distress. He made a very strong point that, as a physician, he would be guided by documented success and treatment effectiveness ahead of public opinion.

This chiding regarding my continued concern over the use of contingent electric shock despite the successes made me stop and reconsider the source of that concern. I realized what I had learned through the use of contingent electric shock to that point: that it was capable of producing very rapid and dramatic changes in behavior at what could be defined as very low intensities (based purely on the infant's response to the stimulation). I also reconsidered the issue of speed of treatment and behavior changes in relation to the seriousness of the behavior. I realized that most people who were concerned with the use of electric shock had two major reasons for the concern. The first was the possible misuse and misapplication of the procedure, and the second stemmed purely from a misunderstanding of the procedure per se.

I became very aware of all the factors that went into making an effective punishment procedure and concluded that electric shock may not be more effective than some other punishment procedures because it is more aversive, but because the application of electric shock is often done in a way that maximizes those other factors contributing to the effectiveness of a punisher or, for that matter, a reinforcer. Specifically, immediacy of application of the contingent stimulus and the client's inability to escape or avoid the stimulus are factors that may be equally as important as the actual intensity of the stimulus. I also realized that the nature of electrical stimulation and the sensation it produces is very different from what is normally encountered in everyday life and that this novel sensation, which is generally described as unpleasant but not necessarily painful, may be the reason for the success (as opposed to some subjective experience of pain). In sum, as a result of my first experience with electric shock, I learned that the procedure offered nothing to be afraid of in an individual treatment application and, if done correctly, could produce dramatic, rapid, and durable behavioral changes.

Another case served to confirm my perceptions that this was not a dangerous procedure and again to make me reexamine the dimensions of perceived restrictiveness of treatment versus treatment effectiveness. A 14-year-old girl with profound mental retardation was referred to us from an institution in a nearby state. The girl suffered from chronic rumination and an unusual self-injurious behavior—self-induced rectal prolapsing. Rumination had been a chronic problem, and her weight at the time of referral was 33 pounds. The girl was also capable of prolapsing her rectum, which she did on a daily basis, to a distance of nearly 14 inches. This behavior, of course, was of concern to her physicians, who feared the damage she might do to her colon and gastrointestinal (GI) tract from the continuation of this behavior. Previous surgery was undertaken to insert a steel wire around the anus in an attempt to prevent her from prolapsing her colon through the anal opening. This had lasted only a day or two before the young girl had produced a break in the steel wire, and rectal prolapsing resumed. More extensive surgery was being considered in order to make it physically impossible to continue this behavior; however, her low weight and poor nutritional status as a result of ruminating argued against such major surgery at that time.

Her caretakers had heard of our treatment for infant rumination and referred her to us. It was made clear to them at the time that we were not a residential facility and that we would not be able to provide long-term inpatient treatment, as we could not provide all the other services that she needed (educational, recreational, etc.). We did agree, however, to accept this patient for an initial trial of contingent electrical stimulation for the ruminating, with the idea that providing documentation of its effectiveness would help to secure permission to continue the treatment in her home site. In addition, weight gain produced by the elimination of ruminating would make the surgical procedure possible. With this as the agreed-upon goal, we began treatment with this girl and within the first day reduced the rumination by more than 99% (Figure 1).

During the 30 days of hospitalization the patient gained weight, and rumination remained at a very low level. It was decided to transfer her back to her home institution, using a differential reinforcement (DRO) procedure in the interim until permission for electrical stimulation could be obtained. Because of the dramatic success of the electric-shock procedure for the rumination, it was decided to reassess whether surgery was really necessary to treat the rectal prolapsing. An alternative of treating it with electrical stimulation was considered, because she had responded so well to treatment for rumination. Rectal prolapse in this case was considered to be a voluntary behavior, self-stimulatory in nature, similar to the rumination.

A request was made for permission to use an electric-shock procedure

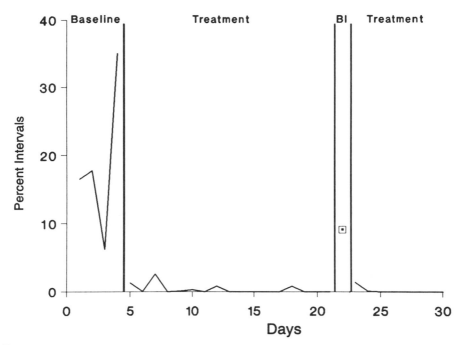

FIGURE 1. Percentage intervals in which rumination occurred during baseline and treatment.

for the rectal prolapsing and to continue the DRO procedure for the rumination as long as it continued to be effective. Several months passed before permission could be obtained for the electric-shock program, and when it was obtained, no behavioral psychologist could be identified in the state who was willing to conduct the treatment. The girl's surgeons were becoming more distressed by the damage she was doing to her lower GI tract and felt that because some weight gain had occurred, surgery should proceed. Unfortunately, the girl died on the operating table, most likely as a result of complications engendered by a weakened health condition.

When my colleagues and I heard about her death, we were saddened on the one hand and angered on the other. Our anger arose from the fact that we were sure there was an effective behavioral, nonsurgical treatment for both her rumination and her rectal prolapsing, and it was only bureaucratic regulations produced by misconceptions and fears that prevented her from receiving this treatment. I remember thinking that this girl's final benefit from having been protected against a restrictive procedure was her death. One can certainly argue that this girl's self-injurious behaviors may have been a result of lifelong institutionalization in a nonstimulating, noneducational environment. Although this may very well have been the case, there was no way to correct that immediately and to make the changes necessary to protect her from serious self-induced or iatrogenic consequences.

One more treatment case served to solidify my attitudes and feelings regarding the limited but appropriate use of electrical stimulation. A 12-year-old female with a long history of severe self-injurious head hitting was referred to us, again with the idea that we could provide an initial demonstration of effectiveness that would then be used by her treatment team to apply for permission to use contingent electrical stimulation in her home institution. This girl's past self-injurious behavior had been so intense as to result in hairline fractures of the skull, frequent open sores to two major target areas on her head, and the necessity to keep her physically restrained much of the time. Her physician was extremely concerned about the potential damage to her skull and the potential for systemic infections because of the near-constant open wounds. Permanent misshaping of the bony structures of her head had also occurred from longtime self-injurious behavior, despite padding, protective helmets, and the like.

Once treatment began, head hitting decreased to a near-zero rate within just a day to two. After 10 days of treatment, during which no head hitting occurred on the last 4 days, the young woman was returned to the home institution. Because the latter had not yet obtained permission to continue the electric-shock program at the institution, she was returned with a set of electrodes attached to her leg and a wire extending several feet from the site where the electrodes were attached. This was done in the hope that the girl would use the presence of the electrodes as a discriminative stimulus to signal that the program was still in effect. Upon returning to the institution, she went 10 days without hitting her head. On day 11, the first instance of head hitting occurred; without the contingent electrical stimulus, the girl immediately returned to her pretreatment rates of self-injurious behavior. Despite the dramatic data supplied from our initial intervention, videotaped evidence of only mild behavioral responses to the shock, and knowledge of the rapid return to baseline levels without the treatment, the state official in charge of making the ultimate decision denied permission to continue the contingent electric-shock treatment program in the institution. It has now been more than 12 years since this treatment occurred, and although the girl has moved from the institution into a community-based group home with ample consultation regarding behavioral and educational programming, she continues to bang her head and still needs a protective helmet.

I recount these experiences because I think they are important in understanding why I was willing to become involved in the development of the Self-Injurious Behavior Inhibiting System and why I have been willing to continue research on this treatment strategy in the face of intense opposition. It is my feeling that through these experiences, I acquired a realistic knowledge of what contingent electric stimulation treatment was, rather than a knowledge based on preconceived notions and fears. I had learned that the alternative of no treatment was frequently much more serious in its long-term consequences than the mild distress engendered by the treatment. In addition, I had learned that the intensity of the electrical stimulation necessary to produce dramatic results could be kept at a minimum if other factors (described earlier) were maximized. The net result of these experiences for me was a commitment to myself never to reject any treatment out of hand until I had thoroughly familiarized myself with all the facts and to proceed on these facts, not my initial emotional reactions. Perhaps this is why I have been so disappointed at the opposition to SIBIS by those who have never taken the time to learn about the device itself or the results of the initial clinical applications. More distressing, perhaps, is the selective willingness to distort the scientific literature in order to bias an audience against this form of treatment. I will expand upon these concerns later in this chapter.

INITIAL INVOLVEMENT WITH THE SIBIS PROJECT

In the course of my duties while working in the university-affiliated program mentioned above, I came to know Leslie and Mooza Grant. The Grants had two daughters, both of whom carried the diagnosis of autism and who were in their early 20s at the time of my first involvement with this family. One of the daughters had a lifelong history of severe head-hitting behavior that resulted in physical damage to her if she was allowed to continue it without restraint. Mr. and Mrs. Grant had been very involved in treatment and educational programming for both their daughters and had consulted with a number of nationally known medical, educational, and psychological authorities regarding the best treatment for them. As a measure of their dedication to children with this type of problem, they organized the American Foundation for Autistic Children and actually ran their own day school for children with autism for a number of years in the suburban Washington, D.C. area.

Mrs. Grant, particularly, is a unique individual who is very resourceful and very diligent in pursuing whatever might be of benefit to her daughters. In the absence of finding any medication, behavioral program, or educational approach that showed any potential at all for decreasing or eliminating her daughter's self-injurious behavior, she was instrumental in the development of a precursor to SIBIS. This device (which was very large, clumsy, and unreliable) utilized the same concept of SIBIS in that it had the capability of detecting a blow to the head and delivering an electrical stimulus as a consequence. The device involved the use of accelerometer switches attached to a helmet or the individual's wrists, which were connected via wires to a somewhat large and heavy battery pack worn on the back. Batteries would quickly run down, and it was necessary for the individual using the device to wear a special shirt in which the wires were sewn into channels to that they would not become entangled.

The Grants felt forced to resort to this type of treatment, as their daughter had been successful in nearly blinding herself, ripping off an ear, and producing near-constant bruises any time she was not physically restrained from hitting herself. The Grants had noted over and over again that their daughter did not seem to want to hit herself and would seek out restraints that had been removed. Indeed, once the device was utilized with their daughter, they saw an immediate and dramatic reduction in the rate of her head-hitting behavior and also noted that she tried to put it back on when it was removed. While she was wearing the device, the rate of head hitting was low enough that no physical restraint was necessary, and thus she was free to use her arms and hands for other activities.

For several years Mrs. Grant tried to perfect this device technologically, but without sufficient financial resources and lacking engineering expertise, she had not succeeded; the device had changed little since its initial development. It should be noted at this point that other researchers (Ball, Sibbach, Jones, Steele, & Frazier, 1975) had tested a conceptually similar device with self-injurious clients and found comparable success in terms of treatment effectiveness, but they also had encountered difficulties with the reliability and durability of the device itself. In the early 1980s the Grants, in their continuing effort to develop a more sophisticated and reliable form of this device, approached the National Aeronautics and Space Administration, whose Technology Transfer Division put them in touch with one of the biomedical engineers at the Johns Hopkins University Applied Physics Laboratory (JHU-APL). When the Grants met with the personnel at the laboratory and spelled out their needs, the engineers assured them that the technology they were describing was readily available, and after further meetings, a decision was made to go ahead with the project.

At this point, Mr. and Mrs. Grant asked me to serve as a behavioral psychology consultant to the project. They were aware that I had experience using electric shock in the cases described earlier, and I was familiar with their daughter and her problems. The understanding was that I would participate during the technological development of the device and provide consultation in regard to specifications that were consistent with application of operant conditioning principles. In addition, it was assumed that I would be involved in the initial clinical application of the device once it was developed by JHU-APL.

I felt the need at the time for other behavioral colleagues to be involved in the process. I also knew that in order to locate a sufficient number of individuals who could potentially benefit from the device once it was developed, I needed to involve individuals from another agency. To this end, I contacted my colleague Michael Cataldo at the John F. Kennedy Institute with the request that he or his colleagues from Kennedy be involved in the project.

Dr. Cataldo subsequently also involved Brian Iwata and Gary Pace; these two individuals served as the primary behavioral consultants from the institute. During the several years of technical development, we, as behavioral consultants, attended periodic (usually every 3 to 6 months) meetings in which we were updated on the progress of the development and our advice was solicited regarding factors such as timing, size, and electrical stimulation intensity. As a result of this process, such features as an internal counter to record the number of electrical stimulations and an external tone signaling the actual delivery of electrical stimulation were incorporated into the plan.

Funds for the development of the project were raised through a private foundation and through medical instrumentation companies who were willing to provide financial support in exchange for the rights to market the final product. At no time during the development of the device or subsequently have any of us who served as behavioral consultants been paid for our consultation time. Expenses related to the planning meetings were sometimes reimbursed and sometimes incurred at our own expense.

Whereas there had been two medical instrumentation companies involved financially and from a planning standpoint in the early stages of development, the company that was awarded the rights to manufacture and distribute the product was an organization, formed for this purpose, called Human Technologies Incorporated (HTI). Once the technological development of SIBIS completed by Johns Hopkins University, its manufacture and marketing came under the auspice of HTI, and those of us who had served as behavioral consultants to the development process continued in that capacity. Again, it was agreed that none of us would receive financial compensation for our consultation time.

As we began to realize the technological sophistication and capabilities of this device, Brian Iwata made an excellent suggestion to incorporate an automated DRO component so that the device would be able to provide automated reinforcement for periods of absence of the self-injurious behavior, to delay the delivery of this reinforcement based on occurrence of the behavior, and/or to provide delivery of the electrical stimulation contingent on self-injurious behavior. It should go without saying that those of us who participated as behavioral consultants on this project never envisioned that SIBIS would be used as the sole treatment for self-injurious behavior in individuals. The device was seen as an integrated component in an overall behavioral and educational treatment program; in addition, we knew this was a device that would be used in only a small number of cases in which self-injury was severe and resistant to other forms of treatment. SIBIS was not developed as an either-or treatment, or with the intent of being used on large numbers of individuals. HTI itself publishes guidelines indicating that the device may be appropriate only for individuals with long histories of self-injurious behavior, with documented medical injuries as a result of the self-injurious behavior, and for whom reasonable attempts at nonaversive behavioral interventions have not proven successful.

The final product—the Self-Injurious Behavior Inhibiting System, as it is officially known—is composed of two main parts. One part, the sensor module, is worn on the client's head. This module is capable of detecting blows to the head through an electronic device that senses vibrations. Once a blow to the head has been detected, a radio transmitter contained in the sensor module sends a coded radio signal to the stimulus module, which can be worn on the client's arm but has generally been attached to the client's leg. The stimulus module contains a radio receiver that receives the radio signal and has the capability of delivering the electrical stimulation. In addition, the stimulus module contains an internal data recorder that keeps a frequency count of the number of electrical stimulations delivered and produces an audible tone with the delivery of each stimulation. The electrical stimulation delivered has a maximum of 3.5 milliamperes delivered at 85 volts. The total duration of the stimulation is 200 milliseconds, or 0.2 seconds. During this time period, however, the electrical stimulation switches on and off in 16 cycles so that the actual time in which electrical current is in contact with the skin is only 80 milliseconds, or .08 seconds (for more detailed descriptions see Linscheid et al., 1990).

Subjectively, the electrical stimulation has been described as similar to a pinprick, or a rubber band being snapped on the skin. In my experience, the majority of people who actually experience the stimulation report that it is milder than they had anticipated. The electrical stimulation does not cause any type of tissue damage at the site. Because the SIBIS electrode is a 1-inch-diameter circle surrounding a central button electrode, current flow is contained within that circle and there is no chance of current flowing across any bodily organs, particularly across the cardiothoracic area. When one compares the shock intensity delivered by SIBIS with published studies utilizing other electrical stimulation, in almost all cases SIBIS utilizes a lower intensity (see Linscheid, Iwata, Ricketts, Williams, & Griffin, 1990). Indeed, I found that when a group of 23 judges were asked to guess based on a 5-second video excerpt of behavior whether an individual using SIBIS had just received an electrical stimulation, the judges were unable to do so at a rate any better than chance guessing (i.e., 50%; Linscheid, 1992).

SIBIS is registered as a Class II medical device with the U.S. Food and Drug Administration. To the best of my understanding, to be registered as a Class II medical device, the device must be shown to be substantially similar to other devices on the market and, through engineering specifications, to pose no physical risk for human use. Indeed, both Butterfield (1975) and federal government regulations for safety indicate that an electric current of less than 5 milliamperes (SIBIS uses 3.5 milliamperes or less) poses no danger to humans. As a Class II medical device, SIBIS can be sold only with the prescription of a medical doctor or licensed psychologist.

INITIAL CLINICAL EVALUATION

In the fall of 1986, the device was ready for clinical evaluation. By this time Brian Iwata, who had planned on doing some of the initial trials, had left the Kennedy Institute to take a position in Florida. Because Florida has a law banning the use of electric shock as part of any treatment program, he was unable to conduct any of the initial clinical evaluations. Other individuals from around the country who knew of the development of SIBIS and who felt it would be appropriate for some of their most difficult treatment cases became part of a network of individuals involved in the initial clinical evaluations.

Also by this time, I had moved into my current position in Ohio and had personally been referred a case of a woman in her 30s who was blind and had been living in an institutional setting for a number of years. The woman, who had high rates of self-injurious head hitting and needed constant physical restraint, was referred to me in 1983 for possible treatment with contingent electrical shock. She had been evaluated by a nationally known behavioral psychologist who had tried, with no success, a number of different techniques to attempt to control her self-injurious behavior. At the time the referral was made, I explained to her caretakers that I was involved in the development of SIBIS but that the device would not be ready for several years. I did indicate that if they were willing to enroll her in the initial clinical evaluation and if her behavior had not responded to other forms of treatment by the time the device was ready, I would be willing to include her as one of the individuals who would receive treatment.

Late in the fall of 1986, it was decided to proceed with treatment for this individual. Baseline data were collected and revealed a head-hitting rate of around 250 hits per minute once physical arm restraints were removed. Initial treatment with SIBIS was problematic; because this the first time the device had actually been used in a clinical treatment setting, we found that there were a number of adjustments that needed to be made to the device in terms of sensitivity, location, and so forth. After about 45 treatment sessions of 10 minutes or less covering a 2-week period, the reduction in rate of self-injurious behavior was only about 50%. At this point, I made the decision to stop the treatment so that the necessary minor adjustments could be made to the device.

While waiting for the company to make these adjustments, the protection agency that served as the guardian for this woman withdrew its permission for her to continue in the treatment program. They had decided to bring in an outside consultant to determine whether the electric-shock treatment program was necessary for this client. This outside consultant recommended a functional communication-based treatment regimen for the client, and therefore the evaluation with this client was never completed. Although the client has shown some improvement (e.g., is out of arm restraints), she continues to engage in head-hitting behavior and is still institutionalized.

Minor modifications subsequently were made to the device, and it was tested by me on three individuals (see the first three cases in Linscheid et al., 1990). Treatment using SIBIS with these three cases proved to be dramatically successful. After completing the first two of these cases, the Johns Hopkins University Applied Physics Laboratory scheduled a press conference to announce the development and marketing of SIBIS in the spring of 1987. At this press conference the engineers presented information regarding the technical specifications of the device, Mr. and Mrs. Grant reported on the historical events leading to its development, and Brian Iwata described self-injurious behavior in general and his experiences with treating such behavior through the John F. Kennedy Institute at Johns Hopkins University. In addition, I presented the initial data from two of our clients.

As a result of the press conference, press releases were picked up by newspapers across the country, and a news report appeared on national television. This seemed to be the initiation point for a flurry of activity by groups that were appropriately concerned regarding the overuse of aversive conditioning procedures. Two groups took the lead in opposing SIBIS: the Association for Retarded Citizens of the United States (ARC) and the Association for Persons with Severe Handicaps (TASH).

To understand fully the concern expressed by these groups, it is important to understand some of the factors occurring in the field of mental retardation and developmental disabilities at the time. Advocacy groups had rightly been concerned about the maltreatment on a number of fronts of individuals with these conditions. Certainly the deinstitutionalization and normalization movements begun in the 1960s were maturing and were having a major effect on service delivery systems throughout the country. In truth, abuse of individuals with developmental disabilities had occurred in a number of areas, one of which was the inappropriate or excessive use of punishment contingencies. To this end, TASH adopted a policy against the use of aversive conditioning procedures and aversive stimuli in 1982, and a similar policy was later adopted by ARC.

I am sure that in the minds of those advocates opposed to the use of any aversive procedures, the national press clippings and releases regarding the introduction of SIBIS were proof of the correctness of their position. In their response, advocacy groups claimed this to be a throwback to medieval times and a threat to the progress made up to that point in the normalization and societal acceptance of individuals with mental retardation and developmental disabilities.

In October 1987, I received a letter from Alan Abeson, the executive director of the Association for Retarded Citizens, indicating that he had been told I was treating individuals with mental retardation using SIBIS. In his letter, Mr. Abeson asked that I cease this evaluation and remove SIBIS from any individuals who were currently using it. In addition, he offered to supply me with the names of consultants and experts in the area of behavioral programming to help these individuals be treated without the necessity of aversive conditioning procedures. My return letter to Mr. Abeson expressed the fact that I also was concerned about the welfare and rights of individuals with mental retardation. In addition, I expressed my concern that nowhere in his letter had he asked anything about the results of this treatment and whether it had been helpful to these individuals. I suggested that it may be appropriate to learn more about the treatment itself, the individuals treated to date, and the results before asking me to stop treatment. I offered to travel anywhere in the United States to present the data that we had collected to date on the individuals treated with SIBIS to the ARC executive board so that they might make an informed decision.

Mr. Abeson did not respond to my letter and offer to present this information. Therefore, to the best of my knowledge, Mr. Abeson (or whoever had decision-making power in the Association for Retarded Citizens) came to whatever conclusions they had regarding SIBIS based on a total lack of information about the device, its specifications, and its treatment effectiveness. I remember thinking to myself that the ARC was taking a stance very much like my initial reaction when I was asked to treat my first infant with rumination—a response based on misconceptions and emotional responses rather than facts.

In April 1988, a number of advocacy organizations (headed by TASH) held a press conference in Washington, D.C., to call for the U.S. Food and Drug Administration to remove its registration of SIBIS as a Class II medical device. The claim was that the device had not been fully tested, that it was not substantially similar to other devices, and that it represented a return to cruel and outdated treatment procedures. At the press conference, literature was circulated suggesting that B. F. Skinner disapproved of the use of punishment procedures, despite the fact that Dr. Skinner prior to the news conference had repudiated that literature as not reflecting his true views. In addition, a lawyer suggested that parents were frequently coerced and forced into using aversive procedures against their will based on a threat by an institution or treatment agency that their children would not be served any longer if they did not give permission for these procedures. When asked whether he knew of any parents who had not freely agreed to the use of SIBIS with their children, he had to respond that he was not familiar with any such instance.

Near the end of the news conference, a father whose two daughters had been successfully treated with SIBIS interrupted the proceedings to express his outrage that these individuals with no direct knowledge of the device or of his daughters' problems would attempt to deny them the only successful treatment of their self-injurious behavior that had been found in their 30-year life span. Several other parents of individuals who had been treated with SIBIS were also present at the news conference and were able to inform the press following the conference of the success that they had experienced with the device and their children.

Most interestingly, a document entitled "Support Document on SIBIS" was distributed at the press conference. This document was later described "as an authoritative summary of available evidence regarding the safety and clinical effectiveness of electric shock to treat self-injury" in an article written for the TASH newsletter (Meyer, 1988, p. 1). A task force of the Association for the Advancement of Behavior Therapy had concluded that contingent electrical stimulation was one of the most widely researched and generally most effective treatment procedures for initially decreasing the rate of self-injurious behavior (Favell et al., 1982); it had been able to identify more than 20 publications documenting this conclusion. The support document on SIBIS, however, while claiming to be an authoritative summary, referenced only three peer-reviewed treatment articles, one nonreviewed book chapter, and one article describing safety considerations when using contingent electric shock with humans. The author of this "support document" apparently had purposely neglected the numerous published articles documenting effective treatment with contingent electric shock.

The support document appeared to use selective research literature to make a case against the use of contingent electric shock, rather than being an "authoritative summary." It was also of interest that Meyer's description (1988) of the news conference failed to report the comments by parents of individuals treated with SIBIS. The national press in attendance was most interested in both sides of the question; apparently, Meyer was not. In addition, the support document suggested that shock has been associated with serious negative side effects. A more thorough and unbiased review of the literature would have revealed that the ratio of positive to negative side effects reported in the literature runs from 5:1 to 11:1 in favor of positive side effects (Carr & Lovaas, 1983; Lichstein & Schreibman, 1976). The support document's seemingly purposeful selective conclusions are representative of the opposition to SIBIS, which in my opinion has been based more on emotion than on fact. Unfortunately, these emotional appeals, disguised as scientific reviews, are directed at people who are least able to acquire the full range of accurate knowledge necessary to come to informed conclusions and most vulnerable to emotional appeal—namely, parents, teachers, and politicians (see Mulick & Linscheid, 1988).

Although 10 or more national organizations joined in the call for an investigation at SIBIS at this news conference, it appears that they were recruited to join this cause by some organizations that were particularly interested in denying parents and trained clinicians the full range of choice in treatment decision making. To the best of my knowledge, there was never a survey of the membership of these organizations to determine whether the members approved of joining in this cause. Indeed, one national organization, the National Association of School Psychologist (NASP), declined to join with the other advocacy groups in this move (NASP, 1988); another, the Autism Society of America, subsequently withdrew its support in favor of a right-to-treatment-choice position.

The controversy over whether aversive conditioning procedures are ever necessary led to the federal government sponsoring a consensus development conference (the NIH Consensus Developmental Conference on Treatment of Destructive Behaviors in Persons with Developmental Disabilities) that was held September 11–13, 1989. Consensus development conferences are utilized by government agencies to garner professional and scientific consensus regarding controversial issues. The outcome of these conferences often guides future research, research funding, and policy development. The general format for the conferences involves the formation of a panel of experts in the field who are not directly involved in the current question at hand, but who have the expertise to be able to evaluate evidence on both sides in as objective a manner as possible. The panel meets, decides what background information is necessary, and asks other experts in the field to prepare background and position statements. This information is reviewed and then the conference itself is held, in which scientific evidence is presented from both sides and public testimony is taken. The panel then prepares a review paper and position statement.

At the consensus development conference, I was asked to present data regarding the clinical evaluation of SIBIS and to submit whatever other materials I wished in support of the use of this treatment procedure. Experts from both sides of the issue presented scientific testimony and data to support their positions, and an open forum in which all parties were given time to address the panel occurred during the meeting. The conference addressed itself primarily to aversive conditioning procedures and their appropriateness, as well as to the use of psychoactive medication, in the treatment of destructive behaviors in persons with developmental disabilities.

The final conference report concluded that such behavior reductive procedures were still necessary in some cases but should be conducted under close supervision and as a part of an overall comprehensive treatment program. Those of us who believe that the reasoned use of aversive conditioning procedures is sometimes necessary were satisfied with this report. We were not seeking an outright endorsement of aversive conditioning procedures independent of appropriate peer review, nor were we seeking from the committee approval of any work or research that we had done. Those opposing the use of aversive conditioning under any circumstances, naturally, were disappointed and angered by the committee's report. They charged that the panel of experts was biased and that they had not been given sufficient notice or time to present their case. Because of these concerns, the final report was delayed, but in its final form, the conclusion that behavior reductive procedures were still necessary under the previously described conditions stood as originally written.

Subsequent to this conference, a number of court decisions have occurred in which SIBIS has been directly involved. In the state of Michigan in 1990, two such cases were ruled upon. In one instance the court ruled that a young girl had the right to wear her SIBIS device during school, as it had proven to be effective in eliminating her self-injurious head hitting and the school had not been able to demonstrate effectiveness in reducing this behavior through educational efforts. In the other case, in which SIBIS was included in a proposed IEP program for a student, the school system had refused to implement the program based on two statutory considerations. First, the state's law against the use of corporal punishment in the schools was alleged to apply to the use of SIBIS, as it delivered what might be considered a punishing stimulus. Second, the school district in question had a specific regulation against the use of contingent electric shock (defined as the use of cattle prods).

In this second case, after hearing testimony from both sides, the hearing officer ruled that SIBIS would not be banned by the state's corporal punishment law, as it was a treatment procedure. In addition, the hearing officer ruled that the district's regulation against the use of electric shock was not valid because it could deny the right to effective treatment to a client. At present, the individual is being treated under a program that does not involve the use of contingent electrical stimulation, based on the court testimony of a number of consultants that nonaversive procedures would result in a 90% reduction in his rate of self-injurious behavior in 6 months and that all forms of physical restraint could successfully be removed from this client in a year. At the time of the writing of this chapter, the year is approximately half over, and a hearing officer ruling prevents discussion of the data and effectiveness of the program to date.

This will prove to be an interesting case, as the school system is investing a significant amount of resources in the program and has two of the nation's most outspoken opponents of aversive conditioning serving as consultants. Recently, TASH honored the school district's superintendent and the lawyers who opposed the inclusion of SIBIS in the student's program with a special award. I thought it most interesting that they did not wait to see if the strictly nonaversive program worked for this student; it suggests that they are more interested in winning a battle than actually seeing this student's self-injury eliminated. Will they take the awards back if the program fails?

SUMMARY

The development of a technology that uses aversive conditioning procedures, when evaluated purely on a research dimension, has been shown to be

dramatically effective in the reduction and elimination of self-injurious behavior in clients with long-standing histories of this affliction. The introduction of this device came at a time when there was an appropriately growing
concern about the overuse of operant conditioning punishment procedures.
Therefore, SIBIS as a device in itself became the focus of a great deal of
controversy. At present, with the publication of an article detailing initial
applications of the device in five cases (Linscheid et al., 1990), there is reason
to believe that SIBIS can be effective in accomplishing the goal of rapidly and
safely reducing high rates of self-injurious behavior. In addition, research
suggests that there is an absence of negative side effects and if anything,
there has been documentation of positive side effects from this treatment.

As of this writing, all the parents of individuals who have used SIBIS
support its continued use and have lobbied at regional and national levels
against those who would have it banned. As Brian Iwata indicated in an
excellent presidential address to the Association of Applied Behavior Analysis (Iwata, 1988), it is the role of the behavioral psychologist not to advocate
treatment with aversive conditioning procedures, but rather to supply factual
data regarding its effectiveness in the treatment of these behaviors. It is for all
professionals to ensure that they conduct their treatment programs in an
ethical manner to best serve the client. At present, SIBIS is being utilized on a
daily basis with a small number of clients worldwide, requests for its use by
other clients are evaluated on a case-by-case basis, and to the best of my
knowledge (other than the case of the woman in her 30s described earlier in
this chapter), the utilization of SIBIS has been successful in all cases. A
number of those who were initially treated with SIBIS have already ceased
using the device, as their behavior has come under control of other contingencies and it has been successfully faded. A number of other people are in the
process of having the device faded, and some individuals continue to need
the device on a daily basis in order to control their self-injurious behavior.

Earlier in this chapter, I described my early experiences using contingent
electrical stimulation so that the reader might understand how I became
involved with SIBIS and why I was willing to conduct the research for it. Most
distressing to me has been the assumption made by a number of people, and
often verbalized to me, that I have an interest in SIBIS only out of a disregard
for the welfare and rights of individuals with mental retardation and developmental disabilities. There has been an assumption that anyone willing to
conduct this kind of research must be either ignorant of positive programming procedures, backward in his or her approach to treatment, or uncon-
cerned about the rights and welfare of disadvantaged individuals with
disabilities. There has also been an assumption that a belief in only positive
procedures is equated with caring and that advocacy for the occasional,
restricted use of aversive conditioning procedures when warranted somehow
indicates a lack of compassion. I think it is unfortunate that this controversy
has been relegated to that level. In my nearly 20 years of providing clinical

service to individuals with developmental disabilities and various medical problems and teaching operant conditioning procedures to students, I have met very few, if any, people in professional positions who truly do not care about their client's welfare. The emotional intensity that this controversy has engendered, however, has led educated people to disregard or distort the scientific literature, to make proclamations in the absence of proper knowledge, and to attempt to manipulate the free exchange of information.

As witness to this last point, the American Association on Mental Retardation denied exhibit space at its national convention in 1988 to Human Technologies Incorporated because it was the manufacturer and marketer of SIBIS. In addition, AAMR refused to sell its mailing list to an organization sponsoring a national conference, based on the fact that one of the speakers would be describing research on SIBIS. This type of censorship, condemned by Division 33 of the American Psychological Association in 1989, is just a reflection of the willingness to deny the free exchange of information and to prevent access to this information by members of organizations based on the executive committee's decision that the information may be misused by the membership. I fail to see how limiting the right of any individual to learn as much as he or she can about various treatment alternatives could ever serve the long-term goals of these organizations.

This chapter obviously has left out a great deal of detail regarding all of the areas addressed. It has been my attempt, however, to familiarize the reader somewhat with my experiences in the development and initial evaluation of the Self-Injurious Behavior Inhibiting System. When I think back upon this process and consider the accusations that have been made against me and the aspersions cast upon my character for my willingness to be involved in this type of research and treatment, I find that the gratitude of the parents and the improvements in the lives and opportunities of those clients who have been successfully treated more than make up for all the negative aspects of this process. All of us in the helping professions should draw our reinforcement and support from the success of our treatments and the positive changes we have made in peoples lives, not from following the crowd or taking the popular course.

REFERENCES

Ball, T., Sibbach, L., Jones, R., Steele, B., & Frazier, L. (1975). An accelorometer-activated device to control assaultive and self-destructive behavior in retardates. *Journal of Behavior Therapy and Experimental Psychiatry, 6*, 223–228.
Butterfield, W. H. (1975). Instruments and technology: Electric shock—safety factors when used for the aversive conditioning of humans. *Behavior Therapy, 6*, 98–110.
Carr, E. G., & Lovaas, O. I. (1983). Contingent electric shock as a treatment for severe behavior problems. In S. Axelrod & J. Apshe (Eds.), *Punishment: Its effect on human behavior* (pp. 219–246). New York: Academic Press.

Cunningham, C. E., & Linscheid, T. R. (1976). Elimination of chronic infant ruminating by electric shock. *Behavior Therapy, 7*, 231–234.

Favell, J. E., Azrin, N. H., Baumeister, A. A., Carr, E. G., Dorsey, M. F., Forehand, R., Foxx, R. M., Lovaas, O. I., Rincover, A., Risley, T. R., Romanczyk, R. G., Russo, D. C., Schroeder, S. R., & Solnick, J. V. (1982). The treatment of self-injurious behavior. *Behavior Therapy, 11*, 529–554.

Iwata, B. A. (1988). The development and adoption of controversial default technologies. *The Behavior Analyst, 11*, 149–158.

Kanner, L. (1957). *Child psychiatry.* Springfield, IL: Charles C. Thomas.

Lang, P. J., & Melamed, B. G. (1969). Avoidance conditioning therapy of an infant with chronic ruminative vomiting. *Journal of Abnormal Psychology, 74*, 139–142.

Linscheid, T. R. (1992). Aversive stimulation. In J. K. Luiselli, J. Matson, & N. Singh (Eds.), *Self-injurious behavior: Analysis, assessment and treatment* (pp. 269–292). New York: Springer-Verlag.

Linscheid, T. R., Iwata, B. A., Ricketts, R. W., Williams, D. E., & Griffin, J. C. (1990). Clinical evaluation of the Self-Injurious Behavior Inhibiting System (SIBIS). *Journal of Applied Behavior Analysis, 23*, 53–78.

Lichstein, K. L., & Schreibman, L. (1976). Employing electric shock with autistic children: A review of the side effects. *Journal of Autism and Childhood Schizophrenia, 6*, 163–173.

Matson, J. L., & DiLorenzo, T. M. (1984). *Punishment and its alternatives: A new perspective for behavior behavior modification.* New York: Springer.

Meyer, L. (1988). TASH joins with other organizations to protest electric shock device. *Newsletter of the Association for Persons With Severe Handicaps, 14*(8), 1–3.

Mulick, J. A., & Linscheid, T. R. (1988). A review of LaVigne and Donnellan's "Alternatives to punishment: Solving behavior problems with non-aversive strategies." *Research in Developmental Disabilities, 9*, 317–321.

National Association of School Psychologists. (1988). Resolution concerning aversives not endorsed. *Communique, 16*(9), pp. 1, 13.

Sajwaj, T., Libet, J., & Agras, S. (1974). Lemon juice therapy: The control of life-threatening rumination in a six-month-old infant. *Journal of Applied Behavior Analysis, 7*, 557–563.

Appendix A
The Right to Effective Behavioral Treatment

Over the last several decades, a number of clinical procedures derived from experimental and applied behavior analysis have been developed, evaluated, and refined. These procedures have the demonstrated ability to teach new behavior and alleviate a variety of behavioral disorders. Unfortunately, many who would benefit from behavioral treatment are not receiving it. Behavior analysts have a professional obligation to make available the most effective treatment that the discipline can provide. Toward this end, the following statement of clients' rights is offered to direct both the ethical and appropriate application of behavioral treatment.

1. AN INDIVIDUAL HAS A RIGHT TO A THERAPEUTIC ENVIRONMENT

A physical and social environment that is safe, humane, and responsive to individual needs is a necessary prerequisite for effective treatment. Such an environment provides not only training, but also an acceptable living standard. The dimensions of an adequate living environment are complex and varied; nevertheless, several elements appear essential. Individuals should have access to therapeutic services, leisure activities, and materials that are enjoyable as well as instructive. Thus, client preference, in addition to factors such as age-appropriateness and educative value, is relevant in the selection of activities and materials. An adequate environment also includes parents, teachers, and staff who are competent, responsive, and caring. Such qualities may be characterized in terms of frequent positive interactions that are directed toward enjoyment, learning, and independence. Finally, a therapeutic envi-

Report of the Association for Behavior Analysis (ABA) Task Force on the Right to Effective Treatment. Ron Van Houten served as the task force chair, and Brian A. Iwata served as the council liaison. This report was accepted by the ABA executive council; however, it does not necessarily reflect the view of the majority of ABA members, nor does it constitute official ABA policy. Reprints may be obtained from Brian A. Iwata, University of Florida, Gainesville, Florida 32611.

ronment imposes the fewest restrictions necessary, while insuring individual safety and development. Freedom of individual movement and access to preferred activities, rather than type or location of placement, are the defining characteristics of a least restrictive environment.

2. AN INDIVIDUAL HAS A RIGHT TO SERVICES WHOSE OVERRIDING GOAL IS PERSONAL WELFARE

The primary purpose of behavioral treatment is to assist individuals in acquiring functional skills that promote independence. Both the immediate and long-term welfare of an individual are taken into account through active participation by the client or an authorized proxy in making treatment-related decisions. In cases where withholding or implementing treatment involves potential risk, Peer Review Committees and Human Rights Committees play distinct roles in protecting client welfare. Peer Review Committees, comprised of experts in behavior analysis, impose professional standards in determining the clinical propriety of treatment programs. Human Rights Committees, comprised of consumers, advocates, and other interested citizens, impose community standards in determining the acceptability of programs and the extent to which a program compromises an individual's basic rights to dignity, privacy, and humane care; appropriate education and training; prompt medical treatment; access to personal possessions, social interaction, and physical exercise; humane discipline; and physical examination prior to the initiation of a program that may affect or be affected by an individual's health status. Professional competence aided by peer and human rights review will insure that behavioral treatment is delivered within a context of concern for client welfare.

3. AN INDIVIDUAL HAS A RIGHT TO TREATMENT BY A COMPETENT BEHAVIOR ANALYST

Professionals responsible for delivering, directing, or evaluating the effects of behavioral treatment possess appropriate education and experience. The behavior analyst's academic training reflects thorough knowledge of behavioral principles, methods of assessment and treatment, research methodology, and professional ethics. Clinical competence also requires adequate practicum training and supervision, including experience with the relevant client population.

In cases where a problem or treatment is complex or may pose risk, individuals have a right to direct involvement by a doctoral-level behavior analyst who has the expertise to detect, analyze, and manage subtle aspects of the assessment and treatment process that often determine the success or failure of intervention. A doctoral-level behavior analyst also has the ability, as well as the responsibility, to insure that all individuals who participate in the delivery of treatment or who provide support services are trained in the methods of intervention, to assess the competence of individuals who assume subsequent responsibility for treatment, and to provide consultation and follow-up services as needed.

4. An Individual Has a Right to Programs That Teach Functional Skills

The ultimate goal of all services is to increase the ability of individuals to function effectively in both their immediate environment and the larger society. Improvement of functioning may take several forms. First, it often will require the acquisition, maintenance, or generalization of behaviors that allow the individual to gain wider access to preferred materials, activities, or social interaction. Second, it may require the acquisition of behaviors that allow the individual to terminate or reduce unpleasant sources of stimulation. Third, improved functioning may require the reduction or elimination of certain behaviors that are dangerous or that in some way serve as barriers to further independence or social acceptability. Finally, as a member of society at large, an individual has a right to services that will assist in the development of behavior beneficial to that society.

Decisions regarding the selection of service goals are not based on a priori assumptions of an individual's behavior potential or limitations. It is conceivable that some goals might be achieved very slowly, that others may be only approximated, and that, in the process of achieving still other goals, it may be necessary to expose the individual to either immediate temporary discomfort (e.g., as in teaching physical exercise as a means of promoting health) or future risk (e.g., as in teaching an individual to cross streets or to drive an automobile). Still, unless evidence clearly exists to the contrary, an individual is assumed capable of full participation in all aspects of community life and to have a right to such participation.

5. An Individual Has a Right to Behavioral Assessment and Ongoing Evaluation

Prior to the onset of treatment, individuals are entitled to a complete diagnostic evaluation to identify factors that contribute to the presence of a skill deficit or a behavioral disorder. A complete and functional analysis emphasizes the importance of events that are antecedent, as well as consequent, to the behavior of interest. For example, identification of preexisting physiological or environmental determinants may lead to the development of a treatment program that does not require extensive use of behavioral contingencies.

The initial behavioral analysis is performed in three stages. First, answers to the following types of questions are obtained through interview. Is there any circumstance in which the behavior *always* occurs? Is there any circumstance in which the behavior *never* occurs? Does the behavior typically occur at certain times of the day? Could the behavior be associated with any form of discomfort or deprivation? Could events following the behavior serve as either positive reinforcement (e.g., attention) or negative reinforcement (e.g., escape from demands)? The second stage of analysis, direct observation of the individual's behavior under varied and relevant circumstances, confirms suspected relationships identified during the interview. Finally, the assessment findings are incorporated into a systematic treatment plan.

Successful intervention requires ongoing evaluation in the form of objective data to determine the effects of treatment, to quickly identify unanticipated problems, and, if necessary, to modify the treatment plan. The behavior analyst maintains accountability and solicits timely input into the decision-making process by sharing these data regularly with all concerned parties.

6. AN INDIVIDUAL HAS A RIGHT TO THE MOST EFFECTIVE TREATMENT PROCEDURES AVAILABLE

An individual is entitled to effective and scientifically validated treatment. In turn, behavior analysts have an obligation to use only those techniques that have been demonstrated by research to be effective, to acquaint consumers and the public with the advantages and disadvantages of these techniques, and to search continuously for the most optimal means of changing behavior.

Consistent with the philosophy of least restrictive yet effective treatment, exposure of an individual to restrictive procedures is unacceptable unless it can be shown that such procedures are necessary to produce safe and clinically significant behavior change. It is equally unacceptable to expose an individual to a nonrestrictive intervention (or a series of such interventions) if assessment results or available research indicate that other procedures would be more effective. Indeed, a slow-acting but nonrestrictive procedure could be considered highly restrictive if prolonged treatment increases risk, significantly inhibits or prevents participation in needed training programs, delays entry into a more optimal social or living environment, or leads to adaptation and the eventual use of a more restrictive procedure. Thus, in some cases, a client's right to effective treatment may dictate the immediate use of quicker-acting, but temporarily more restrictive procedures.

A procedure's overall level of restrictiveness is a combined function of its absolute level of restrictiveness, the amount of time required to produce a clinically acceptable outcome, and the consequences associated with delayed intervention. Furthermore, selection of a specific treatment technique is not based on personal conviction. Techniques are not considered as either "good" or "bad" according to whether they involve the use of antecedent rather than consequent stimuli or reinforcement rather than punishment. For example, positive reinforcement, as well as punishment, can produce a number of indirect effects, some of which are undesirable.

In summary, decisions related to treatment selection are based on information obtained during assessment about the behavior, the risk it poses, and its controlling variables; on a careful consideration of the available treatment options, including their relative effectiveness, risks, restrictiveness, and potential side effects; and on examination of the overall context in which treatment will be applied.

CONCLUSION

Behavior analysts have a responsibility to insure that their clients' rights are protected, that their specialized services are based on the most recent scientific and technological findings, that treatment is provided in a manner consistent with the highest standards of excellence, and that individuals who are in need of service will not be denied access to the most effective treatment available. In promulgating the rights described in this document, the field of behavior analysis acknowledges its responsibilities by reaffirming its concern for individual welfare and by prescribing the means by which behavioral treatment can be delivered in the most beneficial manner.

Appendix B

Association for Behavior Analysis Position Statement on Clients' Rights to Effective Behavioral Treatment

Formal methods of behavior change, derived from the field of behavior analysis and referred to here as Behavioral Treatment, provide an effective means for establishing new patterns of adaptive behavior and alleviating a number of debilitating behavioral disorders. As uses of behavioral treatment become more widespread, particularly in clinical, educational, and other settings that serve dependent populations, it is necessary to take steps to ensure that clients' rights are protected, that treatment is based on scientific findings, that service is provided in a manner consistent with the highest standards of excellence, and that individuals who are in need of service will not be denied access to the most effective treatment available.

The Association for Behavior Analysis issues the following position statement on clients' rights to effective behavioral treatment as a set of guiding principles to protect individuals from harm as a result of either the lack or the inappropriate use of behavioral treatment.

The Association for Behavior Analysis, through majority vote of its members, declares that individuals who receive behavioral treatment have a right to:

1. *A therapeutic physical and social environment.* Characteristics of such an environment include but are not limited to: an acceptable standard of living, opportunities for stimulation and training, therapeutic social interaction, and freedom from undue physical or social restriction.

2. *Services whose overriding goal is personal welfare.* The client participates, either directly or through authorized proxy, in the development and implementation of treatment programs. In cases where withholding or implementing treatment involves potential risk and the client does not have the capacity to provide consent, individual welfare is protected through two mechanisms: Peer Review Committees, imposing professional standards, determine the clinical propriety of treatment programs; Human Rights Committees, imposing community standards, determine the accep-

373

tability of treatment programs and the degree to which they may compromise an individual's rights.

3. *Treatment by a competent behavior analyst.* The behavior analyst's training reflects appropriate academic preparation, including knowledge of behavioral principles, methods of assessment and treatment, research methodology, and professional ethics; as well as practical experience. In cases where a problem or treatment is complex or may pose risk, direct involvement by a doctoral-level behavior analyst is necessary.

4. *Programs that teach functional skills.* Improvement in functioning requires the acquisition of adaptive behaviors that will increase independence, as well as the elimination of behaviors that are dangerous or that in some other way serve as barriers to independence.

5. *Behavioral assessment and ongoing evaluation.* Pretreatment assessment, including both interviews and measures of behavior, attempts to identify factors relevant to behavioral maintenance and treatment. The continued use of objective behavioral measurement documents response to treatment.

6. *The most effective treatment procedures available.* An individual is entitled to effective and scientifically validated treatment; in turn, the behavior analyst has an obligation to use only those procedures demonstrated by research to be effective. Decisions on the use of potentially restrictive treatment are based on consideration of its absolute and relative level of restrictiveness, the amount of time required to produce a clinically significant outcome, and the consequences that would result from delayed intervention.

The above statement is an abbreviated version of a report by the Association for Behavior Analysis, Task Force on the Right to effective Behavioral Treatment (members: R. Van Houten [chair], S. Axelrod, J. S. Bailey, J. E. Favell, R. M. Foxx, B. A. Iwata, and O. I. Lovaas). The complete report can be found in *The Behavior Analyst* (1988, Vol. 11, 111–114) or the *Journal of Applied Behavior Analysis* (1988, Vol. 21, 381–384); or a copy may be ordered from the Association for Behavior Analysis, Western Michigan University, 258 Wood Hall, Kalamazoo, MI 49008-5052.

Author Index

Subject Index